FILTER YOUR WATER NOW!

The Shocking Truth
about Water Pollution:
How to Protect Your Family
and Prevent Disease!

All people and creatures depend upon clean water.
For human health, animal health
and planet wellbeing,
we must end water pollution.

Prepare to Rise!

Thank you for buying this book.

Copyright © 2024 Joanna Kappele
Adore Your Planet

For more information, please contact us at
hello@adoreyourplanet.com

Our books are printed through
Prepare to Rise, the publishing department of
Adore Your Planet, a 501c3 nonprofit.
We provide bulk book deals for schools, nonprofits,
and community groups. You can reach us at:
Hello@adoreyourplanet.com

Published by Prepare to Rise
ISBN 978-1-7330884-80
Edited by Joanna Kappele

All Rights Reserved. No part of this publication can be reproduced, stored in a retrieval system, or transmitted, in any form or by any means, electronic, mechanical, photocopying, recording, or otherwise, without the prior permission of the author and publisher.
The information you've been looking for.

With Gratitude

Many thanks to all who've encouraged and supported me along this long and interesting path that led to this much anticipated book. Thanks also to all the health and environmental heroes and nature lovers who help keep the light shining on issues of such importance. May this work contribute to those who came before me and bring us a healthier happier world.

Table of Contents

Introduction   i
    Clean Water and Health
    Origin of the Clean Water Act:
    A dedication to JFK and Rachel Carson   ii

SECTION ONE
Filter Your Water: Overview   1
    1. What's in H2O   3
    2. Boil your water   4
    3. Bottled water   5
    4. Filter your water   6
        Water Filter Chart   8
    5. Water in your town   9
    6. Well water   10
    7. Clean Water Act   11
    8. Water health   13
    9. Water Shortage   16
    10. Health Wake Up Call   19
    11. Climate Wake Up Call   21
    Chart: Ground Water Contaminants   22

SECTION TWO
Water Contaminants Exposed A to Z   33
    1. Agriculture Runoff   34
    2. Aluminum   37
    3. AMR   38
    4. Ammonia   40
    5. Arsenic   41
    6. Atrazine   42
    7. Bacteria & Parasites   43
    8. BPA, BPS, Badge   45
    9. Benzene   50
    10. Biosolids   51
    11. Bromine   54

12. Building Supplies	55
13. Chlorine	56
14. Chloramines	58
15. Chlorpyrifos, CPF	59
16. Chromium-6	63
17. Cleaning Products	65
18. Coal Ash	66
19. Cosmetics	69
20. DBPs	72
21. Dicamba	75
22. Dichlorobenzene (p-DCB)	76
23. Dioxin	77
24. Emerging Contaminants	79
25. Ethanol	80
26. Ethylene Glycol	81
27. Factory Farms	82
28. Fertilizer Runoff	84
29. Flame Retardants	87
30. Fluoride	91
31. Fracking	95
32. Gen X (PFAS)	98
33. Glyphosate	99
Herbicides Special Report	101
34. Hand Sanitizers	102
35. Heavy Metals	103
36. Landscaping	104
37. Lead	105
Lead Water Lines Special Report	108
38. Manganese	111
39. Mercury	113
40. Microplastics	116
41. Nanoparticles	118
42. Neonicotinoids	121
43. Nitrate	123
44. Nitrogen Fertilizer	124
45. Nitrous Oxide	126
46. Nutrient Pollution	127

47. Oil Drilling	128
48. Oil Refineries	129
49. Oil and Gas Pipelines	131
50. Oil Spills	134
51. Packaging Waste	137
52. Paraquat and 2,4-D	139
53. Perchlorate	140
54. PERC and TCE	141
55. Pesticides	142
56. PFAS, Forever Chemicals	149
57. Pharmaceuticals	151
58. Phosphates	152
59. Phosphate Fertilizer	153
60. Plastic	155
61. Plastic Pellets	159
62. POPs	161
63. PPCPs	162
64. Power Plants	163
65. Radiation	164
66. Road Salt	166
67. Sewage	167
68. Stormwater	169
69. Styrofoam	172
70. Sunscreen	173
Safe Sunscreens Chart	174
71. Surfactants	176
72. TCP 1,2,3	177
73. Teflon, Gen X	176
74. Textiles	177
75. Train Derailments	178
76. Vinyl Chloride	179
77. Waste	182
78. Window Cleaner	182
79. Xenobiotics	183

SECTION THREE
In Danger: Human Health and Planet   187

- Animals in Danger   189
- Ecosystems in Danger   193
- Waterways in Danger   196
- People in Danger   219
  - Water Pollution   220
  - Midwest Farming   222
  - Human Health   223
  - Iowa Cancer Surge   224
  - Heavy Hitters & Disease links   227
    1. Carcinogens   229
    2. Endocrine Disruptors   231
    3. Heavy Metals   233
    4. Neurotoxins   234
    5. Reproductive Toxins   236
    6. Respiratory & Digestive   237
    7. Toxic Substances   238

SECTION FOUR
Solutions Department: Water   241
Protect Your Family

- Keep water Clean   242
- Filter Your Water   243
- Conserve Water   244
- Protect the Oceans   245
- Holding Industry Accountable   248
- Water Filters   249
- Nontoxic Cleaning   251
- Nontoxic Home   252
- Nontoxic Gardening   253
- How to shop for non-toxic products   255
- Water Quality Matters   258
- Heal the Ozone Layer   259
- Priority List   260

Healing with Water   261
- Hydration   262

- Water Therapy — 263
- Water is Energy — 265
- Alkaline, Ozone, Hydrogen Water — 266
- Health suggestions Cancer Panel — 267
- Healing in the Kitchen — 269
- Holistic Healing, Nutrition — 270
- Healing Animals — 275

Government — 277
- Communication — 278
- Phone List — 279
- Accountability — 280
- CDC and HHS — 281
- FDA and USDA — 282
- Department of the Interior — 283
- The EPA — 284
- **EPA Water Contaminants Chart** — **286**
- **Laws** — 301
    - How Laws Are Made — 302
    - Regulations — 303
    - Air — 304
    - Animals — 304
    - Environment — 305
    - Pesticides — 307
    - Toxic Substances — 310
    - Water — 311
- Global Agreements — 313
    - Montreal Protocol — 313
    - Stockholm Convention — 314
    - Kyoto Protocol — 314
    - Paris Climate Accord — 314
    - Kunming-Montreal Biodiversity — 314

Shopping Guide — 315
Endnotes — 320
Index — 351

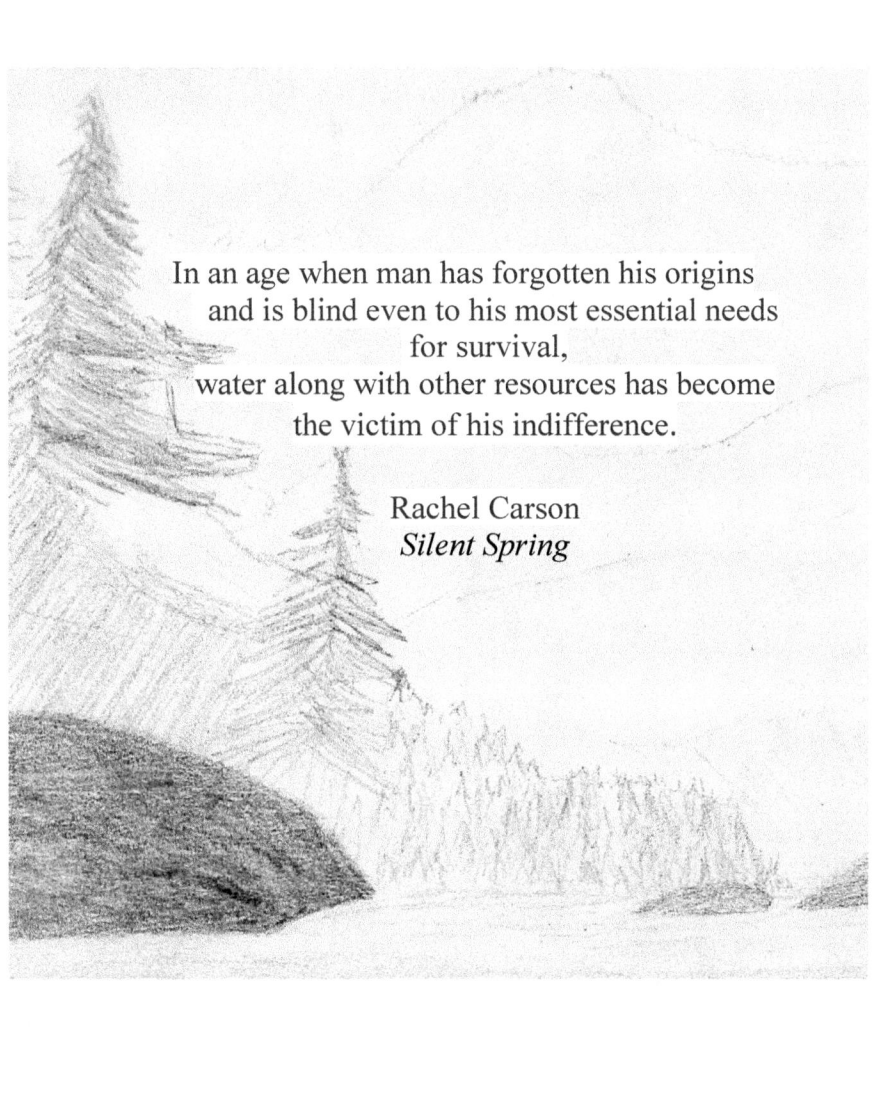

> In an age when man has forgotten his origins
> and is blind even to his most essential needs
> for survival,
> water along with other resources has become
> the victim of his indifference.
>
> Rachel Carson
> *Silent Spring*

Introduction
Clean Water and Health

It's 2025, a time ripe with technological advances, yet we have not conquered the damaging contaminants getting into our drinking water. Instead, they're conquering us. Cancer rates are surging and diseases once reserved for the elderly are striking the young. These growing epidemics are not random, but rather the result of contaminants in our environment. In America, we are enduring the consequences of a failed system that allows agricultural and industrial waste to flow unchecked into our drinking water sources. Those who we think are protecting us, are not. These same factors are spurring the climate crisis that is already worsening water quality in other regions of the world.

For too long now, water pollution has been affecting human health, continuing on uninterrupted day and night. We have reached a climax in disease trends not expected for a civilized society. For our health, our loved ones, and our planet, it's essential we stop allowing industrial pollution into our waterways. It's time to take charge and get things in order.

This book provides the path to a different reality, a better world, a healthier world. Within these pages you'll find vital information on protecting your health, identifying the worst water pollutants, filtering your water, getting the lead out, and ultimately taking care of your health and your family.

Together we can eliminate pollution and protect everyone—children, people, animals, pollinators, this book will show you how. Let's sleep under the stars and watch the moon years from now as we tell stories of how we overcame the industries that sought to destroy our health and planet earth.

Our task right now is to band together and do what must be done to save our drinking water, and in so doing, save each other. Armed with facts and vital health information, you'll be well prepared. We must curtail toxic releases into the waterways, as well as help manufacturers find health-friendly, earth-friendly materials to use in making their products. We can do this. With a little time and effort, and a good plan, great things can be achieved. Believing we can is step number one.

ORIGIN OF THE CLEAN WATER ACT
A Dedication to JFK and Rachel Carson

This book is written with special thanks to President Kennedy and Rachel Carson for their contribution to making water cleaner and safer.

JFK was greatly moved by Rachel Carson's writings, and specifically, the findings in her earth-shaking book, *Silent Spring*. This led to a partnership of sorts that inspired an awakening for our nation. For not only was conservation needed as stewards of the land, but people were mostly unaware as to how their own health might be impacted from contaminated water. Rachel was intent to change all that. Through Ms. Carson's writing and President Kennedy's position as leader of the free world, the problem of water pollution and the diseases it caused was finally getting the attention it deserved.

The President's fierce determination to protect our natural resources led to major changes in our country's approach to water pollution. In his first meeting with congress, water pollution was at the top of his agenda. He was determined to clean up the nation's waterways and stop polluters as much as he was determined to get a man on the moon. His persistence led to the passage of the Federal Water Pollution Control Act Amendments of 1961.

In all of his ambitions, he never stopped short of what was best for the nation and what was best for our health. Thankfully his mission to establish and strengthen environmental health protections was carried forward by President Johnson and Nixon after him. A short excerpt from JFK's Natural Resources address to Congress follows.[1]

February 23, 1961 Natural Resource Address to Congress (excerpt)

To the Congress of the United States: [2]
"From the beginning of civilization, every nation's basic wealth and progress has stemmed in large measure from its natural resources. This nation has been, and is now, especially fortunate in the blessings we have inherited. Our entire society rests upon --and is dependent upon--our water, our land, our forests, and our minerals. How we use these resources influences our health, security, economy, and well-being.

"But if we fail to chart a proper course of conservation and development--if we fail to use these blessings prudently--we will be in trouble within a short time. In the resource field, predictions of future use have been consistently understated. But even under conservative projections, we face a future of critical shortages and handicaps. By the year 2000, a United States population of 300 million--nearly doubled in 40 years--will need far greater supplies of farm products, timber, water, minerals, fuels, energy, and opportunities for outdoor recreation. Present projections tell us that our water use will double in the next 20 years; that we are harvesting our supply of high-grade timber more rapidly than the development of new growth; that too much of our fertile topsoil is being washed away; that our minerals are being exhausted at increasing rates; and that the Nation's remaining undeveloped areas of great natural beauty are being rapidly pre-empted for other uses.

"Our Nation has been blessed with a bountiful supply of water; but it is not a blessing we can regard with complacency. Pollution of our country's rivers and streams has--as a result of our rapid population and industrial growth and change--reached alarming proportions. To meet all needs--domestic, agricultural, industrial, recreational--we shall have to use and reuse the same water, maintaining quality as well as quantity. In many areas of the country, we need new sources of supply but in all areas we must protect the supplies we have. Current corrective efforts are not adequate. Industry is lagging far behind in its treatment of wastes."

President John F. Kennedy emphasized the urgency of addressing water pollution, and in his last few years he didn't waste any time. Through Kennedy's persistence, the passage of The Federal Water Pollution Control Act Amendments of 1961 came swiftly. "This marked a significant shift in the federal government's role in combating water pollution. The amendments broadened the scope of the Act to include almost all of the nation's waters and expanded federal abatement authority. The Act allowed for federal intervention in intrastate cases upon request of the Governor, acknowledging the national nature of the water pollution problem. Additionally, the amendments enabled municipalities to request federal assistance in combating pollution, albeit with the concurrence of the governor and state water pollution control agency.

"The Federal Water Pollution Control Act Amendments of 1961 reflected the growing recognition of water pollution as a national problem requiring a strong national program. The amendments strengthened the federal government's role in combating water pollution and set the stage for continued progress in addressing this critical issue."[3]

Today calls for a return to this kind of impassioned time. A time when government includes people, when the President and his Directors fight the polluters and protect the people's health. Never before have we had such rogue industries disrespecting the health of the people, and blatantly polluting waterways everywhere. The 1960s was not a good time for America's environment, but today is far worse. Back then you didn't see government agencies giving the worst polluting industries 'waivers' to keep polluting. You didn't see the absurd abundance and wide array of disease-causing toxins spread throughout the environment like we have today. You didn't see the rapid and declining fall of biodiversity, huge numbers of animals and plants quickly vanishing from the planet.

Now more than ever, it's urgent we return to the basics, of working together, of putting pollution rules in place and adhering to them. It's going to take a unified effort, but together we can restore our waters' health, people's health, and the planet. America really is a beautiful place, let's keep it that way.

> We must think and act not only for the moment but for our time. I am reminded of the story of the great French Marshal Lyautey, who once asked his gardener to plant a tree. The gardener objected that the tree was slow-growing and would not reach maturity for a hundred years. The Marshal replied, "In that case, there is no time to lose, plant it this afternoon!"
>
> President John F. Kennedy
> March 23, 1962
> Berkeley, California

SECTION ONE

Filter Your Water
Overview

Roughly 70% of the Earth is covered in water. Not all that is fresh water though-- only about 2.7% of all that water is drinkable. In the big scheme of things, that's a small amount of water for all the people around the world to share. With so little water available for our consumption, it's ever more important to keep the world's water as unpolluted as possible.

Was it planned by the universe, or is it just coincidence that humans are also 70% water. We need water to maintain our energy and health, hydration is paramount to keeping fit and well. Yet, not just any water will do, it must be clean water!

Every living thing needs water to survive. Without water, none of us could live for long. Water keeps us hydrated, keeps us healthy, keeps our bodies and minds functioning properly. Plants and animals also need water.

WATER IS H2O
Water is comprised of Hydrogen and Oxygen, that's why water is known as H2O. Two Hydrogen (H) atoms combined with one atom of Oxygen (O) make one water molecule.

WATER CONTAMINANT OVERVIEW
Types of Water Contaminants:
- Heavy Metals: Lead, manganese, cadmium, chromium
- Neurotoxins: Lead, cyanobacteria, pesticides, chromium 6...
- Chemical Toxins: Plastic, Petrochemicals, Pesticides, Dioxin,
- PFAS: Teflon and its cousin, Gen X, Biosolids,
- Reproductive Toxins, Carcinogens, DBPs, EDCs
- Endocrine Disruptors (EDCs), BPA, phthalates, herbicides,
- DBPs: chloroform, trihalomethanes, iodoacids, MX, BDA
- Farm Chemicals: Weed Killers, Insecticides, Herbicides,
- Agricultural Runoff: Sewage, Fertilizer, Nitrate, Pesticides,
- Industrial: Perchloroethylene, PCBs, Heavy Metals, Benzene,
- Bacteria, Microbes, Mineral deposits, Protozoa, Viruses
- Sewage and Biosolids: Heavy Metals, PFAS, pharmaceuticals
- Plastic: Plastic, Petrochemicals, Pellets, Toxins, Carcinogens
- Oil and Gas: Spills, Pellets, Pipelines, Petrochemicals, Pesticides

What's Creating the Worst Water Pollution:
1. Agriculture: Runoff, Weedkillers, Insecticides, Biotech, GMOs, CAFOs, Synthetic Fertilizer, Nitrate, Raw Sewage, Biosolids
2. Big Chem Industries:
    a. Plastics and Petrochemicals and Pharma and Pesticides
    b. Surfactants (toxic accelerant chemicals)
    c. Toxins: PFAS, Flame Retardants, Perc, **Nanoparticles**
3. Waste Treatment: Untreated raw sewage releases Biosolids, PFAS and disease-causing microbes harming us
4. Energy, Fossil Fuels, Green Energy
    a. Oil Drilling, Gas, Mining, Fracking, Refineries, Ethanol, Pipelines, Spills, Accidents, Leaks
    b. Power Plants: Biomass, Coal, Gas, Oil, Nuclear
    c. Electric car batteries, lithium mining, SF6!
5. Food Packaging, Plastic, GRAS, EDCs, Nanoparticles
6. Manufacturing, mineral mining, burn pits, military ammunition
7. Paper Mills-landfills, hazardous waste sites,
8. Stormwater Runoff
9. Vehicles: Boats, Auto industry, Trains, Planes, Rockets!
10. Military, Ammunition, Fireworks, and anything I forgot to list

1. What's in H2O?

Aside from hydrogen and oxygen, there are many other things that get in water. Water health depends on what's in the water, and that question depends on where you're located.

From tap water to the lakes and rivers tap water comes from, there's a lot in the water besides water. Water quality comes down to a number of factors in the environment. This book will help explain types of contaminants that can be found in our drinking water today. Armed with this knowledge, together we can unite in saving people, the animals and the planet from further destruction. Together we can turn the tide and guarantee children and future generations have clean water for years to come. Together we can prevent unnecessary disease and extinction of our most beloved animals. It starts with caring and knowing what we're dealing with. So let's start by assessing the situation. Pollutants getting in the water cause disease. Where's the pollution coming from? Why isn't the pollution stopped?

With this book you'll discover:
- The extent of water contamination
- How contaminants get into the water
- What contaminants are in your town's water, or your well
- Methods to protect yourself and your family
- Filtering and purifying methods for water
- What bottled water is best if you need bottled water
- How to choose the best filter for your home or business
- Who's in charge of stopping water pollution
- How to end water pollution and help people & planet be healthier

Contaminants come in many different forms. Some are natural, some are manmade Some are from single identifiable source (point source), some are from unknown sources (non-point source). For some, multiple locations could be contributing, which makes it difficult to distinguish what entity is especially at fault. Most you can filter out. Some don't get filtered out so easily. Some need more than one filter to be removed. Good minerals you don't want to entirely remove.

Boil Your Water

Boil water advisories happen when water systems lose pressure or when a toxic presence has been identified in the water. Microbes and bacteria and gross stuff can linger in water when systems are down. This is where boiling comes in handy. Boiling water for at least one full minute helps inactivate many of these organisms.

Yet, boiled water may still not be great for drinking unless it's filtered also. At times like these, bottled water is preferable and recommended for drinking purposes. Boiling water will help remove volatile chemicals but not all toxins. Boiling can actually concentrate some chemical toxins while others become air-borne in steam.

DIRECTIONS FOR BOILING WATER:
Bring water to a rolling boil for at least 1 minute. Cool before using.

WATERBORNE PATHOGENS
"There are many disease-causing organisms that we can be exposed to through ingestion and contact with contaminated drinking water. The more common pathogens found in drinking water are as follows:
- **Protozoa and Parasites:** microorganisms that can live in water, animals, people, the environment.
- **Bacteria:** Bacteria are usually killed by chlorine treatment. Most bacteria will be removed by microfiltration.
- **Viruses:** Viruses are rapidly inactivated by chlorine, but their small size, typically less than 0.01 microns, allows viruses to pass through 1micron filters. Viruses are usually controlled with chemical disinfection."[4]

How to Remove Chemicals
Purify your water and filter toxic chemical contaminants out with carbon filters or reverse osmosis. These filter systems can fit on your counter or faucet, under the sink, or in pitchers. There are ion exchange water softeners if you have your own well, and there's whole home filters available that are great if you can afford them.

3. Bottled Water

The Good Things About Bottled Water:
- It can save your life
- It helps tremendously when contaminated water is present
- It helps provide water when it's unavailable otherwise
- It's convenient
- It's there when we need it

The problems with bottled water come down to:
- Plastic disposable bottles –Choose Glass bottles
- Endocrine disruptors in plastic
- How long water's been in the plastic--over 6 months, discard*
- Water can have many undisclosed contaminants in it (some bottled water can be straight tap water, unfiltered!)
- Transport and shipping expense of water
- Corporations taking and bottling water from communities
- Corporations taking H2O from towns with water shortage

Best (rated independently)
- Those bottled in glass not plastic
- Mountain Valley glass bottle has high ratings
- Topo Chico, Core Hydration, Just Water
- Fiji: High in Silica but recently recalled for high manganese

Good
- Smart Water
- Deer Park – BPA free bottles

Not so Good[5]
- Aquafina—is just bottled tap water[6]
- Dasani – many samples found to contain Bromate
- Nestle/Blue Triton – sourced unsustainably

DISCARD BOTTLES OVER 6 MONTHS OLD
* If your water bottles are older than 6 months old, they're absorbing BPA and toxins from the plastic. Throw them away.[7]

4. Filter Your Water

The President's Cancer Panel reported in 2009:
"Filtering home tap or well water can decrease exposure to numerous known or suspected carcinogens and endocrine-disrupting chemicals. It is preferable to use filtered tap water instead of commercially bottled water, unless the home water source is known to be contaminated."[8]

Do you assume tap water is safe to consume?
If you answered yes, please review this book. Tap water everywhere is tainted with health-harming substances be it from the products we use or from industry. Decades of pollution is catching up with us. Due to a mixture of industry carelessness, government missteps, lack of leadership, pollution in many forms continues daily.

Purifying and filtering water is relatively easy. This is how you can reduce your exposure to many of the health-harming contaminants mingling in our water. Shower filters also help lower your exposure to contaminants. If you're lucky enough to have a whole home filter system, all the water in your household is purified. With all filters, regular maintenance and replacing filters is necessary.

When it comes to filters, the two main types are Reverse Osmosis (RO) and Carbon. There's also ion exchange, ultraviolet light, and in Europe they use ozone to disinfect as well. Most RO systems are installed under the sink to the water line. Carbon is available in more options: countertop, faucet, pitcher, and combo undersink. RO is used in whole-home systems where the water line enters your house. To determine which one is right for you, consider: What's your main concern, what style will fit in your kitchen, and what's your budget? Aside from the initial cost, note filter price and maintenance expenses. At the end of the day, any filter is better than none but some are superior to others.

WHY FILTER?
- The USDA estimates 50 million people in the United States obtain their drinking water from groundwater that is contaminated by pesticides and other agricultural chemicals."[9]

Filter Type	Pros	Cons
Activated Carbon, Carbon Block	99% contaminants, incl PFAS, heavy metals	Nitrate and fluoride remain
Reverse Osmosis R.O.	Removes Most pollutants incl fluoride and nitrate	Wastes the most water
Pitcher Filters	Most remove 60- 80% ZeroWater up to 99%[11]	Nitrate and other contaminants remain
Water Softener Ion Exchange	Removes Nitrate	Removes essential minerals
Distillation	Believed to removes all contaminants, Requires evaporation	Removes all minerals, Doesn't taste good

- Nitrates are accumulating in water from municipal water filtration methods that use chloramines,[10] and from nitrogen fertilizer. Remove nitrate with RO or ion exchange

Filters that Remove Nitrate and Groundwater Pollutants:
- Reverse Osmosis: Yes
- Ion Exchange Water Softeners: Yes
- Zero Water Pitchers: Yes, filter + ion exchange

Other good filters include:
- Berkey Gravity Filters: Fluoride filters can be added on

Reverse osmosis: "removes contaminants by forcing pressurized water through a semi-permeable membrane covered in microscopic pores. These pores act like a sieve, separating the pure hydrogen and oxygen from the water's contaminants. The membrane has such a fine micron rating that it can rid the water of ions, like nitrates. The clean, treated water passes through the membrane and collects in a storage tank, contaminants are rejected by the membrane and flushed down the drain in the brine."[12]

WELL WATER: COMMON POLLUTANTS

If you have your own well, you alone are responsible for maintaining the quality of water in your well and testing it for contaminants. There are agencies who'll do the testing for you. Call your local town's water dept for help. Annually test for: Nitrate, Pesticides, Arsenic

WATER FILTERS
COMPARING WATER PURIFACTION SYSTEMS

TYPE	LEAD	NITRATE	PESTICIDES	FLUORIDE	PFAS	BPA	Microbes	Chromium 6	Price
R.O.	yes	yes	yes	yes	99%	yes	yes	yes	$$$
Carbon	yes	no	yes	no	yes	yes	yes	yes	$$
Ceramic	yes	no	yes	yes	yes	yes	yes	yes	$$
UV Filters	no	no	no	no	no	no	yes	no	$$
Ion Exchg	yes	90%	yes	95%	yes	yes	yes	yes	$$
Distillation	yes	yes	yes	yes	yes	yes	yes	yes	$$
boiling	no	no	no	no	no	no	yes	no	$
UNDER SINK or COUNTERTOP- (Reverse Osmosis and/or Carbon)									
WATERDROP	yes	yes	yes	95%	99%	yes	yes	yes	$$$
PUR RO	yes	yes	yes	95%	most	yes	yes	yes	$
CLEARLY	yes	yes	yes	95%	most	yes	yes	yes	$$
Cloud	yes	yes	yes	95%	99%	yes	yes	yes	$$$
HYDROVIV	yes	no	yes	no	most	yes	yes	yes	$$
GRAVITY (CARBON BLOCK or CERAMIC, COUNTERTOP)									
BERKEY	yes	no	yes	yes	most	yes	yes	yes	$$$
Berkefeld	no	no	yes	no	most	yes	yes	yes	$$
Epic Nano	yes	80%	yes	yes	yes	yes	yes	yes	$
FAUCET									
waterdrop	yes	yes	yes	yes	yes	yes	yes	yes	$$$
PUR faucet	yes	yes	yes	yes	yes	yes	yes	yes	$
Zero Water	yes	yes	yes	yes	yes	yes	yes	yes	$$
FRIDGE									
Hydroviv	yes	no	yes	no	yesish	yes	yes	yes	$$
waterdrop	yes	yes	yes	yes	yes	yes	yes	yes	$$
PITCHERS									
Zero Water 5 stag	yes	98%	yes	yes	yes	yes	no	yes	$
Epic Pure	yes	no	yes	yes	yes	yes	no	50%	$
Brita	no	no	no	no	no	no	no	no	$
Brita Elite	yes	no	some	no	yes	yes	no	yes	$
Pur Pitcher	yes	no	some	no	some	some	no	yes	$
Clearly Filtered	yes	no	yes	no	yes	yes	no	yes	$$
TRAVELERS									
Berkey	yes	no	yes	no	yes	yes	yes	yes	$
Epic	yes	no	yes	no	yes	yes	no	yes	$
SHOWER FILTER									
Jolie	yes	no	yes	no	yes	yes	yes	yes	$
Berkey	yes	no	yes	no	yes	yes	yes	yes	$
WHOLE HOME									
Spring Well	yes	yes	yes	yes	yes	yes	yes	yes	$$$$

5. Water in Town

For those that have public water, your town issues a water quality report once a year. If you have your own well, please see the next page. Keep in mind not all contaminants will be included in the annual report, for most toxins in water aren't regulated by the EPA or required to be monitored. Many towns, however choose to test for contaminants over and above the EPA regulated contaminants.

The Environmental Working Group (EWG) goes the extra mile and tests for those suspected of causing disease. If you go to their website, just enter your Zip Code and you'll get a list of any contaminants that are at unsafe levels. The EPA has a MCL (maximum contaminant level) threshold of safety noted in ppb (parts per billion) for regulated contaminants. The EWG uses this as their baseline. You'll find out if there are contaminants of concern, what's over the EPA guidelines, as well as any alerts for those that aren't currently regulated by the EPA that pose a danger. Go here: EWG TAP WATER DATEBASE

EPA LIST OF CONTAMINANTS
The EPA list of Regulated Contaminants and unregulated contaminants can be found at the back of this book. Discover more about these monstrous pollutants in the next section of this book beginning on page 22 and the big daddy EPA list beginning on page 286.

YOUR TOWN'S PUBLIC WATER SUPPLY
To get an idea what's coming out your kitchen tap, tap below to get info about what's in your town's water. Just enter your zip code when prompted: **www.ewg.org/tapwater/**

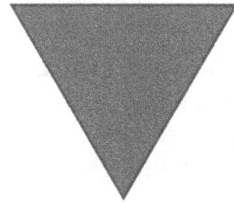

What's in Your Water

6. Well Water

WELL OWNERS HOTLINE: (888) 395-1033, wellcarehotline.org
Over 23 million households have private wells. Those who live in the countryside, or outside of town usually have their own well.

Testing Your Well Water
If you have your own private well, you have to test it yourself to find out what contaminants it may contain. Some counties provide free well testing. This is very important so please take the time to do it yearly. You must protect your health from contaminants in water.
Also, you can call your local water utility or health department to see who they recommend. You can also look up your county or nearby towns through the Environmental Working Group Go Here, and see if there are any water pollutants in your community's public water system. There's also a podcast for well water owners which you might find interesting, www.**drinkingwaterpodcast.org.**

Filter Well Water
Everyone needs to filter their water, even well owners. Wells can easily absorb toxins both natural and manmade from ground water, lawn chemicals, fertilizer, pesticides, arsenic, nitrate and nitrite. Please use filtered water for cooking also. Some people even filter their shower water.

Water Softeners
Some say Water softeners are ok, and then there's others who say they can increase your sodium levels. Perhaps what we really don't know comes down to the interaction between contaminated well water and the salts in softened water, and further, does the impact of water softening affect one's disease risk from water contaminants?
"Domestic well owners commonly have water softeners. The calcium and magnesium ions that make water hard are replaced by sodium ions that are obtained from resin in the softening equipment. Iron and other heavy metals are usually removed in the exchange process. When the resin reaches capacity and can no longer remove calcium and magnesium ions, it needs to be regenerated."[13]

7. Clean Water Act

The objective of the Federal Water Pollution Control Act, commonly referred to as the Clean Water Act (CWA), is to restore and maintain the chemical, physical, and biological integrity of the nation's waters by preventing point and nonpoint pollution sources, providing assistance to publicly owned treatment works for the improvement of waste- water treatment, and maintaining the integrity of wetlands.[14]

Water Pollution

The most serious and harmful sources of water pollution are caused by industries, government, and ultimately, people. How can people be so discourteous to pollute or litter? Do we not each have the responsibility to take care of our planet? This means to keep it

> "Pollution is nothing but the resources we are not harvesting.
> We allow them to disperse because we've been ignorant of their value." –
> R. Buckminster Fuller

clean. Why does anyone pollute? Why do corporations and industries pollute? Is it because they're lazy, or too cheap to dispose of waste properly, or secretly have a motive to poison us? Is the big factory owner too much a penny pincher, or just too blind to see the big picture and the value in installing the proper equipment that prevents air and water pollution? Those days of covering up irresponsibility are over. I know we can all do better. Maybe if we can't control our trash, we shouldn't be in business

In this interconnected world, pollution travels be it by stream or river or by wind and dust, toxins get carried everywhere. The EPA was created to protect our water sources, our air sources, and ecosystems throughout the country. While climate change occupies everyone's mind, toxic polluters are still up to their same old tricks. Can't industry do better? Can't America do better? People used to care and be responsible, and be proud that their family set an example—that their company was a good company. Can't we be that way again? Or do we have to save a dollar at any cost, even if it means poisoning the water supply or fish down the stream.

History of the Clean Water Act

> See more EPA, pages 284-298

Growing public awareness and concern for controlling water pollution was reignited by President Kennedy and Rachel Carson's research and breakthrough book, Silent Spring. As soon as Kennedy was signed in as President, he got busy with tackling water pollution. Through his effort the Federal Water Pollution Control Act Amendments of 1961 were Passed *(see intro pages ii -iv)*. Throughout 1963, President Kennedy crusaded for environmental awareness and protection for future generations. This caused a stirring in human consciousness worldwide and eventually led to the 1965's Water Quality Act, and also the Refuse Act of 1970. In 1972, President Nixon signed the Federal Water Pollution Control Act Amendments, which were amended in 1977, this is when it became known as the Clean Water Act (CWA). Prior to the 1960s, there were earlier attempts for water protection: Rivers and Harbors Act of 1899, and the Federal Water Pollution Control Act of 1948.[15]

"The Act established the basic structure for regulating discharges of pollutants into the waters of the United States. It gave EPA the authority to implement pollution control programs such as setting wastewater standards for industry. The Clean Water Act also continued requirements to set water quality standards for all contaminants in surface waters. The Act made it unlawful for any person to discharge any pollutant from a point source into navigable waters, unless a permit was obtained under its provisions."[16]

The Safe Drinking Water Act

SDWA was originally passed by Congress in 1974 to protect public health by regulating the nation's public drinking water supply. The Safe Drinking Water Act (SDWA) is the main federal law that ensures the quality of Americans' drinking water. Under SDWA, EPA sets standards for drinking water quality and oversees the states, localities, and water suppliers who implement those standards. SDWA authorizes the EPA to set national health-based standards for drinking water to protect us all against both naturally-occurring and man-made contaminants that can be found in drinking water. The EPA, states, and water systems work together to make sure that these standards are met.

8. Water Health

70% of our planet is covered with water. Only 2.6% is fresh water and 2% of that is trapped in ice and glaciers. That means less than 1% of earth's water is accessible and available for drinking![17] **With so little water to go around, we all need to do our share in taking care of it. That equates to adding as little pollution to it as possible. Industry as well as people everywhere must find better, cleaner methods for doing just about everything.**

Wastewater treatment facilities are currently unable to filter out all pollutants. Already, we can see the polluted Mississippi creating an ever-expanding dead zone in the Gulf of Mexico. Every one needs to be responsible with water.

Pollution seeps into our water in innumerable ways. Pollution is classified as either **Point Source**—meaning it comes from an exact identifiable place like a factory or discharge pipe, or **Non-Point Source**—meaning it's hard to pinpoint the source as in the case of rain that washes pollutants together (runoff), or like persistent organic pollutants that travel far and wide.

> **Water Consumption**
> **PEOPLE:** For good health we need to drink about 0.5 gallon (2 liters or 8 glasses) of water each day. Two more gallons (8 liters) are used for drinking and cooking. A person can live one month without food, but only one week without water.
> **HOMES:** Each person in the United States uses about 90 gallons (341 liters) of water a day for cleaning and gardening.
> **FACTORIES:** Factories use enormous amounts of water to produce goods. It takes 60,000 gallons (227,000 L) of water to make a ton of steel.
> **FARMS:** Farms use water to irrigate land for growing crops and to raise livestock. It takes 115 gallons (435 liters) to grow the wheat for one loaf of bread, and 4,000 gallons (15,000 liters) to produce one pound of beef.
> The National Geographic
> www.nationalgeographic.com

Without question, water is our most precious and valuable resource. Without water, life cannot exist. Currently, many organizations are working to ensure that we have clean water for generations to come. Support them as much as you can.

The Unmentionables: PPCPs: EMERGING POLLUTANTS

Pharmaceutical and personal care products (PPCPs) are an ever-growing body of new pollutants flushing into our waterways. Scientists worldwide have only just begun to study the consequences of PPCPs accumulation. Because of the resilient nature of these types of compounds, they are found in both untreated and *treated* water! Our water treatment facilities are simply incapable of filtering out these types of mixtures. Most prevalent chemicals found include: anti-inflammatory drugs, sex hormones, oral contraceptives, anticonvulsants, beta-blockers, antidepressants, bronchodilators, lipid regulators, antibiotics, hypnotics, sunscreen products, and synthetic fragrance. Because these things are normally not administered or ingested in combinations like these, scientists are testing aquatic creatures to determine long-term effects. Even more reason to avoid tap water. Learn how to keep your water clean at www.reverse-osmosis-water-filter-guide.com.

Toxic Byproducts resulting from Chlorine and Ammonia

Current chloramine processes utilized throughout the country to purify public water supplies result in toxic carcinogenic byproducts in our drinking water. To avoid these, people need to purify the water as it comes out of their tap. Perhaps we can push for a better nontoxic program at the municipality level that will create more efficiency and less expense and less toxicity to us the end users.

OZONE DISINFECTION

"Ozone disinfection is the least used method in the
U.S. although this technology has been widely accepted in Europe for decades. Ozone treatment has the ability to achieve higher levels of disinfection than either chlorine or UV, however, the capital costs as well as maintenance expenditures are not competitive with available alternatives. Ozone is therefore used only sparingly, primarily in special cases where alternatives are not effective." [18]

SOLUTIONS

- Contact your elected officials. Encourage them to introduce legislation that will ban toxic industrial waste from entering our water resources.
- Like Europe, we can use better filtering processes like ozone[19] to provide clean and safe drinking water that's free of DBPs.
- Keep toxic chemicals out of the water and out of your body
- Let's work together to insist industry complies with zero toxic water pollution discharges that the government enforces!

KEEPING WATER CLEAN

- Keep litter, pet wastes, leaves, and debris out of street gutters and storm drains—these outlets drain directly to lake, streams, rivers, and wetlands.
- Apply lawn chemicals sparingly and according to directions.
- Dispose of used oil, antifreeze, paints, and other household chemicals properly, not in storm sewers or drains. If your community does not already have a program for collecting household hazardous wastes, ask your city to establish one.
- Clean up spilled brake fluid, oil, grease, and antifreeze. Do not hose them into the street where they can eventually reach local streams and lakes.
- Control soil erosion on your property by planting ground cover and stabilizing erosion-prone areas.
- Encourage local government officials to develop construction erosion and sediment control ordinances in your community.
- Have your septic system inspected and pumped at least every three to five years so that it operates properly.
- Purchase household detergents and cleaners that are low in phosphorous to reduce the amount of nutrients discharged into our lakes, streams and coastal waters.

www.epa.gov/owow/nps/whatudo.html

9. Water Shortage

In areas suffering with drought and water shortages, fear of not having water can keep people awake at night. Yet there can be enough water for all if we start being wiser about water as well as stop polluting it.

From the Southwest to Canada to China, drought conditions demand urgent action. Sometimes governmental policies may be making things worse by preventing water from reaching places it's needed most. In some of the driest places when it rains, you think they'd collect it. But that's not always the case. California for the most part doesn't direct the rain to reservoirs, but lets it flow out to the ocean.[20] In times of drought, one would think rain like that would be collected.

> 70% of freshwater is used for Agriculture. In Arizona, that figures rises to 74%.
>
> Source: World Bank[21] ADWR[22]

ProPublica explains the reasons for Arizona's water situation in Holy Crop, *How Federal Dollars are Financing the Water Crisis in the West.*[23] Here are some nuggets from this report:

> The depth of the troubles seems to stem from the mismanagement and siphoning of the Colorado River. Further, the government's subsidies to farmers to grow crops needing a lot of water in the dry arid southwest is at the heart of it. Explosive urban growth matched with the steady planting of water-thirsty crops – which use the majority of the water – don't help.
>
> The federal subsidies that prop up cotton farming in Arizona are just one of myriad ways that policymakers have refused, or been slow to reshape laws to reflect the West's changing circumstances. Provisions in early–20th-century water-use laws that not only permit but also compel farmers and others to use more water than they need are another. "Use It or Lose It" is the cynical catch phrase for one of those policies."

"Water scarcity is further complicated by the massive amounts of water needed to grow crops. Around 70% of freshwater globally goes to agriculture, and about one third of the world's cities already

compete with agriculture for water, according to the U.N. report. Competition will only increase as the urban demand for water is predicted to grow by 80% within the next three decades."[24]

150 years ago, John Wesley Powell, the geologist and explorer, traveled the Colorado River in an effort to gauge America's chances for developing its arid western half. His report to Congress reached a chastening conclusion: There wasn't enough water to support significant settlement. For more than a century, Americans have defied Powell's words, constructing 20 of the nation's largest cities and a vibrant economy that, among other bounties, provides an astonishing proportion of the country's fruit and vegetables.[25]

Bottling Water
Behind water shortages everywhere there seems to sit a corporation siphoning springs and fresh water lakes for bottling. Blue Triton (formerly owned by Nestle) is perhaps the biggest of the perpetrators pumping vital water resources out of nature to fill up their plastic water bottles. This process of taking water is often with little thought of replacing stock or compensating the community from which the gold is taken. In some places like California and Colorado they're harvesting water in areas suffering with drought conditions. They take the water by truckloads for processing and packaging. These then get shipped across the country leaving a disastrous footprint in its wake. There has to be a better way to maintain nature's balance and provide water to people.

Bottled Water: Savior in Emergencies
Bottled water is a savior in emergencies, water shortages and natural disasters. But must we bottle it in plastic? Can the companies at least move away from plastic or find a nontoxic biodegradable similar breakproof bottle?

What is the answer?
- Conserve water use
- Grow native plants and trees that grow well in your climate
- Plant vegetation that doesn't need a lot of water
- Save rain. Get a rain barrel or some buckets out there
- Purchase water in glass bottles rather than plastic.

~ Conserving Water ~

- Shorten your shower time if possible
- Turn off the tap when brushing teeth
- Fix leaky faucets and pipes
- During rain storms, avoid laundry or dishwashing to help prevent sewer systems overflowing.
- In your yard and garden, plant native plants that don't require constant watering. Better yet go for those that can withstand drought conditions and are pollinator friendly.
- Save and collect rain water for reuse. Get a rain barrel to capture water coming off the roof and create a raingarden in your yard with bioswales and landscaping to prevent water from going into the sewer system.

STORMWATER RUNOFF
Landscaping is key. We can develop urban systems and bioswales that capture stormwater runoff rather than letting it run down the sewer. Perhaps towns can host a contest to see who can design the most efficient, durable and functional systems. Mimicking wetlands will filter it too!

> **Water**
> **Potable**: water is drinkable; safe for people and animals
> **Non-potable:** not for drinking or cooking: good for gardening, irrigating, washing the car, laundry

GROW SENSIBLE CROPS FOR YOUR REGION
In drier climates, people and farmers must switch to planting crops that are native to the region and less water intensive. The Government needs to stop incentivizing farmers to do such. Farmers should plant what's sensible for the area geographically. Let's get the Farm Bill fixed so this nonsense isn't carried forward to yet another administration. Funding should go instead to saving animals and preserving biodiversity.

IRRIGATION:
- Irrigation can be done conservatively with Drip Irrigation
- If there are ways to redirect rainwater for irrigation in California, for health's sake that must become a priority weighted against awkward environmental policy preventing it.

10. Health Wake Up Call

According the United Nations, 2 billion people worldwide lack access to clean and safe drinking water.[26] What's wrong with us that we allow this? As we unravel the sources and causes for water pollution and scarcity, we will manifest the solutions to solving our expanding health crisis.

Between the pollution and the exposures in our environment, lies the cause for many diseases triggered by factors other than genetics. Most cancer is now known to be the result of factors in our environment. Once we understand the cause, there is great hope for recovery and healing. It's of the utmost importance that we tackle the sources of pollution now. Whether it's in the water, air, or our food, the most sinister of pollutants and toxic substances must be withdrawn from use.

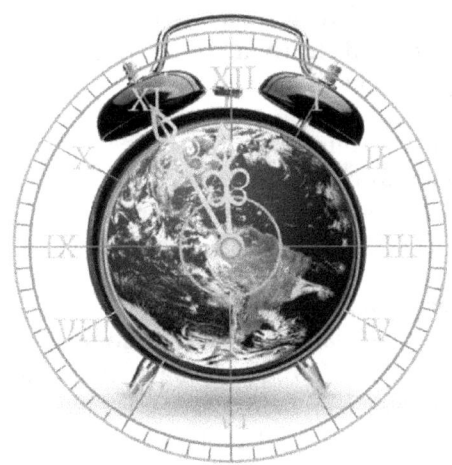

Today's Health Emergencies include:
- Rising rates of early onset cancer[27] in adults under 50
- Rising rates of colon cancer and lung cancer
- Rising rates of Alzheimer's and Dementia
- Rising rates of antibiotic-resistant diseases
- Rising rates of diabetes and metabolic syndrome
- Rising rates of childhood cancer, autism, and allergies

President's Cancer Panel Report 2008-2009
"The entire U.S. population is exposed on a daily basis to numerous agricultural chemicals, some of which also are used in residential and commercial landscaping. Many of these chemicals have known or suspected carcinogenic or endocrine-disrupting properties. Pesticides (insecticides, herbicides, and fungicides) approved for use by the U.S. Environmental Protection Agency (EPA) contain nearly 900 active ingredients, many of which are toxic. Many of the solvents, fillers, and other chemicals listed as inert ingredients on pesticide labels also are toxic, but are not required to be tested for their potential to cause chronic diseases such as cancer. In addition to pesticides, agricultural fertilizers and veterinary pharmaceuticals are major contributors to water pollution, both directly and as a result of chemical processes that form toxic by-products when these substances enter the water supply. Farmers and their families, including migrant workers, are at highest risk from agricultural exposures. Because agricultural chemicals often are applied as mixtures, it has been difficult to clearly distinguish cancer risks associated with individual agents."

"The good news is that a large number of cancers can be prevented. It is estimated that as many as two-thirds of all cancer cases are linked to environmental causes. This number may even be higher. Many of these are linked to lifestyle factors that can be modified."[28]

The President's Cancer Panel Report 2008-2009[29]
"A precautionary, prevention-oriented approach should replace current reactionary approaches to environmental contaminants in which human harm must be proven before action is taken to reduce or eliminate exposure. Though not applicable in every instance, this approach should be the cornerstone of a new national cancer prevention strategy that emphasizes primary prevention, redirects accordingly both research and policy agendas, and sets tangible goals for reducing or eliminating toxic environmental exposures (that cause cancer)."

SOLUTIONS:
Filter your water. Avoid toxins in water, in air, and in food.
Drink and cook with purified water. Be a leader and help encourage our elected officials to take action, introduce a bill, whatever it takes to help move the process forward effectively. We have no time to lose. We all must help in cleaning up our country's water resources.

11. Climate Wake Up Call

According the United Nations, Global cancer cases are expected to rise around 77 per cent by the middle of the century.[30] Further, "higher water temperatures and more frequent floods and droughts are projected to exacerbate many forms of water pollution – from sediments to pathogens and pesticides."[31] Getting a handle on warming and pollution is of the utmost importance right now. In fact, it may be our only hope to prevent disease, heal disease, and save humanity as we know it.

Today's Climate Emergencies include:
- Air and Water Pollution causing disease & warming
- Water Stress & Scarcity
- Warming Temperatures and Extreme Weather
- Droughts & Wild Fires, Rising tides and Coastal Erosion
- Significant loss of animal and plant biodiversity

"Water scarcity is becoming endemic as a result of the local impact of physical water stress, coupled with the acceleration and spreading of freshwater pollution. As a result of climate change, seasonal water scarcity will increase in regions where it is currently abundant. Poor ambient water quality in higher-income countries is often related to runoff from agriculture."[32]

We must do what we can to slow down warming. The main drivers for warming aside from burning fossil fuels are Big Ag and the toxic chemical industry. Factory farm waste, biosolids, and synthetic fertilizer are killing us and our atmosphere. In fact, chemical fertilizer has a lot to do with depleting earth's protective ozone layer and warming.[33]

The good news is this is all fixable! Getting a hold on climate comes down to accountability—eliminating toxic pollution from industry and Agriculture. Isn't it time these sectors all upgrade to using and creating nontoxic materials in the first place? Isn't it time the EPA enforce Clean Water rules for _all_ industries? If we do not take a stand now & insist our Government step up and end industries' laziness of polluting our planet, the government will leap forward hastiliy with the agenda hatched by the polluters—The vile SRM program. This is an insane scheme to block sunlight from reaching earth[34] by using nanoparticles and sulfur dioxide! SRM is being pushed so that the industry can skip making changes. They're so pathetic! It's up to us to hold them and our government accountable. Let's begin.

SPECIAL REPORT

Chemicals & Contaminants in Groundwater

Contaminated ground water affects our drinking water, which affects our health. This is an emergency. The following list, courtesy of the US Geological Service lists groundwater contaminants, sources, and the health effects exposure can cause.

\multicolumn{3}{c}{Inorganic contaminants found in groundwater}		
Contaminant	Sources to groundwater	Potential health and other effects
Aluminum	Occurs naturally in some rocks and drainage from mines.	Can precipitate out of water after treatment, causing increased turbidity or discolored water.
Antimony	Enters environment from natural weathering, industrial production, municipal waste disposal, and manufacturing of flame retardants, ceramics, glass, batteries, fireworks, and explosives.	Decreases longevity, alters blood levels of glucose and cholesterol in laboratory animals exposed at high levels over their lifetime.
Arsenic	Enters environment from natural processes, industrial activities, **pesticides**, and industrial waste, smelting of copper, lead, and zinc ore.	Causes acute and chronic toxicity, liver and kidney damage; decreases blood hemoglobin. A carcinogen.

Inorganic contaminants found in groundwater

Contaminant	Sources to groundwater	Potential health and other effects
Barium	Occurs naturally in some limestones, sandstones, and soils in the eastern United States.	Can cause a variety of cardiac, gastrointestinal, neuromuscular effects. Associated w/ hypertension &cardiotoxicity in animals.
Beryllium	Occurs naturally in soils, groundwater, and surface water. Often used in electrical industry equipment and components, nuclear power and space industry. Enters the environment from mining operations, processing plants, and improper waste disposal. Found in low concentrations in rocks, coal, and petroleum and enters the ground	Causes acute and chronic toxicity; can cause damage to lungs and bones. Possible carcinogen.
Cadmium	Found in low concentrations in rocks, coal, and **petroleum** and enters the groundwater and surface water when dissolved by acidic waters. May enter the environment from	Replaces zinc biochemically in the body and causes high blood pressure, liver and kidney damage, and anemia. Destroys testicular tissue and red blood cells. Toxic to aquatic biota.

Inorganic contaminants found in groundwater		
Contaminant	Sources to groundwater	Potential health and other effects
	industrial discharge, mining waste, metal plating, water pipes, batteries, paints and pigments, plastic stabilizers, and landfill leachate.	
Chloride	May be associated with the presence of sodium in drinking water when present in high concentrations. Often from saltwater intrusion, mineral dissolution, industrial and domestic waste.	Deteriorates plumbing, water heaters, and municipal water-works equipment at high levels. Above secondary maximum contaminant level, taste becomes noticeable.
Chromium	Enters environment from old mining operations runoff and leaching into groundwater, fossil-fuel combustion, cement-plant emissions, mineral leaching, and waste incineration. Used in metal plating and as a cooling-tower water additive.	Chromium III is a nutritionally essential element. Chromium VI is much more toxic than Chromium III and causes liver and kidney damage, internal hemorrhaging, respiratory damage, dermatitis, and ulcers on the skin at high concentrations.

Inorganic contaminants found in groundwater

Contaminant	Sources to groundwater	Potential health and other effects
Copper	Enters environment from metal plating, industrial and domestic waste, mining, and mineral leaching.	Can cause stomach and intestinal distress, liver and kidney damage, anemia in high doses. Imparts an adverse taste and significant staining to clothes and fixtures. Essential trace element but toxic to plants and algae at moderate levels.
Cyanide	Often used in electroplating, steel processing, plastics, synthetic fabrics, and **fertilizer production**; also from improper waste disposal.	Poisoning is the result of damage to spleen, brain, and liver.
Dissolved solids	Occur naturally but also enters environment from man-made sources such as landfill leachate, **feedlots, or sewage.** A measure of the dissolved "salts" or minerals in the water. May also include some dissolved organic compounds.	May have an influence on the acceptability of water in general. May be indicative of the presence of excess concentrations of specific substances not included in the Safe Water Drinking Act, which would make water objectionable. High concentrations of dissolved solids shorten the life of hot water heaters.
Fluoride	Occurs naturally or as an additive to municipal water supplies;	Decreases incidence of tooth decay but high levels can stain or mottle teeth. Causes crippling bone disorder

25

Inorganic contaminants found in groundwater

Contaminant	Sources to groundwater	Potential health and other effects
	widely used in industry.	(calcification of the bones and joints) at very high levels.
Hardness	Result of metallic ions dissolved in the water; reported as concentration of calcium carbonate. Calcium carbonate is derived from dissolved limestone or discharges from operating or abandoned mines.	Decreases the lather formation of soap and increases scale formation in hot-water heaters and low-pressure boilers at high levels.
Iron	Occurs naturally as a mineral from sediment and rocks or from mining, industrial waste, and corroding metal.	Imparts a bitter astringent taste to water and a brownish color to laundered clothing and plumbing fixtures.
Lead	Enters environment from industry, mining, plumbing, gasoline, coal, and as a water additive.	Affects red blood cell chemistry; delays normal physical and mental development in babies and young children. Causes slight deficits in attention span, hearing, and learning in children. Can cause slight increase in blood pressure in some adults. Probable carcinogen.
Manganese	Occurs naturally as a mineral from	Causes aesthetic and economic damage, and

Inorganic contaminants found in groundwater

Contaminant	Sources to groundwater	Potential health and other effects
	sediment and rocks or from **mining and industrial waste**.	imparts brownish stains to laundry. Affects taste of water, and causes dark brown or black stains on plumbing fixtures. Relatively non-toxic to animals but toxic to plants at high levels.
Mercury	Occurs as an inorganic salt and as organic mercury compounds. Enters the environment from **industrial waste, mining, pesticides, coal,** electrical equipment (batteries, lamps, switches), smelting, and fossil-fuel combustion.	Causes acute and chronic toxicity. Targets the kidneys and can cause nervous system disorders.
Nickel	Occurs naturally in soils, groundwater, and surface water. Often used in electroplating, stainless steel and alloy products, **mining, and refining**.	Damages the heart and liver of laboratory animals exposed to large amounts over their lifetime.
Nitrate (as nitrogen)	Enters the environment from **fertilizer, feedlots, and**	Toxicity results from the body's natural breakdown of nitrate to nitrite. Causes "blue baby

Inorganic contaminants found in groundwater		
Contaminant	Sources to groundwater	Potential health and other effects
	sewage. Occurs naturally in mineral deposits, soils, seawater, freshwater systems, the atmosphere, and biota. More stable form of combined nitrogen in oxygenated water. Found in the highest levels in groundwater under extensively developed areas	disease," or methemoglobinemia, which threatens oxygen-carrying capacity of the blood.
Nitrite combined nitrate/nitrite	Enters environment from **fertilizer, sewage, and human or farm-animal waste.**	Toxicity results from the body's natural breakdown of nitrate to nitrite. Causes "blue baby disease," or methemoglobinemia, which threatens oxygen-carrying capacity of the blood.
Selenium	Enters environment from naturally occurring geologic sources, sulfur, and coal.	Causes acute and chronic toxic effects in animals-- "blind staggers" in cattle. Nutritionally essential element at low doses but toxic at high doses.
Silver	Enters environment from ore mining and processing, product fabrication, and disposal. Often used in	Can cause argyria, a blue-gray coloration of the skin, mucous membranes, eyes, and organs in humans and animals with chronic exposure.

Inorganic contaminants found in groundwater

Contaminant	Sources to groundwater	Potential health and other effects
	photography, electric and electronic equipment, sterling and electroplating, alloy, and solder. Because of great economic value of silver, recovery practices are typically used to minimize loss.	
Sodium	Derived geologically from leaching of surface and underground deposits of salt and decomposition of various minerals. Human activities contribute through de-icing and washing products.	Can be a health risk factor for those individuals on a low-sodium diet.
Sulfate	Elevated concentrations may result from saltwater intrusion, mineral dissolution, and domestic or industrial waste.	Forms hard scales on boilers and heat exchangers; can change the taste of water, and has a laxative effect in high doses.
Thallium	Enters environment from **soils**; used in electronics,	Damages kidneys, liver, brain, and intestines in laboratory animals when

Inorganic contaminants found in groundwater		
Contaminant	Sources to groundwater	Potential health and other effects
	pharmaceuticals manufacturing, glass, and alloys.	given in high doses over their lifetime.
Zinc	Found naturally in water, most frequently in areas where it is mined. Enters environment from industrial waste, metal plating, and plumbing, and is **a major component of sludge.**	Aids in the healing of wounds. Causes no ill health effects except in very high doses. Imparts an undesirable taste to water. Toxic to plants at high levels.
Organic contaminants		
Volatile organic compounds (Benzene	Enter environment when used to make plastics, dyes, rubbers, polishes, solvents, crude oil, insecticides, inks, varnishes, paints, disinfectants, gasoline products, pharmaceuticals, preservatives, spot removers, paint removers, degreasers, and many more.	Can cause cancer and liver damage, anemia, gastrointestinal disorder, skin irritation, blurred vision, exhaustion, weight loss, damage to the nervous system, and respiratory tract irritation.
Pesticides	Enter environment as herbicides, insecticides, fungicides,	Cause poisoning, headaches, dizziness, gastrointestinal disturbance, numbness, weakness, and cancer.

| Inorganic contaminants found in groundwater |||
Contaminant	Sources to groundwater	Potential health and other effects
	rodenticides, and algicides.	Destroys nervous system, thyroid, kidneys, reproductive system, liver,
Plasticizers, chlorinated solvents, benzo[a]pyrene, and dioxin	Used as sealants, linings, solvents, pesticides, plasticizers, components of gasoline, disinfectant, and wood preservative. Enters environment from improper waste disposal, leaching runoff, leaking storage tank, Industrial runoff	Cause cancer. Damages nervous and reproductive systems, kidney, stomach, and liver.

Source: USGS[35]

SECTION TWO
WATER CONTAMINANTS EXPOSED
A to Z

These are the things that make water *not good*. See here what must be removed from water if we are to save our health and the planet.

> Facts are stubborn things; and whatever may be our wishes, our inclinations, or the dictates of our passion, they cannot alter the state of facts and evidence.
> **President John Adams**

1. Agricultural Runoff

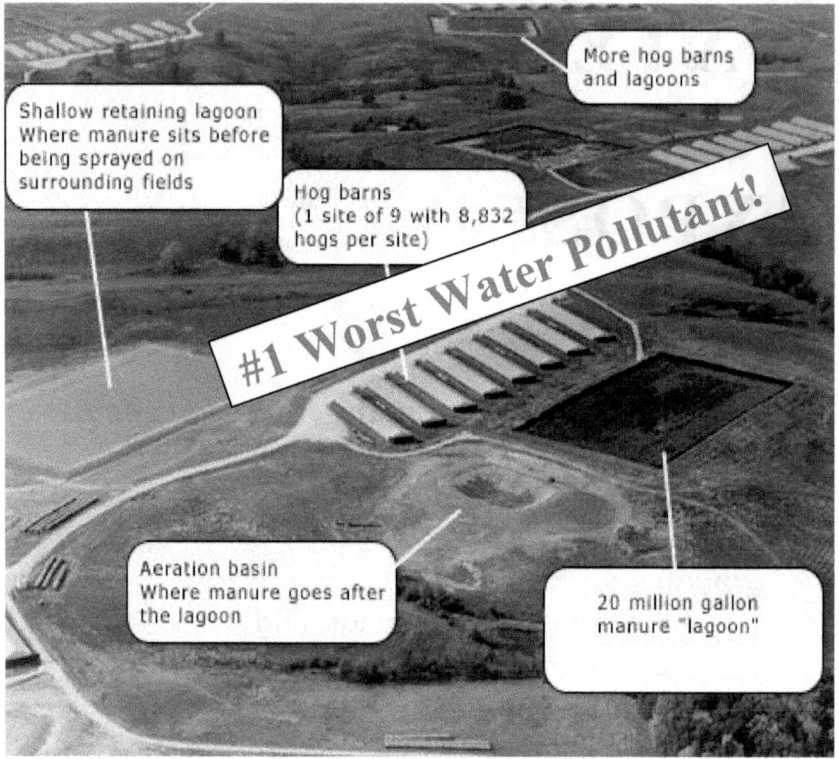

Source: Grace Factory Farm Project, Whitetail Hog Facility in MO. www.factoryfarm.org

Agricultural runoff is a combination of muck and gook from large farms using toxic substances. These farms are on steroids, literally. The big animal factory farms use lots of artificial hormones and other unfriendly toxins to control animals in cramped unfit pens. These farms have a lot of issues, one of them being sewage control. The supersize monocropping farms growing GMOs and conventional crops are killing pollinators and destroying soil with their growing methods. Collectively, these types of farms compromise our drinking water and increase our health risk. They do not embrace the American spirit, honor the earth, or respect human health.

FACTORY FARMS:
America's Biggest Source of Water Pollution![36]

Wherever one looks, from quaint little towns across the country to every big city, water supplies are tainted with pesticides, "dissolved solids", excess nutrients and nitrates from fertilizer runoff. Factory farms contribute to poor water quality mainly because of the untreated, unregulated animal waste. This waste includes genetically modified hormones and blood, antibiotics and feces, GMO animal feed and any parasites or what-have-you the animals may be suffering with. Untreated animal waste from factory farms is a major health threat. One might think agricultural runoff only concerns fertilizer in rural areas. This is not the case, as runoff anywhere affects water everywhere.

Animal Waste from Factory Farms is unregulated and contributes to Antibiotic-Resistant Bacteria.[37]

Untreated animal waste—sewage from CAFOs (concentrated animal feeding operations) and factory farms— is stored onsite in huge manure lagoons that are a major problem during storms. This contributes to very poor water quality for nearby towns and residents affected directly from runoff pollution. We see the results of this in the rise of stomach and intestinal problems, disease, as well as antibiotic-resistant bacteria and fungi.[38] Just this year, Iowa has been crowned as America's Cancer Capital. Could that have anything to do with the fact that Iowa has more factory farms than any other place in the U.S.? **CAFOs in Iowa: 4025!**[39]

Who Will Change It? We Must Regulate the Poop![40]

Sewage from factory farms (or CAFOs) is not regulated by the EPA (Environmental Protection Agency), or USDA (United States Department of Agriculture), or the FDA (Food and Drug Administration). As such, large farms funnel waste from their mega-concrete barns to wide open lagoons on site, often with unlined pits that allow waste to leach into nearby streams and waterways. During storms this is especially troublesome, as this more easily overflows and mixes with stormwater that eventually contaminates the drinking water. This sewage is full of bacteria, microbes, artificial hormones, antibiotics, steroids, disease, blood, GMO animal feed, bioengineered unknown substances. Plain and simply put, animal waste from CAFOS is a hot mess and doesn't do anything good for animals or people who come into contact with it. Why don't we have the government regulating this stuff yet? Better yet, since this waste is a primary driver for methane emissions and warming temps, when are we going to cease allowing mega-farm hell holes to exist?

Pesticides

Along with the fertilizer and sewage in agricultural runoff, comes the toxic herbicides and pesticides as well as the GMO-animal-feed-inspired animal waste. These all then combine in the water to a whole array of debilitating disease inducing substances. Shocking any of us are still healthy! Do we include wastewater from pesticide manufacturing facilities as agricultural runoff as well or is that go into the 'toxic deadly chemicals' pollution category?

Excess Nutrients from Synthetic Fertilizer

Synthetic nitrogen and phosphorous fertilizers are a huge problem for waterways. The runoff causes nutrient pollution that then causes toxic algae blooms, dead zones (eutrophication), and worse Red Tides. as well as sewage sludge and untreated animal waste from factory farms also come along for the ride

State of US FARMLAND

- We must take all strides possible right now to slow down the progression of huge factory farms.
- By restricting and lessening use of synthetic fertilizers, as well as halting the growth of farming that's earth-harming, we can make a huge impact in healing the earth and reversing climate crisis trends.
- Farmers we will help you transition to earth friendly methods of farming that won't harm you or the waterways. Join us at www.adoreyourplanet to learn more. Green farming is less costly for you and far more profitable in every way.
- Many popular lawn and garden products contain Glyphosate, Atrazine and Neonicotinoids. These products are sold at Home Depot and large retailers. Let's stop selling this stuff and let's stop buying this crap!
- Ask your Landscaper not to use these toxins that harm animals.

SOLUTIONS

- Filter your water. Used filtered water (clean water) for cooking and drinking. Give everyone in your household filtered water.
- Let's stop the insanity and get animal waste regulated!
- Let's stop confining large amounts of animals at these horrible farms.

2. ALUMINUM

They call this the Age of Aluminum.[41] Only in the last 100 years has aluminum become part of the human experience. Aluminum is the most abundant metal in the earth's crust, yet, "mining the ore that contains aluminum, called bauxite, destroys forests and grasslands, contaminates water resources, and creates toxic dust and waste."[42] Aluminum pollution in water is not enforced by the EPA.[43] Does anyone really know just how much aluminum we're exposed to these days?

New Exposure Routes Could Amplify Exposure
Aluminum Oxide Nanoparticles (NPs) are new and not just infiltrating water supplies,[44] but are now in products we're using everyday. That could explain the surge in Alzheimer's, and memory-related disorders.[45] They're used in makeup and foundation,[46] drugs, tooth polish, hair products, food packaging, etc. Independent tests have found that due to their microscopic size, nanoparticles are easily absorbed through the skin,[47] through sinus and mucous membranes, epithelial cells and by ingestion. These micro-sized metal particles may potentially accumulate in our memory center—the hippocampus.[48] They "disturb cell viability, alter mitochondrial function, increase oxidative stress, and also alter tight junction protein expression of the blood brain barrier (BBB)."[49]

Sources of Aluminum: Coal fired power plants, incinerators,[50] mining pollution, metal refineries, hazardous waste sites, fireworks, explosives, foil, beverage cans, pots and pans, antacids, antiperspirants, nanoparticle biotech manufacturing,[51] baking powder, buffered aspirin, medicines, vaccines, food additives. "Aluminum salts are also widely used in water treatment as coagulants to reduce organic matter, color, turbidity, and microorganism levels."[52]

Health Effects: High levels of aluminum can harm the brain and nervous system, increase risk of neurodegenerative diseases, memory impairment, Alzheimer's disease, Parkinson's disease, Lou Gehrig's disease (ALS), brain and bone disease in children, kidney disease.

SOLUTIONS:
Filter your water! The FDA must vet all new ingredients and technology designed to go into foods, cosmetics, and drugs. FDA must be more proactive in regulating products containing nanos. The EPA must take a bigger role regulating and preventing aluminum pollution in water.

3. AMR – EMERGING!
Anti-Microbial Resistance

I wish it weren't worth mentioning, however, this book is here to raise awareness about matters in the environment that affect your health and your family, so including this emerging danger is essential.

AMR: is a growing global threat—It's a whole new war we're facing on a tiny level. AMR involves:
- ARB (antibiotic resistant bacteria) tiny germs, bacteria, fungi
- ARG (antibiotic resistant genes)[53]

These tiny invaders are popping up all over the world causing disease that's resistant to medical drug treatment. The conditions at factory farms, including the mismanagement of animal waste and the sky-high use of drugs is to blame. Around the world, the fallout is appearing in diseases that are difficult to heal. Doctors the world over are sounding the alarm. ARG are especially problematic for infants.[54]

The causes of AMR comes down to a couple factors:
1. Overuse and misuse of antimicrobials in animals, people, plants[55]
1. Animal wastewater from factory farms (CAFOs) contaminates water and soil.
2. The dire amount of antibiotics, antifungals, steroids given to animals confined in factory farms and the toxicity of those drugs
3. Biosolids from human waste used as fertilizer on food crops
4. Wastewater facilities are unable to filter the tiny particles of AMR bacteria, fungi, and genes out of water.
5. Animal waste from animals treated with growth hormones being used as fertilizer. "Their abundance in agricultural soils has been increasing since antibiotics were introduced for growth promotion purposes in animal farming, making their way into agricultural fields via manure." [56] Makes one wonder if any dairy products with rBGH or rBST would increase risk of AMR type disease.

"Municipal wastewater irrigation and the use of biosolids and manure in agricultural soils, can contribute to the spread of antibiotic-resistant bacteria (ARB) and antibiotic resistance genes (ARGs) in these soils."

What needs to happen to stop the growth of AMR:
- Wastewater needs to be regulated by the EPA. Untreated animal wastewater cannot be used for fertilizer any longer. Untreated wastewater needs to be handled more responsibly so it no longer has the opportunity to dirty our drinking or irrigation water.

The EPA said in 2005 they'd begin, yet it's nearly 20 years later and people of the US are still waiting.
- Factory Farms transition to better conditions for the animals, and less drugging, and smarter waste management. Or, Confining animals at CAFOs ends.
- The Biosolids industry needs to be halted immediately. There is no good coming from this. WE need to turn poop into fuel, not fertilizer! Keep the toxins out of food and the earth for Christ's sake already! Biosolids is a reckless practice serving the waste water treatment and waste management industries and whoever is reaping benefits in government. Follow the money.
- Biosolids are toxic and polluting food and the good earth. Biosolids are destroying families and farms! Biosolids are interfering with all Americans' pursuit of health and happiness. Our health and soil, our pets and ranches, our good life is threatened by Biosolids. Biosolids are infusing foods and animals and topsoil with persistent toxic chemicals, namely, PFAS. Biosolids are also contaminating farm fields, the food supply, and the water supply with AMR: Antimicrobial Resistant disease-causing bacteria and fungi from sewage.

SOLUTIONS
1. Wash your hands before you eat with soap and water
2. Don't touch your face unless your hands are clean
3. Thoroughly Wash lettuce, fruit and vegetables before eating and preparing.
4. Filter your water. "Dissolved solids" are a sign of microbes in your water. Use filtered water for cooking and drinking, and making beverages.
5. Avoid factory farm food, meat, eggs, dairy
6. Support farmers who treat animals well

4. AMMONIA

WARNING: Never mix ammonia with Chlorine bleach. This causes the release of toxic chlorine gas, which is deadly.[57]
Despite the danger, ammonia is used with chlorine to filter water across America. When mixed with chlorine, Chloramines are created. Today, Chloramines are the most common disinfectant used by cities across the country to purify tap water! Worse, the ammonia in chloramine breaks down to form nitrate, a dangerous water pollutant and carcinogen linked with stomach cancer.

Ammonia is a strong, colorless gas. When dissolved in water, it's liquid ammonia. Poisoning may occur if you breathe in ammonia vapors. Poisoning may also occur if you swallow or touch products that contain very large amounts of ammonia. In drinking water, chloramines break down to cancer-causing Nitrate and Nitrite. Is this why nitrate and nitrite levels have been rising in city water? Nitrate is common in rural areas due to runoff, but its prevalence in cities has only recently been realized.

HOW WE ARE EXPOSED
Contaminated water, cleaning products, food and meat preservatives, meat products treated with ammonia

Pollution Sources: Agricultural Runoff, Water disinfection, Steel Mill waste, Synthetic Fertilizer Processing, Petrochemical Facilities

HEALTH EFFECTS:[58] Cough, Chest pain (severe), Chest tightness, Difficulty breathing, Wheezing; Tearing and burning of eyes, Temporary blindness, Throat pain, Mouth pain, Lip swelling; Rapid, weak pulse, collapse and shock; Altered mental state, Fever, Restlessness; bluish colored lips and fingernails, Severe stomach pain,

SOLUTIONS
- Filter your water for drinking as well as cooking.
- Urge your town to not use Chloramines to purify water.
- Let's get the EPA to unsubscribe from the Chloramines agenda.
- Industry: Ammonia pollution and use must be restricted, or banned

5. ARSENIC

Before being recognized as a carcinogen, arsenic was widely used as a pesticide and defoliant on orchards, cotton and tobacco fields. Extensive contamination remains today. Surprisingly, arsenic can still be found in many types of fertilizer and pesticides, as well poultry given arsenic-based drugs. Due to its persistent nature, arsenic does not go away easily. Today, drinking water supplies, especially from private wells can contain high levels of arsenic.

SOURCES OF ARSENIC
Arsenic can be found in contaminated water, herbicides, pesticides, contaminated soil, rice, wood preservatives, sawdust from wood treated with chromated copper arsenate (CCA), ammunition, firecrackers, glass manufacturing, hazardous waste, superfund sites, dust, smoke, emissions from power plants, areas near oil drilling, mining, and metal work, cigarettes. (Until 2013 poultry feed had arsenic Roxarsone added to it).

HOW WE ARE EXPOSED
You can be exposed to arsenic by drinking contaminated water, eating contaminated food, breathing contaminated air, LED light bulbs[59], being exposed to dust and smoke, CCA wood, eating contaminated meat.

HEALTH EFFECTS: Arsenic damages organs, causes cardiovascular disease, impairs brain functioning, lowers IQs, and is especially dangerous for children and pregnant women.

SOLUTIONS
- Filter your water, reduce contact with arsenic.
- To remove arsenic from rice, rinse with water before cooking. Boil rice like pasta with six cups of water for every one cup of rice to remove an additional 40% to 60% of the arsenic.[60] Or opt for a preparing gluten free quinoa, amaranth, or wild rice instead.

6. ATRAZINE
#2 Worst Weed Killer (Herbicide)

"An estimated 33 million Americans have been exposed to atrazine through their drinking water systems."[61]

Atrazine is one of the most troubling and widespread herbicide chemicals in use. This substance is so dangerous that survival of all species comes into question. Owned now by ChemChina, this weedkiller is destroying the health of people all across the U.S. With continued atrazine use, the future of humanity and wildlife becomes increasingly uncertain.

NRDC's *Poisoning the Well*, explains, "Atrazine is the most commonly detected pesticide in U.S. waters. Though it's been "banned by the European Union since 2003! An extensive U.S. Geological Survey study found that approximately 75 percent of streams and about 40 percent of all groundwater samples from agricultural areas contained atrazine."

Berkeley's Tyrone Hayes first raised concerns abnormal sexual effects displayed in frog populations exposed to atrazine in water. "The herbicide atrazine is one of the most commonly applied pesticides in the world. As a result, atrazine is the most commonly detected pesticide contaminant of ground, surface, and drinking water. Atrazine is a potent endocrine disruptor that is active at low, ecologically relevant concentrations. Atrazine-exposed males were both demasculinized (chemically castrated) & completely feminized as adults with depressed testosterone, decreased breeding gland size, demasculinized/feminized laryngeal development, suppressed mating behavior, reduced spermatogenesis, & decreased fertility."[62]

HEALTH EFFECTS
Birth defects, reproductive effects, chemical castration, feminization, uterine, ovarian cancers,[63] infertility, breast, prostate cancer, liver, kidney, heart damage, cardiovascular damage, muscle degeneration.

SOLUTIONS
Filter your water. Together we can get Atrazine banned in the U.S.

7. Bacteria & Parasites

Disease causing pathogens, viruses, bacteria, fungi, protozoa[64] and parasites easily contaminate water supplies from natural sources, as well as from overloaded septic systems, stormwater and factory farm runoff. A very common source is animal waste from large scale factory farms, which also contributes to the rise of antibiotic resistant bacteria. Untreated human sewage also contaminates water, especially when stormwater systems are overburdened. Most microbes are killed with the chlorine disinfection process, but you still want to filter your water. UV light and Ozone *with* chlorine may be most effective method for destroying all of them.[65] According to Stanford University, "At least 25 percent of cancer malignancies are caused by viruses, bacteria and parasites."[66]

Don't assume water or food is always clean. For example, crabs and crayfish can carry lung fluke which affects 22 million people.[67] Watercress hosts tapeworm eggs.[68] Parasites can live in the human body for years before symptoms appear.[69] Anyone can get infected. The good news is some only last a short time and there are natural medicines to help eliminate them. Some, however, take a persistent effort to remove. According to the CDC, "parasitic infections affect millions around the world causing seizures, blindness, infertility, heart failure and death.[70]" If you feel something's off, don't wait. Go to a qualified doctor to avoid being misdiagnosed.[71]

HOW WE ARE EXPOSED: Unclean water, contaminated surfaces, raw fish, seafood, uncooked meat, unwashed produce, pets, biting insects, eating undercooked pork, bad meat, dirty environments.

HEALTH EFFECTS: digestive disorders, itching, discomfort, liver disease, stomach distress, cancer[72], ulcer, brain infections, headaches, lungs, kidneys, malaria, yeast infections[73], lymph disease, bile duct & bladder cancer,[74] nutritional deficiency, seizures, blindness.[75]

SOLUTIONS Wash hands with soap & water often.
- Heat meat sufficiently, avoid meat and leftovers in danger zone
- Filter your water for cooking and drinking. Freeze fish first.
- Soak & rinse vegetables, lettuces, and fruits before preparing.
- Use herbs and natural remedies to expel parasites and heal body

URGE the NIH (National Institutes of Health) to Develop Cures

TABLE 1 INFECTIOUS AGENTS POTENTIALLY PRESENT IN UNTREATED DOMESTIC WASTEWATER

Organism	Disease Caused
Bacteria	
Escherichia coli (enterotoxigenic)	Gastroenteritis
Leptospira (spp.)	Leptospirosis
Salmonella typhi	Typhoid fever
Salmonella (=2,100 serotypes)	Salmonellosis
Shigella (4 spp.)	Shigellosis (bacillary dysentery)
Vibrio cholerae	Cholera
Protozoa	
Balantidium coli	Balantidiasis
Cryptosporidium parvum	Cryptosporidiosis
Entamoeba histolytica	Amebiasis (amoebic dysentery)
Giardia lamblia	Giardiasis
Helminths	
Ascaris lumbricoides	Ascariasis
T. solium	Taeniasis
Trichuris trichiura	Trichuriasis
Viruses	
Enteroviruses (72 types, e.g., polio, echo, and coxsackie viruses)	Gastroenteritis, heart anomalies, meningitis
Hepatitis A virus	Infectious hepatitis
Norwalk agent	Gastroenteritis
Rotavirus	Gastroenteritis

Source: Adapted from Crites and Tchobanoglous, 1998.
Source: EPA Wastewater Treatment, Ozone Disinfection[76]

8. BPA, BPS, Badge

BPA and BPS contaminate waterways and drinking water worldwide.[77] These water contaminants are potent carcinogen and endocrine disruptors. BPS is used as a substitute but it's actually more toxic to the reproductive system. BADGE is another substitute, but worse than both! All these substances cause metabolic disorders, obesity, and cancers.[78]

"BPA Impairs body's ability to stop tumor spread!"
Bisphenol A (BPA) is a plasticizer used in forming hard plastic. A similar group of substances, phthalates, are used in softening plastic.

"Estrogen receptors (ER)are found in reproductive organs and other cells like the cardiovascular system, liver, pituitary, bone, and central nervous system."[79] 80% of Breast Cancer tumor growth and spread begins with increase of ER. The chemicals leach into food or liquid substance within the container. Bisphenol-S, the alternative to BPA may be even more harmful contributing to abnormal brain development.

HOW ARE WE EXPOSED
BPA can be found in adhesives, epoxies in construction materials, plastic in food packaging, receipt and credit card paper, plastic thermoses, tickets, labels, anything printed on thermal paper, plastic bottles, coatings, can lining, plastic straws, glue, stickers and Making matters worse, hand sanitizers intensify BPA absorption! Avoid hand sanitizers, Use soap and water.

HEALTH EFFECTS
Increases risk of breast cancer, prostate and testosterone cancer, reduces fertility, causes obesity, abdominal fat, hard to remove visceral fat, birth defects, miscarriages, hyperactivity, immune system problems. especially harms child development, normal growth is disrupted and sexual development can be stalled

The good news, is that BPA will flush and wash out of your body when exposure ceases. This means, reducing your exposure takes immediate effect and helps your body return to normal. But for those who continue being exposed on a daily basis there is not much relief.

March 1, 2024: EU prepares for banning 99% of all uses of BPA that make contact with food, including plastic and coatings used to line cans. FDA, are you paying attention?[80]

HAND SANITIZERS INCREASE ABSORPTION OF BPA!
Please Don't Use Hand Sanitizers or touch receipt paper often. Receipts and hand sanitizers increase exposure of BPA. "We found that when men and women held thermal receipt paper immediately after using a hand sanitizer with penetration enhancing chemicals, significant free BPA was transferred to their hands and then to French fries that were eaten, and the combination of dermal and oral BPA absorption led to a rapid and dramatic average maximum increase."

Using FDA's own exposure estimates, the average American is exposed to more than 5,000 times the safe level of BPA![81] "Without a doubt, this constitutes a high health risk! Given the magnitude of the overexposure, **we request an expedited review by the FDA** of the food additive petition because the proposed amendments to the agency's rule are intended to significantly increase the safety of the food supply (and restore) the proper functioning of the (human) immune and reproductive systems, (and) allow the immune system to more successfully respond to exposure to pathogens in or on food."[82]

The FDA is failing our health, despite repeated attempts to ban BPA, the FDA continues to allow its damning usage. Why?!! Can we really tolerate this assault to our health, to our water, to our animals any longer? If you think this is intolerable, please join in helping us change it. The FDA must step up and protect the people.

The People Have Spoken!
January 27, 2021: A petition was filed with the FDA's Office of Food Additive Safety to ban approvals of BPA with expedited review. Petitioners included the Environmental Defense Fund (EDF), Clean Water Action, and Breast Cancer Awareness asking for expedited review to ban approvals of BPA.

EXPEDITE
• to accelerate the process or progress
• to speed up
• to finish promptly, quickly please

Here it is 2024, and still crickets from the FDA. How many people are affected by cancer, or by disease caused by these BPA products, how many of those diseases may have been prevented had BPA already been banned? How many are we capable of saving if we BAN BPA TODAY?

BADGE: Artists, Painters, Handymen, Crafters

Made by the devil's people, BADGE is a super toxin found in epoxy resins, adhesives, paint, and woodworking materials.

BE CAREFUL HANDLING EPOXY ADHESIVES!
Badge is a chemical cousin to BPA, but less stable.
Badge can cause: Diabetes, Cancer, and Reproductive Harm.

WHAT PRODUCTS CONTAIN BADGE:
- Epoxy resins used in woodworking
- Glue and Adhesives!
- Filler substances!
- Many paints!
- Nanoparticles!
- Boat repair and refinishing
- Powder Coatings in auto and metal finishings
- Food storage products, metal can linings

FACTS ABOUT BADGE
- BADGE is unregulated by the FDA
- Warning labels are not required by the FDA on any products containing BADGE

FACTS ABOUT BADGE (continued)
- Workers and Artisans are at risk.
- There are no Regulations for workplace exposure to BADGE!
- It's Bullshit that this stuff is in products threatening human health
- It's a toxic water pollutant increasing risk of disease for every person or animal that consumes it.
- The FDA has to step up and Ban Badge and BPA and all its related compounds immediately

Source of Information for BADGE: EHN[83]

SOLUTIONS
- Avoid plastic containers, avoid handling receipts printed on thermal paper, anything coated or contaminated with BPA.
- Buy BPA-free products (many items labeled as "BPA-free" still contain Bisphenol-S, which is just as bad as BPA☹
- Help nudge the FDA to expedite this matter. Write or call Dr. Kristi Muldoon Jacobs, Director of the Office of Food Additive Safety. You can get cues from the following page. Thanks for standing up for human and animal health!

CONTACT THE FDA!

- BPA, BPS, and Badge threaten our health with disease.
- Manufacturing with toxic plasticizers, BPA, BPS, and BADGE must be banned.
- BPA is in the environment and getting into our bodies through food packaging, foods, and contaminated water.
- People and animals deserve a world free of thes toxins.
- BPA is a toxic substance that never should have been approved for use in food or materials that can lead to dermal or oral exposure
- The FDA approved BPA and they can unapprove it pronto.
- The FDA has the power to remove BPA from the market place
- While BPA remains in use, our drinking water will contain it

Ten years ago, the FDA withdrew approvals for BPA from baby bottles, sippy cups and baby formulas. We are grateful for that, but there's more work to do still! Everyone deserves to be safer.

HOW WE ARE EXPOSED: BPA can be found in Polycarbonate, hard plastic water bottles, adhesives, paint, woodworking materials, construction materials, food packaging, straws, paper receipts and anything printed on thermal paper, plastic bottles, plastic or metal food packaging, metal can coatings, plastic packaging, and resins.

- Woodworkers, handymen, construction workers, crafters, students, and DIY artists shouldn't be exposed to Badge!
- Wash hands with soap Avoid hand sanitizers unless free of triclosan and benzene.[84]
- Filter your water. Avoid receipts, plastic, and epoxy adhesives.
- Food Manufacturers: Please stop using them in your products! Make your own company smarter and healthier for all of us. We'll buy more from you!

TO voice your thoughts about BPA, please write to:
Dr. Kristi Muldoon Jacobs, Director
Office of Food Additive Safety
Center for Food Safety and Applied Nutrition
5100 Campus Drive
College Park, MD 20740-3835

THE FDA
The U.S. Food and Drug Administration

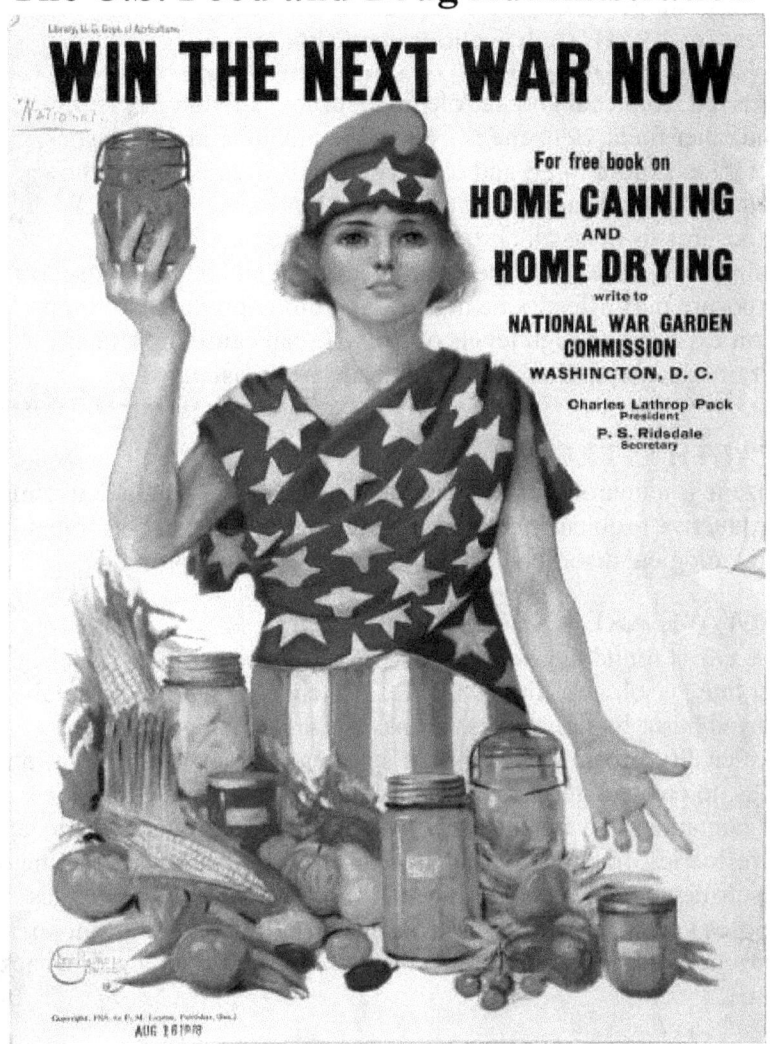

Established 1906
The FDA manages substances used in:
**Food, Food Packaging,
Cosmetics, Drugs, Vaccines**

9. BENZENE

Benzene is an industrial byproduct, volatile organic chemical (VOC), and a carcinogen. Benzene's derivatives include styrene (Styrofoam), toluene, and PAHs (polycyclic aromatic hydrocarbons).

> Derived from coal and petroleum, benzene is found in gasoline and other fuels. Benzene is used in the manufacture of plastics, detergents, pesticides, and other chemicals. Research has shown benzene to be a carcinogen (substance that causes cancer). With exposures from less than five years to more than 30 years, individuals have developed, and died from, leukemia. Long-term exposure may affect bone marrow and blood production. Short-term exposure to high levels of benzene can cause drowsiness, dizziness, unconsciousness, and death. **www.osha.gov**

HEALTH EFFECTS
Benzene is a neurotoxin and carcinogen. It causes anemia, leukemia, reproductive problems, headaches, nausea, neurological disorders, immunological disorders, and cancer.

HOW WE ARE EXPOSED
Benzene is found in pesticides, styrofoam, hand sanitizers, fuels, gasoline, gasoline additives like BTEX, char-grilled foods (notably charred burnt foods), waxes, resins, oils, inks, paints, adhesives, plastics, Styrofoam and rubber; it's used to extract oil from nuts and seeds, to create detergents, pharmaceuticals, dyes and explosives; it can contaminate water sources, leaks from underground storage tanks; oil refineries, fracking sites, petroleum and gas facilities, gasoline & diesel-fueled vehicles contribute benzene to the air. Pumping gas exposes you to benzene vapors, as does inhaling cigarette smoke. Benzene is a known carcinogen that is present in fracking flowback water."[85]

SOLUTIONS
- Filter your water for drinking and cooking.
- Reduce your exposure to benzene. Let's ban benzene additives.
- BTEX (benzene toluene ethylene xylene) fuel additive increases air pollution &causes mental, behavior and health abnormalities.

10. BIOSOLIDS
Sewage Sludge is Not Good for Us!

People throughout the world may need to reuse and recycle things a bit more these days, but some ideas take it a little too far. Take Sewage Sludge for instance, otherwise known as Biosolids. This is human waste that's been treated and then repurposed for fertilizer use! Initially imagined as an efficient way to reinvigorate soil with minerals, the fertilizer is more like a curse that won't go away. It's loaded with forever chemicals PFAS, heavy metals, carcinogens, hazardous waste, microplastics, pharmaceuticals, and a whole lot of bad bacteria, viruses, pathogens, and parasites! We don't want disease causing parasites or pathogens added to the land! Please halt this practice!

FARM LAND BECOMES CRAP LAND

Today, Sewage Sludge is applied to about 20 million acres of farm fields across the US. Since 2016, that's about 19.1 billion pounds of Waste Excrement.[86] What health effects this causes is wildly unknown. Where it's been applied, tests are finding PFAS are in everything from drinking water and soil to the animals and grains, the vegetables, fruit, milk, and eggs.

HOW DO THEY CONVERT WASTE INTO BIOSOLIDS

At facilities with modern technology, like Boston's Deer Island plant[87], waste can be treated to be super clean. And that's great in countless ways! However, even after all the great cleaning at a super facility like Deer Island, at least one pesky group of contaminants remains—PFAS, the most dreaded forever chemicals that include Teflon. These substances just don't go away easily. Wherever these biosolids have been spread, PFAS contamination is prevalent. Scientists are starting to peer into the long-term effects for human and animal health. Evidence from isolated tests on rats shows liver damage and other organs effected. "It's not one or two PFAS compounds that pose the risk, but the flood of PFAS chemicals, both legacy or emerging, that continue to accumulate in the environment."[88]

HEALTH EFFECTS

Liver damage, kidney cancer, testicular cancer, increased cholesterol, weight gain, obesity, increases risk of high blood pressure, change in liver enzymes, Birth defects, delayed development, newborn death.[89]

HOW WE ARE EXPOSED
Drinking water contaminated with biosolids, eating contaminated food. Biosolids are in use in over 40 States! We need organized federal monitoring of where biosolids are going and a citizen protection plan! Thank God biosolids are not allowed on organic farm land!

1000s of Toxins, at least 352 Hazardous Pollutants!
Right now, universities and public health scientists are conducting research while the EPA moves like a snail on this issue. Instead of taking the helm, the EPA Biosolids Program is struggling with funding and leadership. One would think they'd treat this issue with urgency. The danger PFAS contamination poses to our health is a 911. In their own audit, the EPA determined they were unable to adequately assess the health impacts of 352 hazardous pollutants present in biosolids. Further, they recommend the Office of Water and Office of Enforcement and Compliance get involved.[90] Not a bad idea to get some serious folks involved and get the job done.

SYNAGRO BEING SUED! Synagro, owned by Goldman Sachs, is the largest distributor of biosolids across the U.S. They're currently being sued[91] by Texas farmers, but this is just the tip of the iceberg.

HISTORY OF BIOSOLIDS and K061
The practice of using Sewage sludge biosolids for fertilizer started in the 1970s, it was touted as a simple fast way to get minerals and nutrients back into the soil. Though disease risk was evidenced in the early 2000s, in 2024 biosolids are still being spread by the tons daily. It seems only a few countries aren't allowing this. IT's really crazy, this is concentrated poop and a whole bunch of toxins, many yet identified. Now that PFAS issue has become so clear, in 2022 Maine declared a Statewide ban on sewage sludge for fertilizer. At this time, Maine is the only State with a ban.

Fertilizer has a twisted history. In 1997, Patty Martin, former mayor of Quincy, Washington, discovered that fertilizer used throughout the United States was contaminated with heavy metals, arsenic, dioxin, mercury, lead, and other hazardous materials. Apparently, it began with the refineries and steel mills, iron smelting, and chrome plating are now involved. To avoid costs of disposal, these industries huckstered their waste materials as fertilizer. The EPA learnt of it, then made it legal. It's now legally known as K061 Waste.

Things got even more interesting after the late great Adrienne Anderson, an environmental professor at University of Colorado in Boulder was consulting for Denver waste management. In 2005, she discovered that Superfund waste from Lowry Landfill was being pumped to Denver Metro Sewage Plant and mixed with Biosolids and then resold as fertilizer! [92] This is radioactive waste we're talking about together with heavy metals and all types of hazardous compounds. Rather than take action, the EPA legalized a new category of Fertilizer: Biosolids with hazardous waste or anything else the cat dragged in.

Fast forward to today

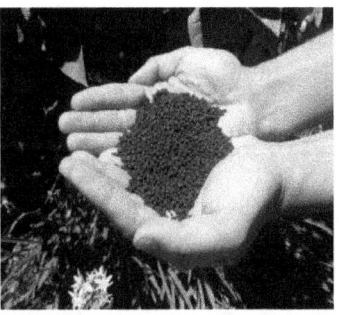

Now, though the practice is contaminating land and waterways and certainly influencing colon and gut disease rates, the practice of spreading Biosolids on farm fields is more popular than ever! Government, municipalities, and large industrial farms can't get enough of it! If this doesn't give you reason to shop organically, I don't know what will.

Photo: Synagro Biosolids turned into Pellets

Until Congress updates the Clean Water Act to regulate the discharge of these chemicals, "it is incumbent upon states to require wastewater treatment plants to use the industrial equivalent of a Brita filter or charcoal treatment to remove parasites, dangerous bacteria, PFAS and other chemicals of concern. To make this additional treatment less expensive, new evidence shows biosolids could be converted to charcoal and then used to remove chemicals from wastewater. Treatment technologies such as membrane bioreactors may also be part of the solution for reducing costs, and tighter regulations could spawn additional innovation."[93] Holy Crap! Thinking like Buckminster Fuller, wouldn't it be more sensible to turn biosolids into fuel instead of fertilizer!

SOLUTIONS
- Eat organicallly to avoid Biosolid filth in your food!
- Let's save everyone & ban biosolids in the U.S.!
- Toxins, microbes, parasites and PFAS in biosolids make it harder for people to avoid disease.
- In 2022, the State of Maine banned the use of Biosolid fertilizer[94]. The rest of the country should follow suit immediately.

11. BROMINE

Bromine gets in our water through disinfection and flame retardant fire-resistant chemicals. Biomass burning places bromine atoms in the atmosphere causing both depletion of the earth's protective Ozone Layer, and magnification of toxic mercury deposits in marine fauna and fish.[95] Scientists attribute the increase of flame retardant chemicals (bromine) in drinking water to dust, fabric and laundry waste water.[96]

Additionally, bromated flour and vegetable oil is carcinogenic and banned in other countries but still allowed in the US. Why? "The FDA should fulfill its responsibility to protect the public's health," said Michael F. Jacobson, Ph.D., executive director of Center for Science in the Public Interest. "Instead of meeting privately with industry, the FDA should ban bromate immediately."[97]

Bromine and Pharmaceuticals
While for years, iodine was the go-to ingredient for any beneficial medicine company, today's pharmaceutical industry has replaced iodine with bromine, chlorine and fluorine. These substitute halogens actually deplete iodine out of the body! "Drug makers attach these halogens to drugs because they help the drug cross through fatty tissues, like cell walls. Without it, drugs would just stay in the blood stream and not get into the tissues. They could use iodine which is very nutritious but they choose the other halogens so they can *patent* the new drug formula."[98]

HEALTH EFFECTS
Bromine damages kidneys. It also contributes to memory and hearing loss, nerve disorders, birth defects, it's a thyroid toxin and likely carcinogenic.

HOW WE ARE EXPOSED: drinking contaminated water, flame retardants, water aboard Navy ships and oil drilling platforms,[99] swimming in bromine-sanitized spas and pools, brominated bread

SOLUTIONS
- Drink filtered water and cook with it too! Remove it from water with carbon block or reverse osmosis filter. Use non-bromine sanitizers, and non-bromated flour when baking.

12. Building Supplies

Anything that goes down the drain, contaminates water. The Construction sector has many materials that can damage water health if and when they get washed or flushed down the drain. This is why it helps to use earth friendly building materials.

When you're sourcing materials, opt for ones that truly are earth friendly, contain less toxins or no toxins at all. These materials include:
- No VOC Paint, Stain
- Sealants, Acrylic
- Adhesives and Mastic
- Degreasers (toluene, methylbenzene)
- Industrial Cleaning Fluids
- Strippers
- Caulk
- Cement
- Concrete
- Drywall
- Gypsum
- Silicone

Today we have advanced technologies in appliances and HVAC equipment to reduce toxic load on the environment as well as provide energy and cost savings. Now lets get the toxins out of the glues and caulks and paints so we can all enjoy cleaner water and a healthier world.

PROTECTING WATER SOURCES
Through considerate and careful disposal, we all can better protect our water sources and protect the animals and ecosystems.

SOLUTIONS
- When working with these materials please be careful and dispose of unused materials ethically and responsibly.
- Try to use earth friendly materials as much as possible.
- Resist rinsing used paint brushes in the sink, instead use a bucket or jar with as little water as needed.

13. CHLORINE

Chlorinated Water increases Risk of Cancer!

While chlorine has some usefulness in deactivating microorganisms, it has many negative side effects that can impact our health. Of most concern regarding drinking water is the exposure to disinfection byproducts. Chlorine water disinfection processes create a wide variety of DBPs (disinfection byproducts) that remain in unfiltered drinking water. These DBPs are very problematic.

DBPs result from chlorine disinfection. Scientists are discovering new DBPs all the time. The most dangerous to date include THMs--Trihalomethanes, chloroform, haloacetic acids, MX, and BDA—all substances that increase risk of cancer and heart attacks! Chronic exposure should be avoided. "Chlorine causes excess free radicals. Free radicals lead to cell damage. Once the cells are damaged, serum cholesterol levels rise leading to atherosclerosis, hardening of the arteries and plaque formation. Chlorine can cause all these problems related to heart disease and can also be a cause of cancer. The plaque in atherosclerosis is essentially a benign tumor in the blood vessels. With cancer, free radicals create malignant cells. In the chlorination process itself, chlorine combines with natural organic matter, such as decaying vegetation, to form potent, cancer causing trihalomethanes or haloforms. Trihalomethanes, commonly abbreviated THM's, collectively include such cancer-causing agents as chloroforms, bromoforms, carbon tetrachloride and many others." [100] THMs in particular should be avoided though the EPA allows 80ppb. A safer level would be none at all!

Since our public water supply is sanitized with chlorine, we ingest a bit of these toxins when we drink or cook with tap water, unless it's filtered. Since THMs are abundant in hot water steam,[101] and are absorbed by the skin,[102] it's useful to install a reverse osmosis under your sink so the hot water is purer. A shower filter is essential as well.

Safe Alternatives

Chlorine alternatives exist and in fact are used in other countries. These include ozone[103] and ultraviolet light, though alone neither is good enough for full water purification. A system still needs reverse osmosis, ion exchange, or carbon to remove the full gamut of pollutants. According to the EPA, ozone treatment is more effective at eliminating pathogens, viruses and bacteria than chlorine, however, ozone costs more. Compared to chlorine, neither ozone nor UV light create harmful byproducts. Europe has been successfully using ozone water treatment methods for Decades.[104] Yet, the US is not moving away from chlorine. As of 2004, the EPA transitioned from chlorine to chloramines (chlorine mixed with ammonia) to treat water. Scientists at the University of Illinois in Urbana, Illinois, discovered that using chloramines to treat water created the most harmful disinfection byproduct they'd ever seen! Additionally, the ammonia in chloramines breaks down to nitrate in water, which studies show increases risk of prostate cancer,[105] as well as stomach, kidney and colon cancer![106]

After studying the array of DBPs in America's drinking water, scientists at John Hopkins University concluded, "we need to evaluate when chlorination is really necessary for the protection of human health and when alternative approaches might be better,"[107]

HEALTH EFFECTS
Chlorine byproducts increase risk of cancer; particularly colon and rectal cancer[108], bladder cancer, skin cancer, harm to fetal development,[109] stimulate production of free radicals; interfere with the health of blood vessels, cause atherosclerosis, plaque formation, heart attacks, and strokes[110]; anemia; brain abnormalities, miscarriages.[111]

HOW WE ARE EXPOSED
Unfiltered tap water; hot water steam, artificial sweeteners that contain chlorine- Splenda; using cleaning products that contain chlorine.

SOLUTIONS
- Don't drink chlorinated water.
- FILTER YOUR WATER, install a shower filter also.
- Don't ever drink unfiltered hot tap water! Don't use it to make beverages or soup. It's good for washing hands only.
- Use chlorine free cleaning supplies. Look for unbleached, oxygen or hydrogen peroxide-bleached paper products. Several companies like Seventh Generation have a variety of products.
- Don't buy chlorine-bleached paper or paper products as chlorine bleaching causes dioxin pollution
- POOL OWNERS, Use UV and ozone rather than chlorine or bromine to sanitize your pool or hot tub, or make it salt water.
- EPA: its time to rethink chlorine and end support of the chlorine industry with its toxic mercury pollution and carcinogens! Bye bye

14. Chloramines

Chloramines, also referred to as Monochloramine, are widely used today to disinfect public water supplies. It's estimated over 80 million people in the US drink water disinfected with chloramines. This is troubling, for chloramines break down into nitrate. Nitrate is an ever growing concern across the country in both rural and urban areas. Nitrate is despised for causing cancer as well as toxic algae blooms.

Chloramines are what results when chlorine and ammonia are brought togeher. Their relationship provides little benefit for people or planet. The fact that the EPA is choosing to allow this substance certainly raises eyebrows. Mixing chlorine with ammonia creates a deadly gas afterall, that should tell you something!

HEALTH EFFECTS
- Because chloramines cause corrosion in metal, levels of lead and heavy metals increases in drinking water![112]
- Chloramines risk more lead contamination as well as create a very toxic DBP, iodoacids[113] they damage mammalian cells.
- Byproducts of ammonia in chloramines breaks down to nitrate in drinking water[114]—nitrate causes stomach and esophageal cancers!
- Nitrate levels in drinking water across Illinois jumped 43% between 2003 and 2017![115]

HOW WE ARE EXPOSED
Exposure to public drinking water treated with chloramines. Chloramines clearly impact and worsen health for everybody. Why did EPA ever switch to chloramines and why do they continue allowing this substance near our water! If protecting both public health and environmental health is EPA's goal, then chloramines must go!
Does the EPA have it in them to make such a bold stand as removing chloramines some may ask. They often take years, decades to review any issue. This is just one too important to delay and dilly dally. Upgrades are sorely needed at water filtration sites, seems like a great candidate project for some enthusiastic students. Why won't the U.S. follow Europe's Lead, with Reverse Osmosis and Ozone Disinfection?

SOLUTIONS Filter your water. Get the nitrate out!

15. Chlorpyrifos, CPF #1 Worst Insecticide

"Chlorpyrifos is a neurotoxic insecticide in the organophosphates class of chemicals that were first developed by the Nazis for chemical warfare, and later adapted for commercial pesticide use after the break-up of the Nazi chemical apparatus."[116]
This little sucker was banned successfully in 2021! Then in 2023, the EPA caved to industrial pressure and now it's back in use! Beware!
Source: Usage Map and info on this page found at Earth Justice [117]

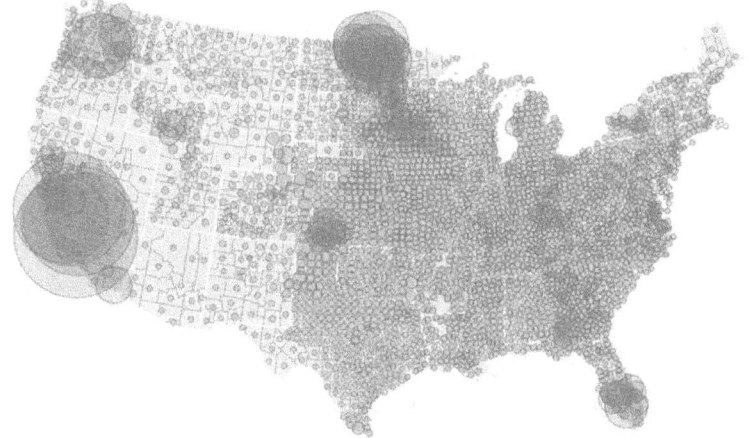

Why is it so Bad? A neurotoxin that harms the nervous system, harms pregnant mothers and their babies, causes neurodevelopmental delays in children, harms brains and damages memory, especially harmful to children, affects learning, causes attention disorders, reduced IQ, low birth weight, delayed development, brain cancer, neurological problems, convulsions, respiratory paralysis, poisoning and death.[118]
Where is it Used: On food crops, Farms, Homes, Golf courses.
It's used extensively for controlling insects that invade crops, roach control in homes and on farms, it can be found in flea and tick collars for dogs and cats.

HOW ARE WE EXPOSED: Residues on common foods, corn soy, wheat, apples, peaches, peppers, tainted drinking water

PERSISTENT TOXIC CHEMICAL
- Chlorpyrifos is a nominee for global elimination under the Stockholm Convention on Persistent Organic Pollutants."[119]
- The EPA has found that a single application is especially harmful to "Endangered Species. Fish, amphibians, birds, reptiles and small mammals, as well as bees and other beneficial insects are vulnerable to the potent insecticide.
- Chlorpyrifos is moderately persistent in soil and can take weeks to years to break down. The insecticide can also reach rivers, lakes and streams, where it concentrates in the fatty tissue of fish. [120]
- Chlorpyrifos can travel long distances to remote areas far from its source. The Arctic Monitoring and Assessment Program reported the presence of chlorpyrifos in a number of locations in the Arctic & subarctic Canadian lakes.

SOLUTIONS
What Must We Do? Ban it immediately. Here's why:
1. All food exposures exceed safe levels
2. Babies are exposed up to 140 times over safe level
3. There is NO Safe level for contaminated drinking water
4. Chlorpyrifos is found at unsafe levels in drinking water, and in the air at schools, homes, and rural, agriculture-based communities
5. Put pressure on USDA and EPA to ban all uses forever more.

FOOD QUALITY PROTECTION ACT
"The 1996 Food Quality Protection Act —(FQPA) passed unanimously in Congress — requires EPA to protect children from unsafe exposures to pesticides. The FQPA requires EPA to ensure with reasonable certainty that "no harm will result to infants and children from aggregate exposure" to pesticides. EPA cannot take industry costs into consideration when protecting children from harmful pesticides, because FQPA is a health-based standard."[121]

USDA: The FQPA directs the Secretary of Agriculture to collect pesticide residue data on commodities most frequently consumed by infants and children. The AMS Pesticide Data Program (PDP) provides pesticide residue monitoring to support this requirement. PDP is a voluntary program for monitoring residues in the nation's food supply.

Since FQPA was passed, PDP has focused its residue data collection activities on foods highly consumed by infants and children.[122]
Beyond Pesticides, November 14, 2023: [123]
One of the EPA's strongest tools for avoiding responsibility is delay, a tactic that kept cancellation of the neurotoxic pesticide chlorpyrifos at bay for 21 years—until May 2021, when a three-judge panel of the Ninth Circuit Court of Appeals, responded to a petition[124] filed in 2007

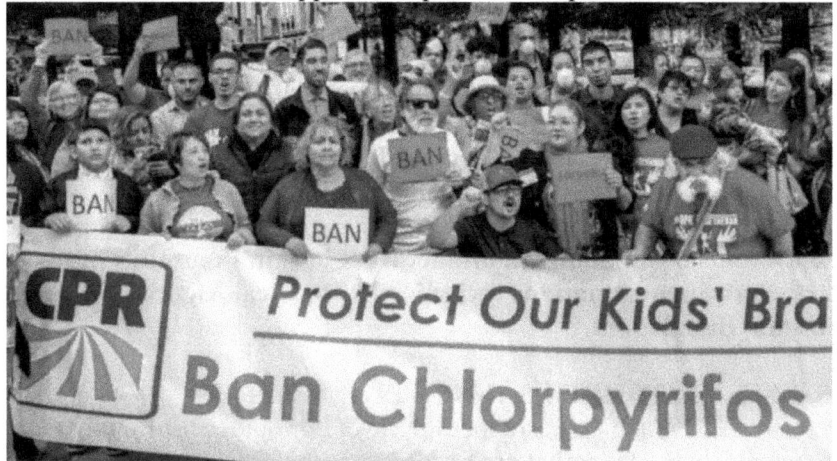

by the Natural Resources Defense Council, Pesticide Action Network, and numerous other groups.

The Ninth Circuit ordered the agency to quit lollygagging and acknowledge chlorpyrifos's threat to human health, something the agency had acknowledged already. Two options were presented to the EPA revoke the "safe" tolerances the agency had set for residue in foods, or demonstrate that they are actually safe. EPA issued a final rule in August 2021 revoking all food tolerances for the neurotoxicant. This proves they could not show it was safe at any level!

OUTRAGEOUS
This was a breakthrough, until February 2022. A different set of petitioners arrived—the sinister pesticide companies, paid U.S. farmer groups, and other countries' agricultural lobbyists—had the audacity to file an action in the Eighth Circuit Court of Appeals.
On November 3, 2023, a three-judge panel of the Eighth
Circuit reversed EPA's decision allowing chlorpyrifos to return!

The EPA allows it's continued use on these Crops:
Apples, Asparagus, Cherries, Citrus, Peaches, Soybeans, Wheat, Sugar Beets, Alfalfa. Please buy organically grown to avoid Chlorpyrifos!

Chlorpyrifos is deadly. It's produced mostly by Dow Chemical (Now Corteva Agriscience since 2019 it's the agricultural division of Dow/DuPont). Chlorpyrifos is a cholinesterase inhibitor, it inhibits acetylcholinesterase (AChE), an enzyme crucial for transmitting nerve signals in humans. This function is very similar in human, animal and insect species, which means the effects of chlorpyrifos on insects are similar to the effects on humans. It has long been evident that the residue tolerances for chlorpyrifos in food products were not protective of human health. [125]

The EU bans it but allows manufacturers to ship thousands of tons yearly to the poorer nations including Costa Rica, Algeria, Tunisia, Pakistan, Bangladesh.[126]

U.S. USES PESTICIDES BANNED ELSEWHERE!
There are 72, 17, and 11 pesticides approved for outdoor agricultural applications in the USA that are banned or in the process of complete phase out in the EU, Brazil, and China, respectively. Of the pesticides used in USA agriculture in 2016, 322 million pounds were of pesticides banned in the EU, 26 million pounds were of pesticides banned in Brazil and 40 million pounds were of pesticides banned in China. Pesticides banned in the EU account for more than a quarter of all agricultural pesticide use in the USA. The majority of pesticides banned in at least two of these three nations have not appreciably decreased in the USA over the last 25 years and almost all have stayed constant or increased over the last 10 years.[127]

IT'S UP TO US: BRING BACK THE BAN!
If we can't count on the EPA, we can work to make it illegal in our own home State. States that have banned all uses include: California, Hawaii, Maryland, New York, Oregon. Put the heat on your State officials to ban it. In the meantime, as always, filter your water!

PROTECT YOUR FAMILY
FILTER YOUR WATER.

16. Chromium-6

Believe it or not, Chromium 6-- also known as Hexavalent Chromium is contaminating drinking water sources nationwide! Yet it's still not regulated by the EPA! Made famous by *Erin Brockovich*, chromium 6 is known to cause cancer. You may recall the story of PG&E's natural gas Compressor Station and the residents of Hinkley, California. "PG&E used hexavalent chromium, also known as chromium 6, to fight corrosion in cooling tower water. The wastewater from the cooling towers was discharged to unlined ponds at the site. Some of the wastewater percolated to the groundwater, resulting in hexavalent chromium pollution."[128]

'Erin Brockovich' chemical taints tap water of 251 million Americans![129]

Chromium 6 is now found in over 89% of water samples tested across the country, and at levels 26 times higher[130] than what California* determined was safe! "In 25 cities where EWG's testing detected chromium-6, it was found in concentrations exceeding California's proposed maximum, in one case at a level more than 200 times higher. Millions of Americans in 42 states drink chromium-polluted tap water, much of it likely in the cancer-causing hexavalent form."[131]

HEALTH EFFECTS
Cancer, kidney, liver failure, stomach cancer, reproductive issues, anemia, gastrointestinal issues, asthma, vertigo, respiratory, nasal problems, ulcers

HOW WE ARE EXPOSED
Oil based paints and dyes contain chromium, steel mills, pulp mills, improper industry disposal, storage leaks, metal, chrome plating facilities, natural means. Go to the: National map of Chromium contaminated drinking water (https://www.ewg.org/interactive-maps/chromium6_contamination/map/)

SOLUTIONS
- Protect yourself: drink, cook, and brush teeth with filtered water.
- If you're using oil or metal paints, use as little water as possible to rinse brushes, squeeze unused paint out of brushes before rinsing, do not pour paint storm sewer, or use hose to rinse brushes outside.

HOW POLLUTERS GET AWAY WITH IT

*California had a Chromium 6 limit[132], set at .02ppb, then cancelled in 2017! *As reported by Michael Hawthorne with the Chicago Tribune*[133] "When a new risk is identified, it can take years before the EPA adds the pollutant to its official list of drinking water contaminants, in part because municipal utilities and industrial polluters fiercely object to changes that could cost them money."

"The Government Accountability Office, the investigative arm of Congress, sharply criticized the EPA last month for failing to add new pollutants to the list during the administration of President George W. Bush. The GAO concluded that the agency has done little to monitor unregulated contaminants in drinking water, and that the lack of data hamstrings the EPA's ability to determine which substances pose the greatest health threats. Industry groups question the validity of research that led the EPA and the National Toxicology Program to identify chromium-contaminated water as a cancer risk. Chemical companies have sponsored their own studies, many of which downplay the potential dangers. Tracing newly discovered pollutants is difficult because local water utilities aren't required to test for contaminants unless they are on the EPA's list. And if a utility decides on its own to conduct testing, it isn't required to divulge the results."

"Bottled water is no different. Food and Drug Administration regulations for bottled water limit most of the same contaminants monitored in tap water but are silent when it comes to hexavalent chromium, drug residues or other unregulated substances. Moreover, some brands of bottled water use municipal tap water supplies." "The argument here is really about the cost of cleanup and treatment," said Thomas Burke, associate dean of the Johns Hopkins Bloomberg School of Public Health and a former New Jersey environmental regulator. "Raising doubt about public health impacts has become a successful strategy for delaying action, especially when huge financial interests are at play. What we really should be talking about is how we can manage these risks."

"The source of chromium in Chicago drinking water is unclear, though federal records show that some of the nation's biggest industrial sources are four steel mills in northwest Indiana that discharge wastewater into the city's source of drinking water (Lake Michigan)." Thank you Michael Hawthorne.

17. Cleaning Products

Have you looked at your cleaning products lately? You might discover all sorts of hazards in your closet—things like bleach, glass cleaner, room deodorizer and harmful shampoos. Keep in mind that for this category of products, not all ingredients will be listed on the label. Considering that children and anyone who spends more time indoors are afflicted with respiratory conditions at an ever-growing rate, you may want to swipe out these toxic products from your home. Converting to toxin-free cleaning products will improve the air quality in your home and help everyone.

- **Chlorine.** When chlorine is mixed with water, ammonia or other substances, dangerous DBPs (chloroform, dioxin, trihalomethanes) are created. These cause cancer, allergies, stimulate production of free radicals, and interfere with the health of blood vessels.
- **Dichlorobenzene.** This is a volatile, organic chemical found in artificial scents and deodorizers. It's now found in the blood of over 95% of children and adults tested in the U.S. Exposure can cause anemia, skin lesions, damage the liver and blood. Most antibacterial soaps and products contain dichlorobenzene!
- **Hand sanitizers and antibacterial soaps**. These products contain triclosan, a registered pesticide molecularly similar to Agent Orange. Look out for it in personal care products like deodorant, blemish gels, toothpaste, dish soap, makeup, first-aid creams, and even sandals, socks and children's toys. Triclosan accumulates in fatty tissue, increases risk of cancer, causes a breakdown in skin cells, increases antibiotic-resistant bacteria, aggravates allergies and weakens the immune response. It's no bueno!
- **Phosphates in Laundry Detergent, Dish Soap and Shampoos:** Look for phosphate-free kinds, this will help our waterways and animals and help prevent toxic algae blooms and dead zones.
- **Window Cleaners.** These cleaners usually contain both ammonia and butoxyethanol—These are very toxic chemicals that harm blood cells, lungs, the kidneys and the liver.
- **Artificial fragrance and scents**—these are endocrine disruptors.

SOLUTIONS

Go nontoxic with natural solutions that are chlorine free, ammonia free, toxic free! See DIY recipes next page. Buy nontoxic options at the store.

18. COAL ASH

"**Coal ash is the second largest stream of industrial waste in the US at approximately 130 million tons produced per year!** Toxic Coal Ash currently is stored in over 310 active on-site landfills and 735 active on-site surface impoundments. These are large facilities. Landfills average over 120 acres in size and 40 feet deep while impoundments average over 50 acres in size and 20 feet deep."[134] The past century's demand for coal has destroyed ecosystems throughout mountain and Appalachian communities, harming water supplies, forests, animals and ecosystems. As the use of coal is declining, fracking and biomass are filling the gap with detrimental effects as well. Sustainable energy production with wind, water/hydro and solar energy are up and coming thankfully. Methods used for both Fracking and Biomass, as well as facilities and their power plants come with a slew of serious flaws. If somehow these energy means can be conducted with methods that don't harm the planet or people, perhaps they could continue. But for now, both fracking and biomass are causing more harm than good committing crimes against public health and earth's precious natural resources.

SECTION 404: EXEMPTIONS

Between the mountain top explosions and extraction processes, to the dirt and debris dumped in nearby streams and wetlands decimates water quality and harms animal life. Scandalously passed under the Bush and Cheney administration, the slick exemption maneuver under Section 404 of the Clean Water Act allows energy companies to fill in precious wetlands. What's even more pathetic is that many of the coal companies skipped town after the coal was gone leaving massive superfund and brownfield sites behind for the residents and towns to deal with. That's just not right.

COAL ASH WASTE PONDS

property, The wastewater produced from processing coal contains carcinogens and heavy metals; yet the coal companies, and apparently the government thinks it's okay to store this toxic brew near local towns and water supplies. One of the largest coal ash accidents occurred at the Tennessee Valley Authority Kingston's plant when the retaining wall in the waste retention pond broke. This nightmare accident displaced people, killed countless wildlife and fish, and nearly destroyed Tennessee's Dan River. Spills and seepages like these occur often at waste ponds, contaminating water supplies and impacting the health of all who have contact. The fact is we need energy facilities to power our modern world, to keep our lights on, our homes heated, and our computers running. However, the energy industry has to become earth friendly as well as health friendly. I think we can all agree that coal, natural gas, petroleum and biomass power plants cause far too much harm to continue on as is.

Nuclear power is in its own category altogether. For while facilities can be so clean while operating, if anything goes wrong the aftermath can be quite disastrous. And what of the end life for the waste material? So much still to resolve concerning our energy production.

December 22, 2008 Tennessee Valley Coal Ash Spill[135]

Over 500 million gallons of wastewater containing toxic radioactive coal ash, spilled when its containing dam broke. Accidents like these are preventable, just like oil spills and pipeline breaks. If the fracking, oil, and coal facilities would simply adopt strategies for safety and pollution prevention, most of our environmental tragedies could be avoided. We can stop the damage if we demand businesses and our government be more responsible. Coal ash from coal mining has been contained in ash ponds that are typically unlined and at risk of collapse. These ponds have let unregulated hazardous waste and toxic metals seep into the groundwater, contaminating drinking water. All too often these ponds spilled into nearby rivers and wetlands, harming people and wildlife.

MERCURY: TOXIN FROM COAL

"Mercury is one of the most serious contaminants threatening our Nation's waters because it is a potent neurotoxin in fish, wildlife, and humans. It is a global pollutant that ultimately makes its way into every aquatic ecosystem through one of two routes: Point-source discharges or atmospheric deposition. Atmospheric deposition is the primary source of mercury to most aquatic ecosystems. According to the U.S. Environmental Protection Agency (USEPA), emissions from coal-fired power plants are the largest source of mercury to the atmosphere. Mercury is deposited from the atmosphere primarily as inorganic mercury. Methylation—the conversion of inorganic mercury to organic methylmercury—is the most important step in the mercury cycle because it greatly increases toxicity and potential for accumulation in aquatic biota. Nearly all of the mercury found in fish tissue is methylmercury."[136]

HUMAN HEALTH EFFECTS[137]
COAL ASH POND CONTAMINANTS

POLLUTANTS	HEALTH EFFECTS
Aluminum	Lung disease, developmental problems
Antimony	Eye irritation, heart damage, lung problems
Arsenic	Multiple types of cancer, darkening of skin, hand warts
Barium	Gastrointestinal problems, muscle weakness, heart problems
Beryllium	Lung cancer, pneumonia, respiratory problems
Boron	Reproductive problems, gastrointestinal illness
Cadmium	Lung disease, kidney disease, cancer
Chromium	Cancer, ulcers and other stomach problems
Chlorine	Respiratory distress
Cobalt	Lung/heart/liver/kidney problems, dermatitis
Lead	Decreases in IQ, nervous system, development, behavioral problems
Manganese	Nervous system, muscle problems, mental problems
Mercury	Cognitive deficits, developmental delays, behavioral problems
Molybdenum	Mineral imbalance, anemia, developmental problems
Nickel	Cancer, lung problems, allergic reactions
Selenium	Birth defects, nervous system/reproductive problems
Vanadium	Birth Defects, lung/throat/eye problems
Zinc	Gastrointestinal effects, reproductive problems

SOLUTIONS
- Filter water for drinking and cooking; protects kids & loved ones.
- Help the coal communities rebound through supporting the Ohio Valley Environmental Coalition www.ohvec.org.
- Let's insist the Gov repeal permits issued under section 404 that allow mining and drilling contamination to harm wetlands and waterways.

19. COSMETICS

As lovely as skin and hair products may look and feel, they're also washed off with water at some point, and wash down the drain. With the water go the ingredients, both good and bad. This is why ingredients matter. Many toxic substances are added to personal care products and contribute to the toxic water burden. The FDA does not require manufacturers to test, identify, or have FDA approval for ingredients or formulations before their products are sold. Many of these ingredients fall under the "Emerging Contaminants" Category—which include heavy metals, toxic chemicals and whatnot that may all be present without any indication on the label. From the trade secrets to ingredients comprising less than 1%, many fall under the vague *"and other ingredients"* category.

Mercury can be used as a preservative and is found commonly in mascara and eye makeup. In 2007, Minnesota became the only State to fully ban the presence of mercury in cosmetics.

Microbeads are tiny plastic beads that were added to a slew of personal care products, including cosmetics, toothpaste, cleansers, sunscreen. Many manufacturers have since discontinued using them, however they may still be in some products. Once in the water, microbeads cause great harm to animals and people, waterways, and oceans. Avoid products with these microbead words on the label[138]: polyethylene (PE), polyethylene terephthalate (PET), Nylon (PA), Polypropylene (PP), Polymethyl Methacrylate (PMMA).

Nitrosamines are carcinogenic, hormone-disrupting compounds easily absorbed through the skin. To see if your cosmetics are tainted, look at the label. Look for **DEA, MEA, TEA**—when these dangerous ingredients interact with other ingredients like **sodium lauryl sulphate** or **sodium nitrate**, nitrosamines form. The late and great Dr. Samuel Epstein noted, "Nitrosamines have been identified as one of the most potent classes of carcinogens, having caused cancer in more than 40 different animal species as well as in humans. The FDA should take regulatory action against companies manufacturing cosmetic products; responsible corporations should remove these avoidable contaminants from their products; and the public should boycott all products containing nitrosamines."[139]

PFAS: Many types of makeup and personal care products found to contain high levels of PFAS[140], though none were listed on the label. Those included waterproof makeup, concealers, liquid lipstick, mascara.

Preservatives are a red flag These are disguised most commonly as Parabens, which may be labeled as butyl, isobutyl, methyl, propyl and ethyl. They are endocrine disruptors—they mimic and interfere with natural hormone levels. The foundation, Breast Cancer Action is trying to ban them from cosmetics as they are frequently found in breast cancer tissue.

Propylene Glycol:(see Ethylene Glycol) the active ingredient in anti-freeze, is yet another ingredient to run from. Commercially, it's used to break down proteins and cellular structure. As a surfactant, propylene glycol actually enables other toxic ingredients to penetrate the skin further.

Quaternary compounds[141] and **Diazolidinyl Urea** both break down to Formaldehyde, a carcinogen and common skin allergen and irritant.

Talc is also problematic, as it has been identified in connection with lung and ovarian cancer. Use products made with cornstarch instead.

EXEMPT FROM LABELING

The Material Safety Data Sheet warns against skin contact for these products, yet you won't find a warning on any skincare package that contains them. According to the present FD&C Act of 1938, "In cosmetic and cleaning products, ingredients can be exempt if:
- **less than 1% concentration**
- **Color additives**
- **Other ingredients (formula and trade secrets)**

The name of an ingredient as a trade secret need not be disclosed on the label. In lieu of declaring the name of that ingredient, the phrase "and other ingredients" may be used at the end of the ingredient declaration.[142] No telling how deep this rabbit hole goes.

HEAVY METALS ALLOWED IN COSMETICS
Mercury in cosmetics: Mercury compounds are allowed in cosmetics only as preservatives in eye area products. They may be used only in a very small amount—Mercury is not allowed in any other cosmetic products except in a trace amount of less than 1 ppm and only if its presence is unavoidable under good manufacturing practice (GMP)

Lead in Cosmetics: FDA has published draft guidance for industry that recommends a maximum level of 10 ppm for lead as an impurity in cosmetics. This guidance applies to cosmetic lip products (such as lipsticks, lip glosses, and lip liners) and externally applied cosmetics marketed in the U.S.[143]

WHAT WON'T THE FDA ALLOW?
Thankfully, we do have a few ingredients the FDA won't allow [144]:
- Bithionol: photocontact sensitization
- Chlorofluorocarbon Propellants: depletes earth's ozone layer
- Chloroform: causes cancer
- Halogenated Salicylanilides (di,tri,metabromsalan and tetrachloro-: Serious skin disorders
- Hexachlorophene (HCP): toxic, easily penetrates skin, avoid lips and mucous membranes (used as preservative)
- Mercury Compounds: not allowed except in eye makeup at no more than 65 ppm, Neurotoxin (used as preservative)
- Methylene Chloride: causes cancer
- Prohibited cattle materials due to mad cow disease, bovine spongiform encephalopathy
- Vinyl Chloride: causes cancer and other problems
- Zirconium substances: lung toxin, cause granulomas in skin

SOLUTIONS
- What's in your bathroom cabinet? Take time to examine your favorite brands: www.ewg.org/reports/skindeep
- Choose products with natural ingredients, for you & the planet.
- Keep your family safe and away from products with toxic ingredients
- Don't buy products containing plastic microbeads! No Plastic!
- For your own sake, your family's health and every creature's well-being, the world must curtail its use and consumption of products made with health-harming substances. We must insist manufacturers adhere to stronger rules. This is where the FDA needs to step up. If Harvey Wiley, the Father of the FDA, were alive today, surely he would remove heavy metals in products!
- At the end of the day, keeping our water supply safer reduces our risk of disease. Be part of the solution and help the planet by choosing more natural products for your life, your skin, hair, home and family.

20. DBPs: Disinfection Byproducts

Before the water comes to your kitchen, it goes through a filtering process in your city. This is the case if you live in a town that provides your water. If you have your own well, however, you pretty much have to filter it yourself. Municipal public water facilities use a mix of toxic chemicals to purify water for delivery to your home. Today, most U.S. cities use chloramines to purify the water. This is a mixture of chlorine and ammonia. These two chemicals may minimize water-born bacteria and viruses but they create Disinfection Byproducts (DBPs) that remain in the water. You can remove them by filtering your water at home. Some filters are better than others at removing DBPs.

Tap water nearly everywhere is contaminated with DBPs. If you don't filter they will remain in your drinking water. The health effects of combined DBPs is still under investigation. The problem with DBPs begins with chlorine. When chlorine is mixed with water that contains any type of organic matter, such as leaves or dirt, cancer-causing halocetic acids, MX,[145] and trihalomethanes like chloroform are created. These substances travel with the water to your home. Imagine, we're exposed to trihalomethanes whenever we're exposed to hot water steam. This means taking showers or doing the dishes can be hazardous to your health. Then there's MX! Scientists have learned that the gene-mutator MX is 170 more potent and dangerous than chloroform!

With chloramines you get ammonia. Using ammonia in any amount to prepare water for drinking is plain wrong. Though approved by the EPA, this method creates iodoacids. Iodoacids have been identified by Michael Plewa, a genetic toxicologist and his team at the University of Illinois, as **the most toxic** disinfection byproduct ever! "Iodoacetic acid is the most toxic and DNA-damaging to mammalian cells in tests of known DBPs."

But that's not all, when chloramines "decompose, ammonia is released and oxidized to nitrite and nitrate. This process, known as nitrification, is believed to be facilitated by ammonia-oxidizing bacteria (AOB), which use the ammonia as an energy source. These bacteria are commonly found in drinking water systems, and nitrification occurs when conditions allow their numbers to rise."[146] This might explain the increase for nitrate and nitrite in urban water.

BDA: In 2020 researchers from John Hopkins discovered a brand new DBP-- called BDA. BDA is a complex chemical with chlorine attached. "BDA is a very toxic compound and a known carcinogen that hasn't been detected in chlorinated water before."[147] BDA forms when chlorine mixes with pharmaceuticals and ingredients in personal care products. Only in the past 25 years have scientists noticed the uptick of pollution caused by PPCPS (pharmaceuticals and personal care products) in water.

"The discovery of these previously unknown, highly toxic byproducts, raises the question how much chlorination is really necessary."[148]

Water Treated with Chlorine and Chloramines Contains:
- BDA — Carcinogen
- Chlorine — Biocide, poison, heart attacks, stroke
- Chloroform — harms nervous system, liver, kidneys
- Halocetic Acids — carcinogen
- Trihalomethanes — carcinogens absorbs through skin also
- Chloroform — carcinogen
- Nitrate/Nitrite — carcinogen
- Iodoacids — Damages DNA
- MX — carcinogen

If bromine is used:
- Brominated DBPs — carcinogen

HEALTH EFFECTS
When combined, all these disinfection byproducts contribute to disease, cancer, allergies, production of free radicals, they weaken normal blood vessels, contribute to heart attacks, strokes and anemia, as well as cause nervous system disorders, birth defects and miscarriages.

HOW WE ARE EXPOSED
Drinking or eating something cooked or made with unfiltered water.

Trihalomethanes
Trihalomethanes are the most common form of disinfection byproducts. They form when chlorine mixes with organic matter. We can be exposed through drinking water, skin contact, and inhaling hot water vapors. Trihalomethanes are reproductive toxins and carcinogens implicated in bladder, colon, and rectal cancer.[149] The best filters to remove Trihalomethanes include Reverse Osmosis and Activated Carbon.

CHLOROFORM:
Chloroform is a specific trichloromethane DBP. Chloroform is both a naturally occurring and manmade substance. When chloroform enters the body, it is carried by the blood and it is temporarily stored in fat cells, the liver, and kidneys. Once the exposure has ended, the chloroform volatilizes and is released into the air we exhale, as well as in our urine and waste products.[150]

"Chloroform is a by-product of the strong chemical oxidation of organic material associated with water and wastewater treatment, wood pulp chlorination, in chemical syntheses for refrigeration (Fluorocarbon- 22), and in plastics manufacturing. The primary source of chloroform in public water supplies is the disinfection process."

Chloroform:
- Harms the liver and kidneys
- Harms the Central Nervous System
- Harms the Brain
- Harms Children in the Womb
- Causes Birth Defects
- Neurotoxin
- Damages Skin
- Probable Carcinogen

"There is no specific federal drinking water standard for chloroform, but there is a federal drinking water standard for trihalomethanes."[151]

SOLUTIONS
- Purify your water with a good filter.
- Use filtered water for drinking as well as cooking.
- Give your children and pets filtered water as well.
- Filtering water helps reduce your and your family's exposure to toxic Disinfection Byproducts.
- Don't put pharmaceuticals down the drain.
- Use natural nontoxic personal care products
- Use nontoxic cleaning products in your home and work place. Every little bit does help.

21. DICAMBA!

DICAMBA = Colon & Lung Cancer![152]

The EPA first approved Dicamba's use in 1967. The
Dicamba is used on these Crops[153]:Asparagus, Corn, Wheat, Barley, Sugarcane, Sorghum, Fallow, Pasture, Hay, Oats, Millet, Triticale, Grass grown for seed, as well as GMO dicamba tolerant soybeans, and dicamba tolerant (DT) cotton. This weedkiller is also sold for landscaping uses on lawns, golf courses, sports fields, and parks.

Increased uses began after FDA approved Dicamba tolerant GMO soybean and GMO cotton. These majority of these crops are grown in Iowa. In 2024, the Courts withdrew over-the-top uses for Dicamba on GMO crops. Over the top means after the shoot has emerged from the soil. In case you buy roundup for home use, you should know dicamba is added to residential lawn Roundup products.[154] It's also in a lot of other lawn and garden products.

HOW WE ARE EXPOSED:
Dicamba drifts, volatizes readily into the air, onto neighboring fields and playgrounds, yards, schools, fields, everywhere including into the water. Dicamba residues infiltrate the food it's sprayed upon. "Dicamba volatilization is known to greatly increase with temperature, especially at temperatures above 80-85°F, and dry conditions increase the severity of dicamba damage."[155] According to the FDA who approves GMO crops and seeds: Most GMO soy is used for animal feed (for animals at CAFOs, poor things), and making soybean oil, used as an ingredient for processed foods: lecithin, emulsifiers, and proteins! GMO cotton becomes cottonseed oil for restaurants and packaged food industry.[156] We must break these chains and become the land of the free once again! No dicamba, no disease!

Health Effects:
Colon Cancer, Lung Cancer, neurotoxicity, kidney and liver damage, birth defects, reproductive damage, respiratory illness, antibiotic resistance in humans, harms birds, ecosystems, fish and aquatic animals, nontarget species, pollinators, causes abnormal cell division and growth.[157], alters animal liver function to promote tumor growth and cancer.[158] My sweet dog Oscar died of cancer. Now I wonder what pet foods are contaminated with residues of dicamba?!

22. DiChloroBenzene (p-DCB)

Banned in the EU since 2005, the pesticide P-CDB is widely used in America. It's found in multiple products as an insecticide, repellant, fumigant, disinfectant, deodorizer, and fungicide. Beware!

HOW ARE WE EXPOSED
Contaminated water, air fresheners, hand sanitizers, polluted air, scented trash bags, deodorizers, artificially scents, mildew proof products, fumigants, insect sprays and repellants, pesticides.

HEALTH EFFECTS
P-CDB is an endocrine disrupting chemical (EDC), it causes metabolic dysfunction, reproductive problems, extended exposure increases risk of endocrine-related disease, hormonal changes, increases risk of endocrine-related cancers in women: breast, uterine and ovarian.[159]

"Endocrine disruption is an ever-present, growing issue that plagues the global population. Overall, endocrine disruption can negatively impact reproductive function, nervous system function, metabolic/immune function, hormone-related cancers, and fetal/body development. Thus, the connection between cancers and EDCs has a historical establishment. The International Agency for Research on Cancer (IARC) and the U.S. National Toxicology Program (NTP) classify many EDCs as possible carcinogens based on epidemiological studies identifying instances of kidney, ovarian, testicular, prostate, and thyroid cancer, as well as non-Hodgkin lymphoma and childhood leukemia.

However, the variations in EDC exposure levels and duration can make it challenging to investigate among humans. The U.S. Environmental Protection Agency (EPA) fails to evaluate the depth and scope of chronic health and environmental concerns regarding exposure to EDCs. In addition to cancers, exposure to EDCs has links to infertility, early puberty, other reproductive disorders, diabetes, cardiovascular disease, obesity, attention deficit hyperactivity disorder (ADHD), Parkinson's, Alzheimer's, and more. EDCs can also wreak havoc on wildlife and their ecosystems. Hence, advocates maintain that policies should enforce stricter pesticide regulations and increase research on the long-term impacts of pesticide exposure."[160]

23. DIOXIN!

Dioxins are chlorinated compounds and persistent organic pollutants. They linger persistently in the environment and bioaccumulate as they move up the food chain. Dioxins are part of the 'dirty dozen,' considered by many to be the worst known substances on earth. I first learned about the dangers of dioxin when I worked as a canvasser for Green Peace back in 1989. Furans are similar to dioxins and both are listed in the Stockholm Convention of Persistent Organic Pollutants.

Dioxins are unintentional byproducts of manufacturing, and out of the hundreds of types release, "only some are toxic, those with the chlorine atoms in specific positions."[161] Hundreds of facilities manufacturing chemicals, metal products, and bleaching paper release these chlorinated carcinogenic byproducts into the air and water. Dioxin accumulates in the fatty tissue of animals, and transfers as it moves up the food chain.

Drinking Water: Dioxin can get into drinking water from: (EPA)[162]
- Air emissions from waste incineration and other combustion, with subsequent deposition to lakes and reservoirs
- Deposition from air to soils that erode into surface waters used for drinking water
- Discharges into water from chemical factories.

SOURCES OF DIOXINS AND FURANS
Incinerators, Paper Mills using Chlorine bleach, Power Plants, Chemical Processing, and Metal Manufacturing: Dioxins are a byproduct of burning plastics, especially PVC (polyvinylchloride), hazardous waste, medical waste, cigarette smoke, backyard fires, forest fires.

Paper Industry:
When chlorine is combined with wood pulp in the paper-bleaching process, dioxins and other organochlorines are created. Due to poor regulations, the toxic wastewater is discarded into waterways surrounding the paper-producing facilities. Lakes and rivers near paper mills and polluting industries are most impacted, Delaware rivers and streams earned most polluted in the US status in 2022.[163]

HEALTH EFFECTS
"Known human carcinogens, Atherosclerosis, hypertension, diabetes. Long-term exposures to dioxins cause disruption of the

nervous, immune, reproductive, and endocrine system,"[164] endometriosis, birth defects, and lowered IQ[165].

HOW YOU ARE EXPOSED

Contaminated water, eating contaminated foods, notably high fat dairy and animal fats, breathing contaminated air. Dioxin is relatively low in most drinking water, but it does have a half-life of 7 - 11 years once in your body.[166] As a bioaccumulative toxin, every little exposure adds up. After contaminating the water, land and atmosphere, dioxins easily find their way into grasses and animal feed. Once digested by farm animals, dioxins accumulate in fatty tissue and are transferred to food prepared for human consumption.

> **DIOXIN:**
> Most of us receive almost all of our dioxin exposure from the food we eat: specifically, from the animal fats associated with eating beef, pork, poultry, fish, milk, and dairy products. Because dioxins are widely distributed throughout the environment in low concentrations, are persistent and bioaccumulated, most people have detectable levels of dioxins in their tissues. These levels, in the low parts per trillion, have accumulated over a lifetime and will persist for years, even if no additional exposure were to occur. This background exposure is likely to result in an increased risk of cancer and is uncomfortably close to levels that can cause subtle adverse non-

We must do better. A future with less dioxin depends, according to the WHO,[167] "on strict control of industrial processes to reduce formation of dioxins as much as possible. This is the responsibility of national governments." EPA: please, we need your help here.

SOLUTIONS

- Reduce consumption of animal fats as much as you can.
- Avoid animal fats from factory farms
- Buy paper and tissue products that are chlorine free.
- Encourage the public school system to use recycled paper
- Write to your senators & representatives and ask that tougher dioxin pollution restrictions be put in place in your State, and that corporations be held accountable for cleanup costs! Can we ban dioxins and the chemicals processes that produce them? Restrict use of chlorine in production? We must do everything possible to lessen this horrible health-harming substance.

24. Emerging Contaminants
CECs: Contaminants of Emerging Concern

This subsection of contaminants represents a slew of substances and byproducts that are dangerous for health. These include endocrine disruptors, neurotoxins, reproductive toxins, carcinogens, and heavy metals. Many of the emerging contaminants are found in personal care products, cleaning compounds, surfaces, solvents, nanoparticles, GRAS ingredients, agricultural chemicals, pharmaceuticals, and everyday products.

Many of these are known or suspected to cause cancer, yet they aren't regulated yet by the EPA. Most of these, when comingled with other contaminants have effects not even fully understood yet. Most have never been tested, especially not in combination with other substances. Many other countries have stricter water regulations than the US, and have already banned some of the toxins in this category. The sensible solution is for countries to restrict the use, or outright ban the use of harmful unnatural substances in manufactured products and formulations. Only after thorough testing and proof of safety should any substances be allowed for use in products or formulations.

- Ingredients in Skin Care Products
- Ingredients in Lotions
- Ingredients in Shampoos
- Ingredients in Detergents
- Ingredients in Pesticide formulations
- Ingredients in Cleaning Products
- Ingredients in Pharmaceuticals
- Ingredients in Car Care products
- Ingredients in Air Fresheners
- Ingredients in Textiles and Furnishings
- Ingredients in Perfumes
- Ingredients in Window Cleaner and Stain Removers
- PFAS, PFOA, PFOS, PFCs and products made with them
- Flame Retardant formulations
- Nanoparticles and anything made with them
- Atrazine formulations
- Herbicides and Glyphosate formulations
- Manganese and Heavy Metal formulations, additives

25. ETHANOL!

Ethanol production facilities consume a great deal of precious water in the Midwest,[168] and generate a lot of water pollution that goes into nearby rivers and waterways unchecked. Ethanol farmers use immense amounts of nitrogen fertilizer and animal manure, as well as atrazine and other toxic herbicides. These substances are devastating water quality in farming communities and driving climate change.[169] While the ethanol producers are making a fortune, the people bear the consequences of water shortages, low water pressure in their wells, and carcinogens in their drinking water[170].

The farms and their product contribute to poor air quality as well from cradle to grave. As reported by the American Geophysical Union, "emissions of all volatile organic compounds were five times higher than government numbers, which estimate emissions based on manufacturing information. VOCs and nitrogen oxides react with sunlight to form ground-level ozone, the main component of smog."[171]

Touted as a "green" energy, ethanol comes with too much baggage:
- Corn ethanol growers use tons of Atrazine & Glyphosate[172]
- Ethanol farming destroys native prairie and grassland habitats, already by 2018 having converted 8 million acres of these vital ecosystems to farmland[173]
- Runoff results in more nitrate and carcinogens in water
- More nitrate in water causes toxic algae and dead zones
- Toxic algae blooms are more numerous than ever in Iowa[174]
- Ethanol added to gasoline increases smog and air pollution[175]
- Ethanol in gasoline contributes to trapping heat, warmer temps
- Ethanol raises atmospheric levels of two carcinogens: formaldehyde and acetaldehyde.

"Planting massive amounts of corn to make corn ethanol is not just a climate disaster. The practice has led to increased fertilizer run-off, polluting local waterways, making water too toxic for swimming and too toxic to drink. The expenses of cleaning farm pollution out of drinking water end up in the water bills of Des Moines residents. They have essentially been footing the bill for corn and ethanol producers for almost a decade." [176]

SOLUTIONS: Filter Your water for drinking and cooking. EPA must curtail the damage, ethanol farming expansion must cease.

26. Ethylene Glycol

Ethylene glycol is a clear, colorless liquid with a sweet smell. One might think the government regulates it, but that is not so. Instead, this and other toxic chemicals are often overlooked. While the EPA may be soft, The New Jersey Department of Health declares, 2-Butoxyethanol be handled as a carcinogen—with extreme caution. It can damage the liver and kidneys. There may be no safe level of exposure to a carcinogen so all contact should be reduced to the lowest possible level.[177]

It goes by many names, beware: PEG--poly ethylene glycol is in many personal care products, monobutyl ether, ethylene glycol butyl ether, ethylene glycol, n-butyl ether, butyl Cellosolve, butyl glycol, butyl Oxitol. This toxic chemical is found in air and water pollution, cleaning products, adhesives in produce stickers, as well as window cleaner, paints, industrial cleaners and solvents. It volatizes from products. Its toxic metabolite, oxalic acid, can cross the blood brain barrier. This is unnatural, but medical uses may be useful depending what substance it carries with it into the brain.[178]

FOOD STICKERS: The Food and Drug Administration (FDA) has approved ethylene glycol as an indirect food additive, for use only as a component of **packaging adhesives**.[179]

HEALTH EFFECTS
Reproductive toxin, depresses nervous system, irritates eyes, nose, and throat, targets kidneys, heart and lungs, liver, lymphatic system, blood, respiratory, nervous system, likely carcinogen.

HOW WE ARE EXPOSED
Antifreeze, Indoor air, VOCs, manufacturing facilities, toxic cleaning products, window cleaner, contaminated drinking water, food packaging stickers

SOLUTIONS
Avoid food stickers and packaging adhesives, cut that area off your apple, wash well any food that had contact with adhesives. Filter your water. Use nontoxic cleaning products or make your own with safe ingredients like vinegar, baking soda, and essential oils.

27. Factory Farms

CAFO: Concentrated Animal Feeding Operation

Reduce Your Family's Risk of Cancer

"Exposure to antibiotics, growth hormones, and toxic run-off from livestock feed lots can be minimized by eating free-range meat raised without these medications if it is available."

President's Cancer Panel Report 2009[180]

Factory farms are miserable places, also known as CAFOs and livestock feed lots. Neglected terrified animals never see the sun, they're confined in small crowded cages their entire life. Many problems arise from these farms. One particularly affecting drinking water and human health is the sewage and animal waste. **Number of CAFOs in Iowa: 4025!**[181]

Factory Farm Water Pollution and Disease

In addition to harming animals, factory farms poison waterways and worsen air quality. They emit more methane than cars and trucks release carbon dioxide. The corporations are incentivized to create a lot of manure to repurpose as Biogas[182], which is yet another driver for warming temps! Industrial-scale corporate farms get away with many abuses that affect our environment and our health. Requirements and regulations don't exist for these farms. There's no tracking or record-keeping system for pollutant emissions, despite the fact that their waste contaminates drinking water sources. Their idea for pollution control is to create massive waste reservoirs on-site. Unfortunately, these often leak and overflow, causing toxic, dangerous bacteria and microbes to infest our rivers, lakes and our drinking water.

Surpassing human waste levels in large cities, factory farm waste is not regulated under the Clean Water Act yet. This waste is dangerous. It contains high levels of phosphorous, nitrogen, heavy metals, antibiotics and hormones, blood, feces, parasites, bacteria, disease. While the manure decomposes, ammonia, hydrogen sulfide and methane gases escape into the air. The amount of methane and ammonia produced is staggering and plays a significant role in atmospheric warming.

> **The USDA**
> Created by President Abraham Lincoln in 1862, the USDA was originally referred to as "The People's Department."

As these putrescent toxins loaded with parasites and bacteria journey into our water supply and food chain, antibiotic-resistant bacteria multiply, aquatic organisms die, and human diseases become more difficult to treat and manage. Iowa has the most factory farms of any State in the US, but Indiana currently holds the lead for most polluted lakes and rivers due to factory farm runoff.[183] This is dangerous and could lead to serious disease surges. Athletes and any seeking health and fitness, as well as children, and the elderly, and anyone healing from disease or cancer of any kind must steer clear of tainted water.

The USDA supervises conditions at Factory Farms. The EPA has the capacity to regulate the waste though they don't. There seems to be a conundrum as it's not point source pollution. But, really is it that complicated to identify the negligent farms? "Though there are many large livestock farms in Indiana, most of the animals are raised under a contract for just a few major companies — like Tyson and JBS." [184]

"Beef produced in the United States is heavily contaminated with synthetic sex hormones, which are associated with an increased risk of reproductive and childhood cancers. Increased levels of sex hormones are linked to the escalating incidence of reproductive cancers in the United States since 1975 - 60 percent for prostate, 59 percent for testis, and 10 percent for breast."[185]

The time has come for a change! The EPA must go after these big corporations and hold them accountable. Force them to break up the huge facilities or figure out a way to contain their waste, STAT! Factory farm products may be cheaper, but at what cost to our health? We must uphold and support Farmers who grow food in union with the earth and universe, not those carelessly unconcerned with our health.

With all the factory farm products people consume and the dirty water these facilities cause, is it any wonder we're seeing disease and cancers more often now? We're exposed to such a wide array of toxins through the water and food and air. Health today really is a miracle. Let's regroup and make this country as good as it can be. Together we can gather and get involved with State leadership to make things better in all the places we live.
- Support local small farms, shop at the farmer's markets
- Buy organic meats, milk and eggs that are mindfully raised.
- Find good sources of meat and dairy: www.eatwellguide.org.
- Let's get all animals included under the Animal Welfare Act.
- Lobbyists have to go! USDA is the People's Department!

28. Fertilizer Runoff

Fertilizer runoff is a significant source of water pollution that harms all life. The toxic algae cyanobacteria caused by fertilizer can kill a dog in minutes.[186] The worst offenders are large scale monocropping farms that don't care about families, or animals, or ecosystem health.

Excessive use of toxic synthetic fertilizer destroys life in the soil, the microorganisms that facilitate nutrient delivery to growing plants. These miracle creatures also bind and hold the soil together. Disrespectfully, these life-making microorganisms are killed off by synthetic fertilizer and toxic pesticide use. Poor soil health results rendering the ground lifeless and sterile, unable to hold onto plants, unable to absorb rain. Thus, when storms come, everything washes away including the topsoil, the toxic fertilizer and the toxic herbicides.

These mega farms grow GMO crops, like soybean and corn for animal feed or ethanol, and food ingredients. Regular farmers are not to blame, in fact they're usually the victims of Big Ag and were duped into growing GMOs.

The real culprit is the industry and all their minions controlling how food is grown today. Synthetic fertilizer, pesticides, biotech and GMO seed are their tools that they market as the only way we can feed a growing population. What they don't tell you is their products will kill civilization. It's a dead end, the more synthetic fertilizer and pesticides a farmer uses, the weaker his soil gets.[187] Weaker soil won't grow healthy plants or nutritious plants, at least not natural nutrients our bodies can absorb. Weaker plants are more prone to disease and bug infestations. Thus, farmers must apply more pesticides and herbicides to help the plants resist bugs that the plants can no longer resist on their own. It's a very sad situation and repetitive cycle doing nothing but fattening the profits for the corporations selling poisons. Instead of being able to rise and prosper, the plants and farmers are left living a substandard life, a poisoned life, a life with no hope as long as the pesticide and fertilizer poisons continue their stranglehold. Unless we break this cycle, the farmers and their families will be robbed of their dreams and hopes. We must help these farmers return to a natural, health-friendly style of growing crops.

Monocropping methods further devastate the soil ecosystem and plant symbiosis—any and all complimentary and symbiotic plant species are eliminated, ejected, wiped out, destroyed in the monocropping processes. The corporate farm's only intention is to make money, to produce as much plant sellable material as possible. They have no concern for quality, nutrition, vitality, true nourishment, human health, animal health, or ecosystem health. The industrial mono-croppers don't want any herbs or other plant life around, they don't care about pollinators, birds, or butterflies. They have absolutely zero concern for preventing erosion, toxic algae blooms, climate change, red tides, dead zones, dead fish. They'll deny science that says their fertilizer is causing climate change-- climate change and warming temperatures are a hoax to them. Who wants to buy products that people like this created? Say no to GMOs in your food! Say no to ethanol.

SYNTHETIC FERTILIZER
Manmade chemically manufactured substance that contains high concentrations of one or more of the minerals (Nitrogen, Phosphorous, Potassium) needed for plant growth.[188]

ORGANIC FERTILIZER
Naturally occurring materials derived directly from plant or animal sources that improve soil structure.
Examples: manure, bone meal, ash, biochar
Compost, ground rock minerals like limestone

HARM TO WATER QUALITY
The truth is more toxic runoff does happen when Roundup and other herbicides are used as in the case with GMO crops. More herbicides, more problems. Double the trouble with the use of synthetic fertilizers. "Continued growth in herbicide use poses a significant environmental problem as large doses of the chemicals can harm biodiversity and increase water and air pollution."[189]

All these toxins are used on the mega farms, the monocropping farms, the GMO and conventional farms, the biotech test fields. The entities who contract farmers and own big farms just happen to not care about the planet, the water, the animals, or our wellbeing. All they're concerned with is money. Usually, these corporations have a pharmaceutical company in their portfolio, so they've got all the bases covered. Sickness means more money in their pocket. They have no incentive to stop using the deadly fertilizers and pesticides. Their business model is working just fine with government contracts and widespread farming of GMOs in America. This is why organic and biodynamic farms and regenerative farmers are so important. These farmers don't and won't use these super toxins.

FERTILIZER, RADIATION, & WARMING

For nitrogen-based fertilizers, the process involves natural gas to create ammonia. starts by mixing nitrogen from the air with hydrogen from natural gas at high temperature to create ammonia.[190]

- Nitrogen fertilizer facilities have grown significantly in the U.S. in sync with the expansion of fracking and lower natural gas prices.[191]
- Nitrous oxide is a major greenhouse gas, 300 x worse than CO2, stays in the atmosphere for 114 years! Major source is fertilizer.

Phosphate mining sites create radioactive pollution that is so harmful the EPA won't let them dispose it anywhere but on site. The result is huge tall gypsum mounds in Florida and Louisiana mostly. These sites build wide open surface pits filled with toxic waste. These so easily leak and spill into the waterways. I do believe these contribute to the Sink Hole and to the worsening nature and frequency of Red Tides.

RED TIDES

2022: "A year's worth of nitrogen – 180 metric tons – was discharged into the bay from March 30 to April 9."[192] Like clockwork, within days algae formed followed soon after by cyanobacteria floating mats. As the algae festered, eventually came the Red Tide. Nitrogen fertilizer release causes toxic algae, the same factors that trigger toxic algae trigger Red Tides.

- Phosphate mining creates severe pollution problems: mounds of radioactive gypsum,[193] poisoning waterways,[194] triggering sinkholes, air pollution: radon, sulfur dioxide & fluoride gas (which gets scraped off wet scrubbers & re-sold to fluoridate water across the U.S.) causes algae blooms and red tides, kills millions of marine animals yearly.

SOLUTIONS
- Filter your water.
- Don't support or eat GMO food, or factory farm food
- In your own garden use natural organic fertilizers.
- Farmers: if you need help converting to organic non-toxic methods, please contact us at hello@adoreyourplanet.com.

29. Flame Retardants

Flame retardant chemicals are now <u>found in nearly every person</u> and animal tested.[195] Since the 1970s they have widely used in consumer products, less so now since health came into focus. Originally, Brominated Flame Retardants, PDBEs (Polybrominated diphenyl ethers) were all that existed. Then came 2004. It was determined brominated versions were so bad, they needed to develop replacements, enter stage left: organo-phosphorus and chlorinated flame retardants. The chemical companies had a field day coming up with various poisonous versions. So now, fast forward to present day, the world is contaminated with hundreds of versions of these persistent toxins. Today, the most common flame retardant compound is known as 'chlorinated tris'.

FLAME RETARDANTS are:
- applied to drapes, window treatments, carpet, flooring
- applied to clothing, pajamas, baby's clothes, upholstery
- used in computers, appliances, Styrofoam, polystyrene foam
- building materials, wire insulation, electronics
- applied to seat covers, cushions, foam padding of all kinds, children's toys, tents, dog and cat toys, vehicle compartments

Although the use of flame retardants is intended to save lives and property, the harm their presence causes makes one question why they're still in use. Evidence shows these chemicals are carcinogenic and potent endocrine disruptors. They persist in the environment and accumulate in every living organism, harming people and animals alike. Only recently have scientists discovered they're accumulating heavily in our drinking water[196], though they are not *yet* regulated by the EPA.

HEALTH EFFECTS
They cause liver, thyroid, and neurodevelopment toxicity. They are known endocrine disruptors, reproductive toxins, neurotoxins, and carcinogens-- particularly suspected to cause breast cancer.[197] Neurologically, they delay and interfere with childhood development: they cause hormone irregularities and poor thyroid gland and endocrine system health; they interfere with the body's ability to control blood glucose levels, and last but not least, they contribute to obesity and weight gain.

Fire Retardants are bio-accumulative toxins, meaning levels within our bodies grow throughout our life. The more we are exposed, the greater the level becomes. The higher the level within us, the greater risk to our health. These pesty substances also off-gas volatile organic chemicals (VOCs) and contribute to lung and respiratory problems. God only knows how many people are affected and unnecessary deaths have been caused by these chemicals.

HOW WE ARE EXPOSED: Contaminated drinking water and Dust are two major sources. Because fire retardants have been used in so many household and construction materials, dust in nearly every home and building contains them. Anything in dust can easily get upon our hands as well as our dinner plates, gaining entry into our mouth and nose simply through our breathing, eating, or touching our face. Products containing them include carpet, furniture, mattresses, drapes, textiles, car seats, building materials, appliances, toys, electronics, televisions, and of course, fire proof uniforms.

Why Are They Still in Use? Flame retardants are a $7 Billion Market.[198] Read about the industry's corrupt lobbyist activity here.

As reported by the Chicago Tribune, "Blood levels of certain widely used flame retardants doubled in adults every two to five years between 1970 and 2004. More recent studies show levels haven't declined in the U.S. even though some of the chemicals have been pulled from the market. A typical American baby is born with the highest recorded concentrations of flame retardants among infants in the world." How can we continue to allow children to suffer with the toxic burden of unnecessary toxic chemicals? This is not a legacy people of the United States choose to keep.

Firefighters

How many men and women firefighters have been affected and harmed by these substances in their uniforms? If these substances in fact don't actually ever stop fire, what sense is there to expose these people to harm just to keep the money flowing to the corrupt industry? Enough is enough.

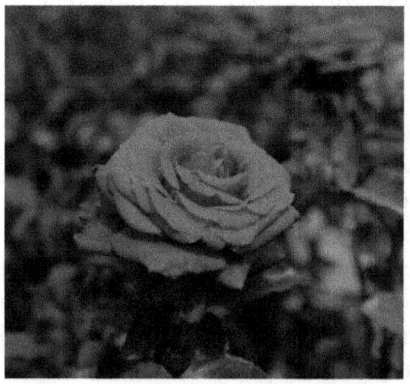

Fire Suppression & Aerial Spraying

Aerial spraying of fire extinguishing chemicals causes immeasurable damage to wildlife and ecosystems. Forests, streams and water sources are hit especially hard. Popular chemicals used on large blazes contain fertilizer and toxins, one of which degrades into cyanide. The residues are highly toxic to fish and frogs, causing cancer, death, and disease, as well as toxic algae blooms from nitrogen, phosphorous and ammonia in the fertilizer. 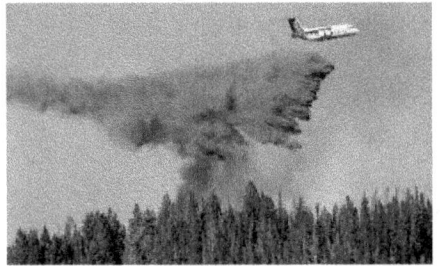 These substances all play a role in disease, air pollution, and climate change. Damage to ecosystems is not discussed enough. Loss of biodiversity will be the death of humanity. Could there be a better way to extinguish wildfires-- or perhaps prevent them from becoming so swift and deadly? What's making them so wildly uncontrollable now, speeding through forests with immeasurable speed, blanketing the majority of the nearby countries with haze and smoke? Does spraying toxins on forests have anything to do with drying out the forests and making them so prone to fire? It's not a big leap when you consider the mass of substances the Forest Service uses in times of emergency, and also every day in their management of forests. Canada isn't much better with their excessive use of desiccating glyphosate on millions of acres of forested land. The stuff dries out plants and trees making them easier to harvest. Well, if the mix is a drying agent, then logically the mix must make trees much easier to burn. When you're camping and gathering wood, you pick the dry sticks for kindling because you know the green twigs won't light no matter how hard you try.

"Millions of gallons of retardant chemicals have spewed from bombers in the last five years, and will continue to flow under the assumption that the toxic effects of the chemicals are less harmful than the effects to wildlife. Indeed, the EPA exempts fire retardant from the Clean Water Act because its use is considered a "cataclysmic release: intended to prevent assumed greater destruction to the environment by wildfire." [199] Considering synthetic fertilizer is made from the same chemicals used to make bombs, is it wise to use this material in anything fire-related? Could the residues left behind be a trigger in the escalating wild fires?

HISTORY OF SPRAYING TOXINS ON FORESTS

The USDA controls the Forest Service, and like the USDA, the Forest Service has a history of spraying pesticides. In America spraying is often followed by rust rot and other fungal killers of trees. In Canada they spray to kill the Aspen trees that are illegal in monocropped forests? Who decided to make forests monocropped? Fields, ok maybe, but forests? That's definitely not natural, no wonder animals are going extinct. Aspens are also naturally fire resistant by the way and happen to act as fire breaks, so could that be yet another reason why today's forest fires are so much worse? Learn more at StoptheSprayBC.com

SOLUTIONS

- Filter Your water for drinking and cooking.
- Avoid purchasing or wearing products with fire retardants
- Remove furnishings containing them and dust your home often
- Filter Your water, drink and cook with filtered water.
- Wash your hands, especially before handling food or eating.
- Keep your house clean and Keep dust to a minimum, use a vacuum with a HEPA filter
- Consider getting a HEPA air filter for your home and office
- If you see "meets flammability standard"--Avoid, Avoid! Instead, look for a tag saying, TB 117-2013, this product has no fire retardants.
- Protect your health with good food: eat dark green leafy greens and cruciferous vegetables, as well as probiotics, essential nutrients, and omega oils. As always, go organic as much as possible.
- Our shopping decisions can influence manufacturing--the less we buy of products containing flame retardants, the greater the chance manufacturers will stop using them on their products.
- Boycott products containing flame retardants.
- Encourage President Biden to add the United States to the Stockholm Convention on Persistent Organic Pollutants, this way we can restrict manufacturers from using flame retardants.
- Manufacturers: A new cotton has been developed to be naturally fire resistant. Perhaps it's time to replace your old fabrics for this.
- Protect forests and nurture them, do no harm

30. FLUORIDE

2024: "US Government reports Fluoridated Water at twice the recommended amount is linked to lower IQ."[200] Fluoride might be the most controversial drinking water additive. While fluoride is touted as the ultimate cavity fighter, it may be nothing more than a horrific industrial assault. Looking at the source of the fluoride will make it easy to see why many consider it unsafe.

> This is against all principles of modern pharmacology. It's really **obsolete**. No doubt about that. I mean, I think those nations that are using it should feel ashamed of themselves. It's against science—anti-scientific.
> **Dr. Arvid Carlsson,** Nobel Laureate in Medicine

Cavity Buster or Industry Spin

As revealed by Harvard's School of Public Health: Cavities overall have decreased throughout the world since the 1970's, even in countries that don't fluoridate their water! "The Cochrane report also concluded that early scientific investigations on water fluoridation (most were conducted before 1975) were deeply flawed. "We had concerns about the methods used, or the reporting of the results, in … 97 percent of the studies," the authors noted. One problem: The early studies didn't take into account the subsequent widespread use of fluoride-containing toothpastes and other dental fluoride supplements, which also prevent cavities. This may explain why countries that do not fluoridate their water have also seen big drops in cavity rates."[201] Maybe this is one reason why students in America are academically falling behind other nations. "China embarked upon a pursuit of water fluoridation for about 20 years before backing away entirely from it in the 1980s. Parts of the country have high levels of naturally occurring fluoride, which one study has linked to developmental difficulties in children."[202] Scientists today are discovering healthy bacteria may really be the reason behind avoiding cavities. "Oral probiotics, contain beneficial strains specific to the oral microbiome." [203]

The World Health Organization:

- "The toxic effects of high fluoride intake are due to the fact that it is a direct cellular poison, which binds calcium and interferes with the activity of proteolytic and glycolytic enzymes.
- Ingested fluoride reacts with gastric acid to produce hydrofluoric acid in the stomach. Thus, acute exposure to

high concentrations of fluoride results in immediate effects: abdominal pain, excessive saliva, nausea and vomiting. Seizures and muscle spasms may also occur. Death due to respiratory paralysis is a possibility."[204]

DANGER: POISONOUS IF SWALLLOWED
Have you ever noticed the warning on your toothpaste tube? Sure, applying fluoride to the surface of teeth may be safe, but as your toothpaste tube states, contact the poison control center *if you swallow it*. If it's poisonous to swallow fluoride in toothpaste, how can swallowing fluoridated water be safe? Is there a limit on how much is safe to swallow? Where's the warning from the EPA or the government who insists on adding this substance to our drinking water! Fluoride accumulates in the pineal and thyroid glands. Scientists now worry that "excess fluoride may be toxic to brain and nerve cells."[205]

How Much Fluoride Are We Consuming?
People are consuming a lot of fluoride and they don't even know it. Many things are made with water, is that water fluoride free? It's added to public water systems, as well as some bottled waters. In the UK they're giving fluoridated milk to school children beginning year 1![206] If it's so harmful you're not supposed to swallow it in toothpaste, how can all this fluoride consumption be good for us? With full disclosure, Cavity prevention? Not sure it's valid—today they say decay can be prevented with healthy mouth bacteria, sufficient nutrients and less sugar. Wouldn't it make more sense and be beneficial for us the drinkers if they added good minerals and perhaps vitamin C to the water?

HEALTH EFFECTS of too much FLUORIDE:
Arthritis, Osteoporosis, bone damage, bone cancer, joint pain and troubles, dental fluorosis, skeletal fluorosis, muscular damage, fatigue, problems, bone changes. There are direct adverse effects on the kidneys by excess fluoride, leading to kidney damage and dysfunction.[207] "In extreme conditions, it could adversely damage the heart, arteries, kidney, liver, endocrine glands, neuron system, and several other delicate parts of a living organism."[208]

HOW WE ARE EXPOSED:
Drinking fluoridated water and consuming products made with it.
PEOPLE on DIALYSIS: DON'T DRINK FLUORIDATED WATER!

THE SOURCE: FLUORIDE COMES FROM WHERE?

Fluorosilicic Acid is the substance added to public water supplies. This toxic acid is derived from the scum washed off wet scrubbers at phosphate fertilizer facilities! This is a sick twist and corrupt as they come. In the 1940s and 50s before pollution control devices were installed, fluorosilicic acid escaped as a gas and was responsible for killing vast amounts of animals, livestock and farm crops near these facilities. This toxic substance contains not just fluoride but also mercury, lead and arsenic. It's hazardous waste and very expensive to dispose of properly. Adding it to water supplies throughout the country is a convenient remedy for the industry to avoid costly disposal.

"Drinking water containing more than 1.5 milligrams of fluoride per liter is consistently associated with lower IQs in kids."[209]

POISON Hotline 1-800-222-1222

THE FLUORIDE MANDATE:

Seventeen (17) States mandate all communities fluoridate water: Arkansas, District of Columbia, California, Connecticut, Delaware, Georgia, Illinois, Kentucky, Louisiana, Michigan, Minnesota, Mississippi, Nebraska, Nevada, Ohio, Puerto Rico, South Dakota.[210]

SOLUTIONS

- **Filter your water.** Some filters filter fluoride, most do not..
- Best filters: Carbon block, reverse osmosis, activated charcoal, gravity filter. Berkey makes special filters to remove fluoride.
- If you have health ailments, joint pain, hip pain, bone pain, arthritis, or kidney disease, avoid fluoridated water.
- If you have your own well, get it tested yearly
- Babies, children and pets can be harmed by water toxins.

COUNTRIES THAT BAN FLUORIDE IN WATER[211]:

Germany	Finland	Estonia	Luxembourg
Austria	Belgium	France	Slovakia
China	Netherlands	Greece	Switzerland
Denmark	Hungary	Iceland	Turkey
Italy	Japan	Mexico	Czech Republic
Sweden	Israel	Portugal	Norway

SPECIAL REPORT
Hazardous Waste

Hazardous waste is derived from extremely toxic substances, like radioactive materials and extreme cancer-causing substances. These must be disposed of in a certain way to prevent harming people, animals, and the environment. Some industries, past and present, who use toxic substances have left a toxic footprint where they manufactured or disposed of the substances. **Map of Superfund Sites**

> Corporation with greatest number of Superfund Sites: **General Electric**

WHAT IS A SUPERFUND SITE?
Superfund is the federal government program to clean up and restore unmonitored hazardous waste sites. These sites are many times abandoned by the corporations and industries that caused them. Sites receive Superfund Site designation because they present an elevated degree of risk to human health, to animals, and to the environment. Typical contaminants found include benzene, cadmium, carbon tetrachloride, tetrachloro-ethylene, lead, mercury, trichloroethene, toluene, PCBs, vinyl chloride, zinc, arsenic.

President Jimmy Carter signed the Superfund Act, otherwise known as CERCLA (Comprehensive Environmental Response, Compensation, and Liability Act) in 1980. This made corporations responsible for cleaning up their mess. Each year the fund was replenished with "polluter pay" or "superfund" taxes instilled upon petroleum products, crude oil, and toxic chemicals. In 1995, Congress failed to renew the tax; between 2001 and 2003, President Bush let Superfund go bankrupt. As of 2022, the Superfund has been restored!

> Hurricane Katrina swept through **54** Superfund Sites.

WHAT IS A BROWNFIELD: A property, the expansion, redevelopment, or reuse of which may be complicated by the presence or potential presence of a hazardous substance, pollutant, or contaminant. It is estimated that there are more than 450,000 brownfields in the U.S.[212]

NATIONAL PRIORITIES LIST (NPL): Sites expedited for cleanup.

31. FRACKING

Across the U.S, fracking sites transform millions of gallons of fresh water daily into toxic wastewater, which they then dispose of underground. This is a major threat to water supplies and threatens us all. The wastewater is loaded with heavy metals, carcinogens, hazardous waste that's also radioactive. Yet, the EPA does NOT regulate fracking wastewater. This means the fracking companies don't need permits to dispose of it, and they're allowed to dump it underground or store it in open waste ponds.

Certainly, the natural gas industry has enough financial resources and subsidies to operate more conscientiously and respect human health and our country's water resources. Why can't this industry be aligned with sensible earth-friendly methods and processes? Is it asking too much to have toxic disease-causing waste water purified or something before its injected underground? Is making the US energy independent worth damaging countless people, animals, and ecosystems?

OVER 1,000 TOXIC CHEMICALS!

Fracking uses lots and lots of dangerous chemicals. Reports conclude up to 1,021 toxic chemicals* are used in fracking! These contaminants remain in the wastewater and all of it is injected underground into disposal wells, or kept in pits. Neither the amount of chemicals, the wastewater, nor the disposal wells are at all regulated by the EPA. Who knows what the fracking industry is keeping secret. According to the NRDC, "fracking wastewater contaminants include*: Barium, Benzene, Bromide, Chloride, Lead, Strontium, VOCs, Toluene, Ethylbenzene, xylene, iron manganese, nitrate, ammonia nitrogen, diesel, ethylene glycol, naphthalene, hydrochloric acid, diethanolamine, formaldehyde, sulfuric acid, thiorea, benzyl chloride, cumene, nitrilotriacetic acid, dimethyl formamine, phenol, Di phthalate, acrylamide, hydrofluoric acid, phthalic anhydride, acetaldehyde, acetophenone, copper, propylene oxide, p-xylene.[213]

CONTAMINATING DRINKING WATER

"Local impacts on drinking water quantity have occurred in areas with increased hydraulic fracturing activity…The aboveground disposal of hydraulic fracturing wastewater has impacted the quality of groundwater and surface water resources. Additionally, the use of lined and unlined pits for the storage or disposal of oil and gas wastewater has impacted surface and groundwater resources. Unlined pits, in particular, provide a direct pathway for contaminants to reach groundwater."[214]

In 2011, the EPA officially connected fracking to underground water pollution and contaminated drinking water. "The contamination contained at least 10 substances known to be used in frack fluids." [215] "A number of studies and publications caution that surface and groundwater contamination remains a risk; some studies document contamination from above-ground chemical spills, leaks, wastewater mishandling and other incidents. How significant these risks are over the long term is presently unclear and in need of continued study."[216]

CAUSING WATER SHORTAGES

Fracking uses so much water that it depletes ground water and drinking water sources. According to the EPA's own study, "withdrawals for hydraulic fracturing can directly impact drinking water resources by changing the quantity or quality of the remaining water. Although every water withdrawal affects water, we focused on water withdrawals that have the potential to significantly impact drinking water resources by limiting the availability of drinking water or altering its quality."

WHEN TOXIC WASTE BECAME NON-HAZARDOUS

This sneaky amendment to the RCRA, Resource Conservation Recovery Act changed everything for the fossil fuel industry. On October 12, 1980, Congress enacted the Solid Waste Disposal Act Amendments of 1980 (Public Law 96-482), which included the Bentsen and Bevill Amendments that exempted drilling fluids, produced waters, and other wastes associated with the exploration, development, and production of crude oil or natural gas or geothermal energy from being considered hazardous waste.[217]

Essentially, this allowed these toxic chemicals and waste products from fracking and drilling to go unregulated. This is no small matter—and one that corporations must have paid for pretty heftily. Who is getting the kickbacks? Why has this amendment and others like it not been overturned yet? The NRDC filed a lawsuit against the EPA in 2016 to get them to review the regulations so the rogue methods employed by this industry will halt.[218] **"The oil and gas companies have a lot of money. In the face of apathy from the general populace, they will get their way."[219]**

HEALTH EFFECTS
Water contaminated with fracking waste contains barium, heavy metals, radioactive material, benzene, ethylene glycol, methanol, toluene. These substances cause poisoning, death, leukemia, cancer, cardiac issues, birth defects, skin ailments, breathing troubles and on and on...

HOW WE ARE EXPOSED
Drinking water from sources that have been contaminated with fracking chemicals, or eating foods made with this water. "The risk to drinking water comes in two major ways. First, water used in the hydraulic drilling process can leak into aquifers and other groundwater supplies. Second, the wastewater that fracking produces can contaminate supplies when waste leaks from landfills that accept oil remains, when waste spills from trucks or pipelines moving it, when equipment fails, or when waste leaks from unlined disposal pits."[220]

WAIVER FOR FRACKING WASTEWATER?
Despite the dangerous chemicals in fracking wastewater, the fracking industry, with the help of lobbyists and a certain Vice President, succeeded in avoiding regulation. In the 2005 Energy Bill, Dick Cheney helped exempt fracking wastewater from the Safe Drinking Water Act and so through this day, the EPA does not regulate fracking hydraulic drilling wastewater. This only strengthened the lack of accountability the oil and

SOLUTIONS
- Filter your water for both drinking and cooking.
- With all the Subsidies to the fracking and energy sector, they have the obligation to be more responsible. Earth is a precious resource and they're mucking it up. The handling of wastewater is completely mind boggling. The injection wells are so deep, how are they monitor adequately for leaks?[221] Nothing good can come from this.
- Join the call to Keep Fracking out of Your Community. Learn how with this guide from the NRDC
- "Even if your state doesn't have a mandatory review process, you can still ask state representatives for strong laws. You can also get involved when regulatory codes are being revised or during comment periods. To know when these opportunities arise, join an anti-fracking group in your state."[222]

32. GEN X: PFAS

Cleverly named to perhaps confuse us. Gen X is a newer dreadful chemical in the PFAS family of forever chemicals. It's a super persistent toxin and carcinogen that's accumulating all over the place, especially in east coast waterways and private wells. It's also known as HFPO-Dimer Acid. Gen X is one of many PFAS chemicals, but it stands out as one of the worst. Originally developed by Dupont in 2009 as a less harmful replacement for Teflon (PFOA), Gen X is turning out to be roughly 10 times worse than PFOA!

For years Dupont and its subsidiary, Chemours have been dumping Gen X and PFOA into the Cape Fear River. Due to severe contamination and health risk, residents of Delaware, North Carolina, and West Virginia avoid tap water in favor of bottled water. In some places where contamination levels are sky high, Chemours is covering costs for those affected and installing whole home carbon filtration systems. To reduce culpability and attempt to hide from responsibility, in 2015 Dupont transferred this fluorochemical division over to its Chemours brand. The toxin is produced now at the Chemours Fayetteville facility, which as of 2022 is expanding operations!

HEALTH EFFECTS
Liver damage, kidney damage, bladder damage, causes reproductive problems and many types of cancer.[223]

HOW WE ARE EXPOSED
Drinking water contaminated with industrial PFAS and GENX pollution is the primary route of exposure.

SOLUTIONS
- Filter your water and reduce your exposure to PFAS
- We must get Chemours, Dupont, 3M and others to stop making PFAS and to clean up all the messes they've created both environmentally and upon human health.
- Find out what's in your tap water, go to: www.EWG.org/tapwater

33. GLYPHOSATE

Glyphosate is a neurotoxin, carcinogen, endocrine disruptor, and one of two most used herbicides in the world (other being atrazine) "It can persist in the environment for days or months, its intensive large-scale use constitutes a major environmental and health problem."[224]

Drinking water sources everywhere are contaminated. AMPA (Aminomethylophophonic acid) is the breakdown product. If you have either glyphosate or AMPA in your water over 10mg/L please get a new source of water.[225]

Unfortunately, glyphosate is implicated in serious health problems for creatures of all sizes, from humans to bees to soil microorganisms. It's sold under many different names, included in heaps of products and brands at your local hardware store.

DANGER: NEUROTOXIN ALERT!
"Glyphosate seems to exert a significant toxic effect on neurotransmission and to induce oxidative stress, neuroinflammation and mitochondrial dysfunction, processes that lead to neuronal death due to autophagy, necrosis, or apoptosis, as well as the appearance of behavioral and motor disorders. The doses of glyphosate that produce these neurotoxic effects vary widely but are lower than the limits set by regulatory agencies."[226]

HEALTH EFFECTS
- Contaminates drinking water
- Carcinogenic
- Endocrine Disruptor
- Disrupts gut microbiome
- Suppresses hormones and thyroid activity
- Disables Apoptosis, body's innate cancer-fighting skill
- Won't let the thyroid absorb the Iodine that it needs
- Causes hormonal anomalies linked with anxiety, depression, insomnia, headaches, stress
- Causes leaky gut and digestive problems
- Harms Pollinators, causes disorientation
- Kills milkweed, the sole food monarchs feed upon
- Probable factor in rising numbers of gluten intolerance

HOW WE ARE EXPOSED

Contaminated drinking water, contaminated foods, GMO foods notably GMO soybeans and corn, landscaping, walking through grass, gardens, golf courses, desiccation, residues from grain, fruit and vegetable crops.

What is the Difference between Glyphosate and Roundup?

Glyphosate is a toxic poison developed in the 1970s by Monsanto. Roundup is a brand of herbicide made by Monsanto with glyphosate and other ingredients including unknown additives and surfactants. Roundup is like glyphosate on steroids. Roundup causes health harm and is more dangerous than glyphosate alone. Monsanto safety tests only ever tested Glyphosate, not the entire Roundup formula.[227] The Roundup products and GMO seeds developed by Monsanto are now owned by Bayer after their merger in 2016.

"Glyphosate infiltrates the brain, and causes neurodegenerative disorders…exposure to this herbicide may have detrimental outcomes regarding the health of the general population."[228] Bayer, who now owns Monsanto-- is claiming they'll remove glyphosate from Roundup formulas, but replace it with Dicamba! OMG! No no no!

SOLUTIONS

- Filter your water
- Reduce exposure to glyphosate (most commonly known as Round*up* herbicide)
- Avoid GMO foods, which contain Round*up* (Glyphosate)
- Protect your babies, pets and everyone in your home by not using glyphosate products on your lawn or indoors
- Ask your hardware store to protect the planet and stop selling Round*up* and other pesticides like Neonicotinoids that harm pollinators. These products have the capacity to put all creatures, including humans on the Endangered Species list!
- Help stop the EPA from allowing more dicamba use on the newly approved dicamba-resistant genetically modified crops! The governments own studies carried out under the Agricultural Health Study[229] recently show that Dicamba causes both **colon and lung cancer**! We do not need to be exposed to this horrible carcinogen on our food or in our water! Farmers and their families don't need to be exposed either! Chinese-owned Bayer can go use it on their country but not ours!! Save American lives and ban Dicamba!

SPECIAL REPORT
HERBICIDES

Herbicides are Weedkillers: poisonous and deadly.
Cause death to: Plants, pollinators, animals, trees, humans
Cause disease to: People, animals, beneficial Insects, aquatic animals, forests, beneficial plants, ecosystems, soil

MOST USED HERBICIDES in U.S:

Atrazine: ChemChina (Syngenta)
Glyphosate: Bayer (Monsanto)
Glufosinate: Bayer (Monsanto). The US is world's largest market for glufosinate, it's used to control glyphosate-resistant weeds.[230]
Enlist Duo: Corteva (Dow)
2,4-D, (Corteva) Dicamba (Bayer)
Paraquat: ChemChina (Syngenta): linked to Parkinson's
Round up: Bayer (Monsanto)

DICAMBA: Causes Colon and Lung Cancer[231]
We must Ban Dicamba!!Recently dicamba-resistant GMO crops were approved for planting in the United States! This is big trouble!!
FDA and EPA: You cannot allow this assault on Americans' health!
Roundup Banned in these Countries: Argentina, Austria, Belgium, Bermuda,Bahrain, Barbados, Columbia, Costa Rica, Czech Republic, Fiji, Germany, Italy, Kuwait, Luxemburg, Malta, Netherlands, Oman, Portugal, Qatar, St. Vincent, Grenadines, Saudi Arabia, Scotland, Slovenia, Spain, Sri Lanka, Thailand, Vietnam[232]
Round Up Ban by 2024: Mexico
Round Up Restrictions: Australia, Brazil, Canada, El Salvador, France, India in 2022 restricted use to pesticide operators.
Round up Ban Cities: California's State University System, Key West, Portland, New York Parks and Recreation, Chicago Public Areas
Atrazine Ban: Austria, Denmark, France, Finland, Germany, Italy, Sweden,
Paraquat Ban: Austria, Brazil, Cambodia, China, Denmark, EU, Germany, Kuwait, Finland, Ivory Coast, Malaysia, Slovenia, Sweden, Switzerland, Syria, UAE, UK,

34. Hand Sanitizers

Most hand sanitizers and anti-bacterial soaps are not good for you, especially not on a daily basis. They contain Triclosan, and most also have benzene.[233] Both are very toxic and cause bad diseases.

BANNED ELSEWHERE BUT NOT HERE!
Triclosan is a registered pesticide[234] molecularly similar to Agent Orange. In 2015 its usage was banned completely in the EU. " According to the European Chemicals Agency (ECHA), 'No safe use could be demonstrated for the proposed use of Triclosan.'"[235] The FDA decided to ban it in a few soap products, but it's still allowed in tons of other products! These include: toothpaste, hand sanitizers, deodorant, blemish gels, dish soap, makeup, first-aid creams, and even sandals, socks, and children's toys, cutting boards, anything marked anti-bacterial surface beware!

Hand Sanitizer formulas contain endocrine disruptors and alcohol amongst other ingredients that collectively don't do your health any favors. Please Note: There are a few all natural nontoxic hand sanitizers out there that do not impart these effects. Studies show triclosan offers no advantage different than soap not containing it.[236]

Triclosan studies show that it accumulates in fatty tissue and epithelial cells,[237] aquatic organisms, causes a breakdown in skin cells, increases antibiotic-resistant bacteria, aggravates allergies and weakens the immune response.

Health Effects of hand sanitizers containing triclosan:
- It's bioaccumulative, it's an endocrine disruptor.
- It's found in breast milk, can cause reproductive problems
- Weakens skin's protective barrier
- Breaches blood-brain barrier
- Disrupts hormones, causes hormone-related health problems
- Increases risk of cancer
- Overuse of antimicrobials causes antibiotic resistance, AMR

SOLUTIONS:
- Wash hands the old fashioned way, with soap and water.
- Avoid anti-bacterial products that contain triclosan!

35. Heavy Metals

Heavy metals are toxic metals. Our bodies need a tiny particular amount of trace minerals and metals in perfect balance for optimal health. Excessive amounts of heavy metals can trigger imbalance and disorders, depleting and preventing other necessary nutrients from being absorbed. This can result in behavioral changes, aggression, anger and violence. We are exposed to heavy metals from a surprising variety of sources and industries including petroleum and steel production.

HEAVY METALS

Aluminum	Arsenic	Beryllium	Manganese	Nickle
Barium	Cadmium	Chromium	Mercury	Methylmercury
Lead	Silver	Selenium	Nickel	Tin
Vanadium	Fluoride	Molybdenum	Iron	

SOURCES OF HEAVY METALS

Mining, contaminated water, dust, smoke, exhaust, fuel additives, particulates and aerosols, contaminated baby Food, vintage plates, cookware with lead and cadmium, glazing on ceramic, contaminated foods, pesticides and fumigants, Cigarettes (and e-cigarettes), burning fossil fuels, incineration, burn pits, fireworks, warfare

NEUROTOXINS affect the brain and nervous system:
HEALTH EFFECTS OF HEAVY METALS:[238]

Brain damage, Cancer, Gastrointestinal disorders, kidney issues, Learning disabilities, neurological disorders, Autism, behavioral changes, lower IQ, mineral deficiency diseases, hormonal imbalance, chronic liver disease, respiratory issues, chronic bronchitis, violence, inflammation in the lungs, kidney disease, organ malfunction, lethargy, weakness, muscle spasms, tremors, aggression, violence, birth defects, immune system damage, skin lesions.

SOLUTIONS

- Avoid contaminated water.
- Filter your Water. Cook with filtered water as well!
- Avoid heavy dust and smoke, use wet-dusting when cleaning your home. Bring plants indoors that absorb air pollution
- Avoid ceramic glazes on plates and mugs, vintage dishes that contain cadmium and lead

36. Landscaping

Lawncare and chemicals used for landscaping easily contaminate ground water, well water, and your drinking water. Growing up my dad loved when our *TruGreen* neighbor came by with his truck. He'd saturate the grass with his brew of lawncare chemicals. If it's not safe to walk on the grass for days, you have to wonder what's in there. To this day I'm convinced those chemicals[239] were involved in my parents' early deaths.

Today these companies continue to swindle lawncare enthusiasts, gardeners and farmers everywhere with their potent blends of fertilizers and pesticides. If you want to protect your family, your pets, and your own health, I strongly suggest finding natural alternatives that do an even better job at keeping your yard and garden healthy. The problem with the toxic chemicals is they not only compromise your drinking water, they weaken your soil, and harm wildlife. This is why it's not surprising to see more trees and plants fall victim to disease [240] wherever toxic lawncare is used. Faithful yard keepers try their best to save their vegetation by reaching for pesticides and herbicides designed to make their plantings more disease resistant. Really all this cycle does is make the chemical companies richer and our plants, our yards, and ourselves weaker and more dependent on the chemicals they're peddling.

The truth is plants of all kinds have an inner defense system capable of maintaining health and defending against disease. This innate system is destroyed and suppressed by chemicals. It's a no-win cycle for the plants. Once you start using toxic synthetic fertilizer, you've unwittingly put your plants at a disadvantage. As these chemicals seep into ground and well water, they put your family at risk. They'll also wash away when it rains and contribute to toxic algae, dead zones, and red tides.

Toxins found in popular lawncare products include development and reproductive toxins, teratogens, endocrine disruptors, neurotoxins, and carcinogens, prop 65 contaminants. For your family, pets and your own health try to switch to natural lawn care products without the health-harming substances we don't need.

SOLUTIONS:
- Use nontoxic products on your lawn
- Filter your water for drinking and cooking.

37. LEAD PB
#5 Worst Water Pollutant

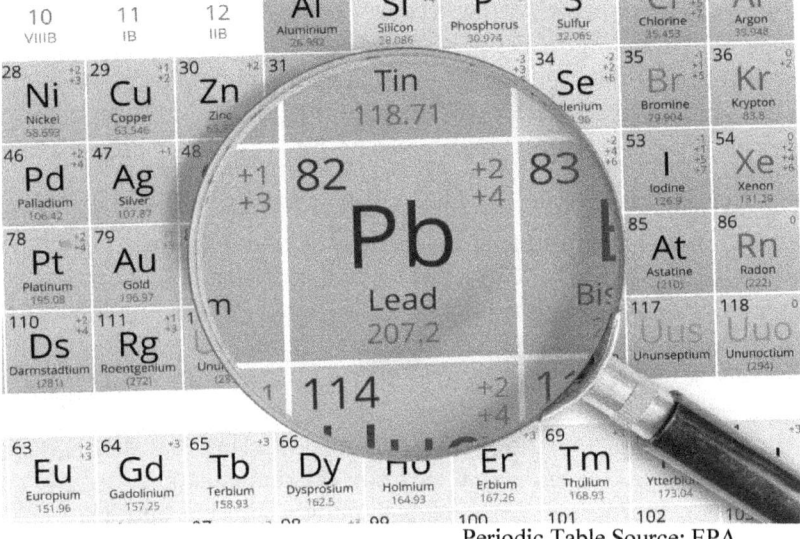

Periodic Table Source: EPA

Lead is a heavy metal and neurotoxin. In 2016, Flint, Michigan put the spotlight on drinking water contaminated with lead. Unfortunately, this problem is more common than one might think.

Water pipes throughout the United States are aging, deteriorating, and have become unsafe. How the lead industry convinced towns throughout the U.S. to install lead pipes in the 1950's could be one of the most deceptive marketing crimes ever pulled off. The Lead Industries Association claimed bankruptcy in 2002[241] to avoid further lawsuits, yet perhaps one day the six corporations[242] that made up the LIA will have justice served. Other cities experiencing a Lead Crisis today include: Jackson, Mississippi, Benton Harbor, Michigan, Baltimore, MD, Phoenix, AZ, Washington D.C., and Chicago, IL. Currently, Chicago is the city with the most miles of lead service lines in need of removal.[243]

FLINT, MICHIGAN

Flint's lead issue became noticeable after corrosive water drawn from the Flint River entered the older pipes. Suddenly lead was leaching into the water. Why did the water from the Flint River get so corrosive to make the Flint disaster happen?

In Flint's case, what allegedly caused the river water to be so caustic has of all things been linked to the use of road salt. As revealed by the National Resources Defense Council, "Road salt is 40 percent sodium ions and 60 percent chloride ions. Water from the Flint River has an unusually high concentration of chloride ions—eight times higher than the tap water in Detroit. According to the Virginia Tech water experts who helped blow the lid off the public health scandal, those high chloride levels are likely responsible for the corrosiveness of Flint River water. Without an aggressive corrosion-inhibiting treatment, like the one Detroit uses, the water readily dissolved lead from the city's pipes."[244]

CHLORAMINES PULLING LEAD FROM PIPES
Another factor causing more lead in water is the way water it's purified. The culprit, Chloramines![245] Chloramines pull more lead and heavy metals into the drinking water. For people in towns afflicted with lead, continue to make use of filtered and bottled water until your lead pipes are removed. As with all water source, it's up to us to keep water clean in the first place; and that means shutting down the sources of pollution. In these cases, we need a national mandate to stop using road salt, something Canada did years ago. Cities must also must stop using Chloramines to filter water! EPA needs to update filtering options.

HEALTH EFFECTS
Since children have lower body weights, lead can affect them more severely. Lead builds up in the body over time. Children with high levels of lead in their bodies can suffer from delayed growth; learning impairment, brain and nervous system dysfunction; behavior and learning problems; hearing problems; and headaches. Adults suffer from kidney issues, damage to the brain and red blood cells, difficulty with pregnancy and reproductive problems; high blood pressure; digestive issues; nerve disorders; memory, concentration issues; as well as muscle and joint pain.[246]

HOW WE ARE EXPOSED TO LEAD
Older Lead Water Lines still in place and in use!
While the government allocated funds to remove lead pipes throughout the country beginning in 2021, in many locations work has not begun and in others, they're only removing partial pipes! They're leaving lead pipes in place, and also removing them cheaply that results in airborne toxins in peoples' homes! See the Lead Line Report on pages 108-110.
Water: older lead plumbing pipes contaminate drinking water. Hot water from the tap can dissolve more lead. Chloramine disinfection pulls more lead out of pipes into the water!

CFL, LED Light bulbs (also contain arsenic, nickel, copper, iron)[247]
Industry Exhaust and Waste: vehicles, mining, steel facilities,
Paint and Paint Chips: Prior to 1978, most paint contained lead.
Dust: Mechanical, Ammunition, industrial dust leeches into water
Lunch Boxes, Art Supplies, Baby Bibs: Some products contain lead, be aware and buy wisely, avoid questionable products **Children:** Dust and paint chips are main route of exposure.

Dust and paint chips in older buildings: Children and babies as well as pregnant mothers and the elderly are particularly susceptible to lead poisoning. If you live in a home built before 1978, lead paint may be present, especially if the home has never been renovated. To reduce your risk, keep dust to a minimum and avoid paint chips.

LEAD IN SCHOOLS & WATER FOUNTAINS
Since they're only removing some of the lead lines, Lead is still contaminating water at schools nationwide. This isn't fair for kids or teachers. Our leadership really needs to start being more efficient.

SOLUTIONS

- Drink and cook with filtered or bottled water. Don't use tap water without filtering. Install a suitable filter for your home, or find a trustworthy source of bottled water.
- Infant formula: heat filtered water on stove or microwave, don't use hot water directly from kitchen sink tap
- Hot Tap Water: Don't drink *hot* tap water. Make water hot by boiling it on the stove or heating it in microwave.
- Install a HEPA air filter to keep air clean.
- On poor air quality days, keep your windows closed and filter any ventilation equipment used. Adjust AC so indoor air is recirculated. Bring plants that filter air pollution indoors (ferns, spider plants, ivy to name a few).
- Dust: Damp dust* your home often, especially if you live in an older home or with stain-resistant carpet. ***Damp Dusting**: Dust with a wet cloth or sponge. Dust will stick to the cloth rather than recirculate through the air
- The most polluting industries are taking us all down the river, worsening water pollution and accelerating disease risk. Industries emitting heavy metals must install pollution control devices. Refineries, steel mills, mining, get your act together and help make this a wonderful and healthy planet for all!

SPECIAL REPORT
Lead Water Lines

Throughout the country water systems are breaking down. Older plumbing pipes are leaching lead into the water. Residents are put on water advisories and bottled water usually comes to the rescue. This is a temporary fix, until the water quality gets back in the "safe" zone. Safe being a bit vague, for the entities determining safety can vary between EPA guidelines and City, Municipal, State and interpretation of government rules.

As years have passed, it seems one town after another has come under crisis due to elevated lead levels in water. Unfortunately, back in the 1950s, lead water lines were installed throughout cities in the US to bring water to the tap. Now all these years later, the pipes' integrity is failing and lead is leaching into the drinking water. If the water is at all corrosive, the situation can accelerate and magnify quickly as it did in Flint, Michigan.

Chicago stands as the city with the most miles of lead pipes still actively used to distribute water. The lead problem can be traced back to the corrupt misinformation campaign promoted by the Lead Industries Association (LIA) in the 1940s and 50s. They convinced city after city that lead was safe, while evidence clearly shows the LIA knew how dangerous lead truly was.[248] Now, conveniently the LIA went bankrupt and isn't taking responsibility for fixing the problem.

> **The Lead and Copper Rule** requires utilities to target and remove only those lines that when tested indicate lead is present. In other words, even if lead lines are present, if the water at the time of testing doesn't show lead over 15ppb, the pipe can remain where it is. Cukoo birds.

INFRASTRUCTURE BILL
The Biden Infrastructure Bill allotted funds to cities across the U.S. to finally remove all these lead service lines. But now new problems are arising. In some places, they're using Cure in Place, a very questionable

technology for a quick fix; and they're not removing all the lines as they need to! It comes down to cutting corners, and a little EPA item called the Lead and Copper Rule.

"PARTIAL" REMOVAL OF LEAD!!

Due to the EPA's own standards, crews around the country are only removing some of the lead lines! This is outrageous! They're actually cutting out sections of deteriorated pipe and leaving the rest of the lead pipe down there.[249] This sounds like the worst way to go about the work. Talk about inefficient! Let's save time and money and do it all at once, not half way. With a little foresight, we can get rid of all the lead water lines and make great strides in preventative maintenance.

"CURE IN PLACE": BAD FOR HEALTH

Another new process has arrived that's causing more woes. At least 50% of cities are using this method because it's cheaper than full out replacement. It's called cure in place or CIPP. Essentially this involves inserting a pliable plastic epoxy resin tube into the old lead pipe. The tube is first usually soaked in vinyl. Once in place the tube is then steam cured to affix to the old lead pipe. As one might guess, the new plastic tube contains toxins like BPA, BADGE[250], Styrene, Benzene, and harmful VOCs, which volatize during the heating process. These fumes are traveling up the lines into homes, offices and schools. People are experience sickness, headaches, nosebleeds, dizziness, loss of balance, poisoning, nausea, unconsciousness, and lingering illness. Some people's symptoms last for weeks or apparently don't go away at all.[251] I don't know what corporation makes these plastic tubes, but this is definitely wrong. When has melting plastic ever been a good idea? People, let's get the job done right. Tell your City to get all the lead pipes out and replace them with safe pipes that won't leak fumes or heavy metals or any toxic substances into the waterways or the air.

SOLUTIONS

Filter your water. When your water is compromised and contaminated, it's vital to use filtered water or bottled water for drinking and cooking. This is especially important for children and any one recuperating. Water filters with carbon, reverse osmosis, or ion exchange do work well. Any filter is better than nothing. Ultimately though the goal must be to replace All the lead pipes in the country, and get the source of lead pollution out of the water. Cities must do their part and promptly and properly remove all lead water lines. No

ENVIRONMENTAL INJUSTICE

Around the world and in America, some of the worst factories and waste sites are located in areas where poverty is inescapable. This positioning exposes those residing in such areas to some of the worst types of pollutants known to mankind. Such toxins can affect learning, behavior, health and wellbeing. It's vital we stop polluting and clean up the pollution, but we also have to stop building polluting facilities in these hard-hit areas that unfairly affects those in poverty. Let's lift them up and help these folks have health and abundance and a clean environment to raise their spirits and their children! We are Americans after all, there's nothing we can't do!

> **Unfair Exposure, Environmental Justice**
> The risk of lead exposure remains disproportionately high for some groups, including children who are poor, non-Hispanic black, Mexican American, living in large metropolitan areas, or living in older housing. While adults absorb about 11 percent of lead reaching the digestive tract, children may absorb 30 to 75 percent. When lead is inhaled, up to 50 percent is absorbed, but less than 1 percent of lead is absorbed when it comes in contact with the skin. The body stores lead mainly in bone, where it can accumulate for decades. "Anyone in poor nutritional status absorbs lead more easily. Calcium deficiency especially increases lead absorption, as does iron deficiency, which can also increase lead damage to blood cells. A high-fat diet increases lead absorption, and so does an empty stomach."

Industries must stop procrastinating when it comes to preventing pollution. If they don't install proper pollution control equipment, why are they still in operation? Some of the areas where toxic pollution unfairly has blanketed residents includes:
- Louisiana: Cancer Alley
- Chicago: Altgeld Gardens
- Niagra Falls, New York: Love Canal

We need accountability, responsibility, and stewardship of the earth. Why do we buy products, why do cities and governments contract with corporations with such a dirty footprint, with such disdain for helping the planet and protecting people's health? Can our health and planet be so easily sacrificed and traded away? Maybe we should all tune in and bring justice upon these corporations who've been harming us all for years with their dirty wastewater, toxic products, and thoughtlessness.

38. Manganese - Emerging!

Manganese occurs in water naturally, but levels wildly increase from toxic pollution. The worse pollution sources include coal, mining, steel production, fracking, and urban waste. When the water travels, drinking water for everyone is compromised. Gasoline MMT additives are another source that contributes to toxic air pollution and smog.

Manganese is a heavy metal and neurotoxin. It's also an essential micronutrient, but overexposure impacts brain health, behavior, and mental health. Overexposure to manganese and lead can turn people into criminals.[252] Despite the danger, the EPA hasn't yet added manganese to its list of regulated substances, though the EPA does have a suggested safe level, its ridiculously high compared to other nations.

Hiding A Growing Mental Health Threat

A 2023 Report by Public Health Watch revealed the industries causing manganese pollution are using their own funded research to sway the EPA and keep the spotlight off this growing health threat.

"The EPA maintains a survey called the Drinking Water Contaminant Candidate List[253] —basically a list of potential contaminants to drinking water systems but which aren't actually regulated. Manganese has been on and off that list for a number of years. And many industries have an interest in manganese: steel manufacturers, coal, and so on. These industries came together to form the Manganese Interest Group, and have argued over time that manganese should not be on the EPA list. They've been important to influencing that process, as well as funding and supporting academic research that questions the need for tighter controls of manganese."[254] This is not in line with American values nor our pursuit for health and a good life.

HEALTH EFFECTS

Despair, irritability, anxiety, depression, mood change, somatization, and obsessive and compulsive behavior. Heavy metal toxins suppress serotonin and dopamine amongst other things.[255] Cognitive problems, hostility, excess exposure can also cause brain neurotoxicity and neuromotor changes, depression, Parkinson's like symptoms,[256], reduced motor skills, slurred speech, and uncontrollable muscle movement; behavior changes, socially withdrawn, slowed reaction, mood changes, aggression, manganism, slurred speech, brain fog.

Mental Health is a serious problem in this country and it hasn't been addressed adequately by our country in decades. This manganese exposure certainly cannot help those already suffering. What effects might be worsened if someone is on medication? What are the full impacts when someone is unknowingly consuming too much of this neurotoxin? How is this affecting our communities and contributing to crime and violence?

HOW WE ARE EXPOSED

Contaminated Water, Air Pollution, Industrial pollution, Pet Coke, Steel drilling, mining, fuel additives. If you notice your water is discolored, or leaves a brownish stain, or smells off you may have too much manganese in your water. This can especially happen if your source is a private well. You should have such water tested; anything above .3mg/L is considered too much manganese.

How America Compares to Other Nations

As data shows, the safe limit 'suggested' by the EPA is 6 times higher than what the EU recommends and far over and above every other country's safe threshold. What is going on here with the EPA! With gun shootings, violence and crime in the world, you'd think the EPA would be doing everything in their power to curtail mental health as it relates to exposures in the environment. They are the Environmental Protection Agency after all.

Doesn't the EPA care about Americans' Mental Health?!!

Authority	Manganese Concentration(ug/L)
U.S. EPA	**300**
Health Canada	120
World Health Organization	80
National Institute of Public Health of Quebec	60
European Union	50

Data Source: Public Health Watch[257]

SOLUTIONS

- Drink, cook, and brush your teeth with filtered or bottled water. If your water is high in manganese, get a shower filter
- At this time there is no Maximum Contaminant Level (MCL) set for manganese, but it is on the EPA's radar.
- Urge the EPA to act on this!

39. MERCURY

In December of 2003, during the Bush Cheney Presidency, the EPA and the FDA declared mercury a **greater danger** than previously believed. Shortly thereafter, however, EPA Administrator at the time, Mike Leavitt, under pressure from lobbyists, *weakened* mercury-related rules and regulations. Mercury officially went from "toxic pollutant" to just a "pollutant" with null regulations. This happened despite the fact that mercury is one of most dangerous neurotoxins facing people and wildlife. In 2011, though the EPA drastically cut mercury emissions from coal-fired power plants, we still have vast amounts of mercury pollution to deal with. Wise nations would start eliminating those sources of pollution.

BIOACCUMULATION
Like other heavy metals, methylmercury bioaccumulates every time it moves up the food chain. Once in our bodies, it settles into our fatty tissue. Because of bioaccumulation, people are advised to rotate fish they eat, as well as restrict frequency of eating freshwater fish.

HEALTH EFFECTS
Kidney damage, liver damage, nervous system damage; causes asthma, muscle cramps and fatigue; impairs health of mothers and fetuses; contributes to brain damage, birth defects, autism, learning disabilities, Alzheimer's and chronic fatigue syndrome; weakens fine motor capabilities; and causes premature death. Learn more from the Children's Environmental Health Network at www.cehn.org.

HOW WE ARE EXPOSED
You can be exposed to mercury through water pollution; air pollution, eating contaminated fish, CFL Light bulbs; through consuming or using products containing mercury, fluorescent lighting, batteries, battery acid, make up, art supplies, pharmaceuticals, metal smelters, cement manufacture, PET Coke, refineries, industrial emissions, landfills, sewage, and dental fillings.[258]

COAL ASH, MINING and POWER PLANTS:
Power plants that utilize coal as their fuel source release greater amounts of mercury than any other industry. In addition, power plants release significant levels of dioxin, CO2, sulfur dioxide, and nitrogen oxide--All climate culprits!

STEEL MILLS pollute our water and our skies with sulfur and mercury, and discharge it into the Great Lakes and other waterways. **TACONITE** Facilities also pollute the air with mercury that eventually settles on land and in water. US Steel is the largest taconite producer. Mining for steel produces vast amounts of toxic wastewater as well.

CHLORINE FACILITIES: Chlorine Factories were developed using a process dating back to 1894. A saltwater solution is pumped through a barrel of mercury to produce chlorine gas and lye. There are nine mercury- chlorine plants in the U.S. & about 51 in the EU—they release two to five *times more mercury* than power plants![259]

Mercury to Methylmercury
Most mercury released to the environment is in the inorganic form, as a result of mining, smelting, and other industrial discharges, or of coal-fired power plants, which in the United States are responsible for 34% of mercury arising from human activities. Bacteria then convert inorganic mercury to organic methylmercury, making it available for uptake into the food chain, where it bioaccumulates and biomagnifies (Lindberg et al. 1987). Food, such as tuna and other types of predatory fish, is considered to be the primary route of exposure for children and adults, while marine mammals remain the main source of exposure for Inuit. This is of particular concern because methylmercury in food is almost totally absorbed into the bloodstream by the gastrointestinal tract.
www.cec.org

SOLUTIONS
- Filter your water.
- Beware of CFL lightbulbs, if they break run out of the room, open a window or get outside, wait 30 minutes to reenter.
- Support companies that utilize clean-energy practices.
- Request mercury-free pharmaceuticals & dental work
- Eat less food contaminated with mercury (for example, limit tuna, swordfish and farm-raised salmon with high levels of mercury).
- See the safe seafood guide at: **Monterey Bay Seafood Watch**
- Contact your representatives, senators, FDA, EPA the President: ask that mercury be reinstated as a hazardous pollutant! Then corporations will have to install equipment to lower emissions.

Fish Consumption Advisory Map

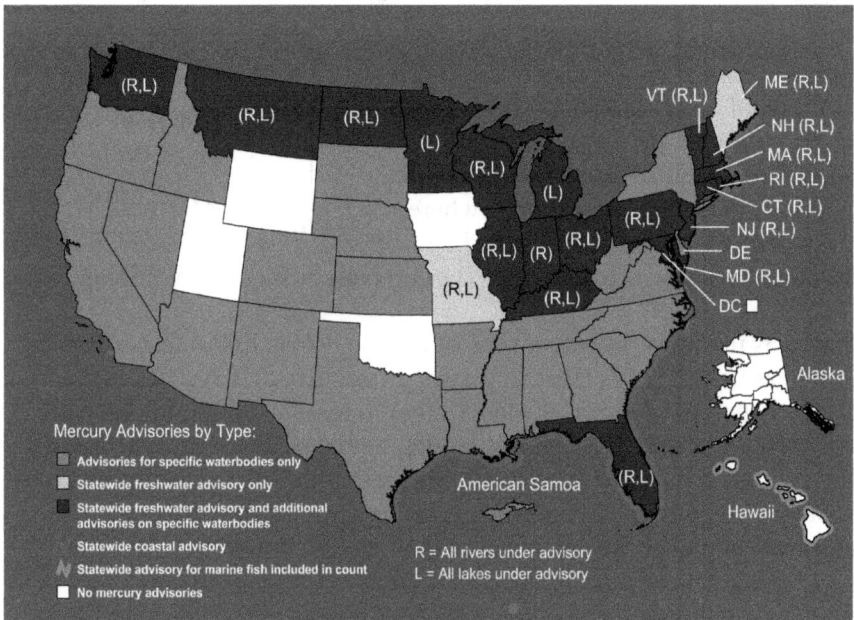

epa.gov/waterscience/presentations/fishslides/2003_files/frame.htm

This map was available back when I started writing this book, but the EPA no longer provides a fish advisories map that I could find. It makes me wonder if that has anything to do with industrial influence from the Energy Sector, Fossil Fuel, Power Plants, etc.

Industrial sites like steel mills emit:
- CO2 (Carbon Dioxide) CO2
- CO (Carbon Monoxide) CO—Deadly!
- Sulfur Dioxide (SO2)- Smog, Acid Rain
- Methane – Ozone Layer Depleter
- Nitrogen -Ozone Layer Depleter
- Hydrogen – used to make ammonia for nitrogen fertilizer
- Mercury – Heavy Metal

Know this: Reducing emissions is not impossible! If the facilities installed *flue gas filters*, for instance, mercury emissions to the air would be significantly minimized. Is that too much to ask of these industries? In case any of you industries need help and guidance as to how to reduce pollution and protect the water and human health, Perhaps this guide will provide some inspiration: How Industries Can Reduce Water Pollution More Effectively. [260]

40. MICRO PLASTICS

Microplastics are ridiculously small pieces of plastic—microscopic pieces no bigger than a small seed is considered microplastic. Plastic will deteriorate but it doesn't biodegrade. With so much use of plastic, microplastic is showing up everywhere. These plastics are neurotoxins and carcinogens. Exposure to them serves no benefit for man or animal.

> "I don't want any plastics!"
> George Bailey,
> *It's a Wonderful Life*

"Plastic is the most prevalent type of marine debris found in our oceans and Great Lakes."[261] Is there any escape from plastic? We've allowed the development of these substances that in reality can remain on earth until the end of time. They don't biodegrade, they don't disappear, they may get smaller and become micro-sized, but they're persistently a problem—relentlessly contaminating every crevice of earth, compromising every living creature that makes contact.

Plastic is a problem for everyone, especially sea creatures where plastic pollution has become so problematic. Once ingested plastic does unmeasurable harm to animals. Because of the minute size of microplastics we unknowingly absorb much more of them than other plastic. Tiny particles are even drifting through the air in dust. The only viable solution humanity has is to reduce production of plastics so we can cease polluting the planet with them. Like dirt stirred up in a pool, once the stirring ceases the dirt settles. When the production ceases and plastic starts to settle, we'll have a lot of work to do.

PLASTICS NOW FOUND IN PEOPLE!

"The world produces about 400 million metric tons of plastic a year, the equivalent of 882 billion pounds, and 80 percent ends up deposited in landfills and other parts of the environment. The smallest particles, the microplastics, range from 10 nanometers — so tiny they are invisible to the human eye — up to 5 millimeters in diameter. Microplastics — including microfibers from clothing — are floating in the air and are found in most of our bottled and tap water, our beer, our sea, rock and lake salt, and our soil."[262] In 2018, researchers discovered microplastics in people's bodies. Up to 9 plastics were found in every person tested, including polypropylene and polyethylene.[263]

STOP USING PLASTIC!
The worst and most notorious plastics littering the planet:
- **Styrofoam (Styrene):** It may be cheap, but styrofoam is not nice. The Chemicals in Styrofoam, styrene, vinyl and benzene, seep into food and beverages-- they're carcinogens, neurotoxins and endocrine disruptors, that harm the liver, stomach, reproduction; they're linked with many health maladies including leukemia and cancers.[264] Don't heat or microwave any foods or beverages in Styrofoam. When a Styrofoam cup is filled with a cold or hot beverage, the chemicals meld into your drink. These are not ordinary chemicals, these are benzene and styrene--potent carcinogenic chemicals that shouldn't be entering your body. Anytime a food or beverage is in contact with polystyrene, contamination can occur-- increasingly so the warmer the food or drink. Styrene does not biodegrade, nor is it recyclable, so anything made from this nasty substance will still be around in 500 or more years.

> Thank you Maine!
> As of May, 2019, Maine became the first State to ban single-use Styrofoam (aka single use polystyrene)! The law takes effect Jan 1, 2021.

- **Straws:** Plastic straws are a menace—made from polypropylene, the plastic can leach into our body, straws harm animals and pollute waterways worldwide. They do not biodegrade.
- **Plastic Bags and Plastic Wrap:** Plastic wrap may be helpful in storing food, but do not heat or cook food with plastic wrap on it, or in plastic containers of any kind.
- **Polycarbonate**
  Don't use polycarbonate containers that contain BPA. They usually have a No. 7, and sometimes a No. 3, on the bottom.
  If you do use polycarbonate containers, don't put them in the microwave. When heated, the plastic may break down over time.[265]

DON'T COOK, MICROWAVE, or HEAT FOOD IN PLASTIC!
Remove food from plastic packaging before microwaving or defrosting. Do not use foam trays and plastic wraps because they are not heat stable and chemicals will melt or migrate into the food.[266]
Collectively we must come up with better solutions for product containers—ones that are plastic-free & free of BPA, endocrine disruptors & other health harmers.

SOLUTIONS: Avoid using plastic. EPA: please ban it all!

41. Nanoparticles NPs
CALLING FOR IMMEDIATE MORATORIUM
EMERGING: NPs Cause Cancer to Grow Rapidly!!

Nanos, or nanoparticles are a new technology of small microscopic particles. They're so plentiful, yet zero safety testing was ever provided by manufacturers nor was even required by the FDA or the EPA.[267] NPs are found in air and water pollution, and NPs are now even intentionally sprayed in the atmosphere.[268] Since 2006 or slightly earlier, they've been added to many common products we buy and eat everyday.

If it weren't for some upsetting research linking nanos with disease, we could forget about all this and let the industry carry on. However, it is time to call a moratorium and halt production! Get the safety testing done. FDA, please wake up! Time to get these biotech sensations out of our food and water supply. A few things scientists have known since 2007 that nanos damage DNA and cause cancer.[269] Recently, they've found NPs not only cause cancer, but also cause cancer to accelerate and grow rapidly! Could this be why cancers lately seem to be growing so much faster! And hitting so many young people out of the blue! We all surely inhaled extra doses of nanos just by wearing masks made with nanoparticle material! See, each additional exposure to a toxin or toxic substance can increase susceptibility to disease.

"Nanoparticles, nanofibers, and other pioneering technologies based on nanomaterials have been introduced in mask production chains to improve performance and confer antiviral properties."[270]

These nanos are not visible to the human eye. They're made of heavy metals: aluminum, sulfur dioxide, iron, and titanium. The whole nanoparticle industry is a bit mysterious. Both production, use, formulations, and the complete inventory of products containing them remains largely undisclosed and unknown. There is zero regulation. Safety testing was not conducted on nanoparticles before they entered the US Marketplace. Today, they're found in thousands of products people use daily.

HEALTH EFFECTS
Titanium dioxide NPs cause[271] chromosomal instability and may lead to lung cancer, disturbance in gastric system, kidney damage, and more! Aluminum oxide nanos could certainly contribute to memory problems and could likely be linked with recent spikes in Alzheimer's[272] and

Dementia! Both zinc oxide and titanium dioxide nanoparticles are bioaccumulative and ridiculously harmful for aquatic species in that they harm coral reefs, reduce reproduction, accumulate in gills, cause behavior changes, bleaches coral, causes mortality in brine shrimp, reduces fecundity of crustaceans, increases uptake of heavy metals, reduces birth rates and impairs growth of zebrafish, reduces immunity of carp, causes respiratory and oxidative stress, damages intestines and gills of rainbow trout. Human health effects include: bioaccumulation, penetration of epidermal cells stimulating release of free radicals, cross blood brain barrier. Nanos may come coated by the manufacturer with aluminum oxide nanos or other materials intended to block undesirable interactions with water and oxygen. Go figure. Sounds perfectly safe to put in countless products, doesn't it? Titanium dioxide nanos when inhaled cause cancer in animals thus take heed and avoid sprays containing titanium dioxide nanos.[273]

REDUCE YOUR EXPOSURE AS MUCH AS POSSIBLE
Nanos are used in Sunscreens, lotions, cleansers, make up, candy, cookies, junk food eating affected fish, food and personal care products, facial cleansers, moisturizers, nail polish, detergents, dish liquid and detergents, cutting boards, gloves, socks, clothing, you name it. These things have no purpose for your health, avoid, avoid, avoid them as much as possible! Especially if you're going in a body of water where they can wash away and harm aquatic animals directly.

SOLUTIONS

- Stay as much away from Nanos as you can. As a precaution, overexposure should be avoided as much as possible.
- Make sure your sunscreen contains no nanoparticles!
- Support Regulation. Under TSCA, Nanoparticles should be restricted or completely Banned. Maybe there are some safe uses in medicine or as pollution control mechanisms[274], but we need to see the safety tests to know for certain. Certainly, there is sufficient cause to put a moratorium on production and use.
- Until safety testing can clear these substances of harmful status, please keep them out of our food, our lotions, our personal products and anything else we use daily.
- Filter your water.
- Companies must be responsible and fully vet and clear the safety of a product before selling it to the public.
- FDA: Put Nanos on pause. Right now, there's no safe Nano.

NANOPARTICLES

SO TINY WE CAN'T SEE THEM

DANGER DANGER!

As reported by the Guardian, "Unlike chemical compounds, nanoparticles cannot be dissolved. Their tiny size gives them, paradoxically, an enormous surface area, which makes them behave differently to "non-nano" versions of the same material. It can make them more mobile, more reactive – and potentially more toxic, depending on shape, size, type, how a substance is released into the environment and its concentration."[275]

"The release of nanos is most likely during manufacture or disposal, but it can also happen when items are washed – which is known to occur with fabrics containing nanosilver. Sewage systems cannot trap them and they end up in the ocean: even advanced wastewater-treatment plants cannot deal with nanoparticles."

ARE THEY SAFE? NO!
Until safety tests prove they don't harm people, let's stop letting manufacturers add them to every big and little product.

WORST EXPOSURE ROUTE: Inhalation is believed to be the most serious exposure route causing memory, brain, lung, sinus problems. Oral and dermal exposures most likely contribute to disease as well.

Companies are eager to sell innovative and fancy products, but they must thoroughly assess their benefits-risks balance at each step of the life-cycle of the products." [276]

EPA and FDA: Please put a moratorium on nanoparticles in consumer products and foods. Please apply the Precautionary Principle to assess whether substances are safe before you allow them in the marketplace. Please require companies to conduct 3rd party safety testing to validate a substance's non-harmfulness before admitting it into the marketplace.

42. Neonicotinoids

Neonicotinoid use is causing honeybee colony collapse as well as loss of wildlife and ecosystem biodiversity. Neonic insecticides are the primary reason for the demise of our essential honey bees! In the United States, neonic use keeps increasing despite being so dangerous it's banned in other countries. Evidence from scientists prove that Neonicotinoids are pushing nearly 1500 endangered species into extinction[277]! This is a violation of the Endangered Species Act as well as a clear threat to both Human and animal health! SOS! Animal and human lives are in danger! This is not a test.

Insect and Animal Armageddon!
The problem is that they kill indiscriminately, exterminating not only "pest" insects but also countless butterflies, bees, and other wildlife. In fact, since their introduction, neonics have made U.S. agriculture nearly 50 times more deadly to insect life![278]

Despite knowing this fact since 2022, the U.S. Government took until June of 2024 to halt approval of any *new* neonicotinoids. That's not enough! What are you doing about the products in use now??? This is what we must urgently stop, across the country, as in everywhere!! They are working on mitigation plans to protect certain species while waiting for the full review and determination, but holy cow this is ridiculous. But at the end of the day, Nobody, not even the government has to take this long to get anything done, there's clearly some resistance in the chain of command. This is a clear indication industry lobbyists stand in the way of our health. All these herbicide companies are getting away with murder, and someone somewhere tied to government is being paid off big time to look the other way.

In the meantime, children, babies, farmworkers and consumers all over America are affected in addition to all the animals. This is wrong. To save species, Clothianidin, Imidacloprid, and Thiamethoxam must be banned without hesitation.[279]

The office of Chemical Safety and Pollution Prevention is in charge and capable of stopping pesticide use. They have the power to call an emergency stop of any substance. An immediate ban. Perhaps it's never happened before, but this product certainly qualifies as a first time for anything candidate! Maybe they're not the ones really in charge. So who is? Let's get to the bottom of all the feet dragging and avoidance of banning substances that cause death and disease to so many living creatures and people we know.

EPA: Carelessly Harming Humans and Animals

Thanks to the NRDC (Natural Resources Defense Council), the EPA was forced step up and initiate long overdue review of Neonicotinoids. "The Endangered Species Act is the country's most important and successful wildlife conservation law. One of the central components of this law is a process called **"interagency consultation,"** which requires all federal agencies to ensure that their actions do not jeopardize the continued existence of threatened and endangered species. Agencies are required to complete this process before they take an action that may affect listed species.

EPA must register all pesticides before they can be sold and used, and this registration triggers the requirement to engage in consultation under the ESA. **But for decades, EPA has approved pesticides while ignoring the consultation requirement, turning a blind eye to the impacts that these chemicals** have on imperiled species.

The Neonicotinoid, Imidacloprid is a good example. EPA first registered pesticide products containing imidacloprid in the mid-1990s—nearly thirty years ago—meaning EPA should have completed the consultation process then. Instead, it continued to register additional imidacloprid products for years, making it one of the most commonly used insecticides in the country.

With no regard for the animals or people these chemicals could be harming, EPA continued to ignore the consultation requirement for imidacloprid products until NRDC sued in 2017 to force the agency to act. In 2020, NRDC and EPA reached a settlement which required EPA to issue a "biological evaluation"—the first step in the consultation process— by July 2022. Without this lawsuit and settlement, it is likely that EPA would have waited significantly longer to begin this process."[280]

SOLUTIONS

- Do not use Imidacloprid or any Neonicotinoid product ever Help ban Neonics, Contact your Reps and Senators. Help reform the EPA so all the toxic pesticides are removed from usage.

43. NITRATE

Each year as springtime rolls around, there's a parade of fertilizer commercials announcing a new growing season. It's a shame so many commercial fertilizer products aren't as safe and as pretty as their packages. These substances are made with hazardous waste and chemicals that harm our health, harm our families, harm animals in the water, and contaminate drinking water. Fertilizer also accelerates warming temperatures by emitting nitrous oxide.

Nitrate is a break down product of fertilizer as well as chloramines. Due to agricultural runoff and water filtration chemicals, the nitrate problem is growing. It's found in drinking water throughout the U.S, both in rural and urban areas.

SOURCES OF NITRATES and NITRITES:
Fertilizers, conventional and factory farms, GMO farms. "Elevated nitrate levels in groundwater are often caused by run-off from barnyards or feedlots, excessive use of fertilizers, or septic systems. Wells most vulnerable to nitrate contamination include shallow wells, dug wells with casing which is not watertight, and wells with damaged, leaking casing or fittings. Nitrate contamination is often regarded as a first sign of deteriorating groundwater quality."[281]

HEALTH EFFECTS: Poisonous; cancerous, stomach cancer, harms thyroid, esophageal cancer, reproductive toxin, bad for babies and pets; causes "blue baby syndrome," deadly if not treated immediately.

HOW WE ARE EXPOSED
Drinking water, beverages or food made from water contaminated with nitrate. Chloramines in water disinfection break down to nitrate.

SOLUTIONS
- Filter your water, for both drinking and cooking.
- Don't use synthetic fertilizers on your lawn or farm
- If you have your own well, be sure to get it tested for nitrate
- Pets need good clean water too
- Remove your shoes when you come indoors

44. Nitrogen Fertilizer

Nitrogen Pollution and Biodiversity Decline

The United Nations Environment Programs advocates for reducing nitrogen fertilizer use. This is why:

"When the availability of nitrogen exceeds plants' consumption, excess nitrogen filters into the environment and aquatic ecosystems. Once there, it can cause a rapid increase of toxic algae, known as algal blooms, which deplete oxygen in water and can create coastal dead zones affecting underwater life.

Nitrogen pollution is the most influential global driver of human-made biodiversity decline after habitat destruction and the emission of greenhouse gases. A landmark global agreement to safeguard biodiversity, finalized in December 2022, includes targets to reduce pollution from all sources so that by 2030, pollutants are not harmful to life and ecosystems.

When nitrogen in its active form, such as in fertilizer, is exposed to soil, microbial reactions take place that release **nitrous oxide**. This gas is 300 times more potent at warming the atmosphere than carbon dioxide. It also remains active in the atmosphere for more than 100 years. Algal blooms in lakes and waterways, often caused by fertilizer run-off, also emit greenhouse gases.

Another issue is agricultural ammonia emissions. This is a gaseous form of nitrogen, which is emitted into the atmosphere from the housing, storage and spreading of animal manure and the spreading of synthetic fertilizer. While ammonia is not a greenhouse gas, when it's released into the air, it acts as a base for emissions of nitrous oxide, a potent greenhouse gas." Source: UNEP[282]

Nitrous Fertilizer: Causes Climate Change

NOW IS THE TIME TO ACT!
BOYCOTT SYNTHETIC FERTILIZER.

Nitrogen Pollution threatens Humanity

Water containing elevated levels of nitrate – a form of nitrogen resulting from animal waste, plant decomposition and fertilizer run-off – raises the risk of cancer in adults,[283] and puts infants at risk of developing methemoglobinemia, commonly referred to as "blue baby syndrome", which can be fatal. High levels of nitrate in drinking water cause stomach and other types of cancer.

DON'T FORGET THE AMMONIA!
Nitrogen fertilizer also releases Ammonia emissions, which further contribute to health problems. "Nitrogen fertilizers are applied to crops to increase yield, but some of that nitrogen is lost to the atmosphere in the form of ammonia. Ammonia is a major air pollutant linked to numerous health issues, including asthma, lung cancer and cardiovascular disease."[284]

Nitrogen Waste Weighs on the Economy
According to UNEP's 2018-2019 Frontiers Report, nitrogen costs the global economy between US$340 billion and US$3.4 trillion annually when taking into account its impact on human health and ecosystems. Most of the UN's Sustainable Development Goals, humanity's blueprint for a better future, are linked with sustainable nitrogen management. Experts say that using the element more efficiently in food production is key to reducing the surplus nitrogen released into the environment.

The industry will tell you the population can't be fed without their fertilizers. But that's not true. Sustainable agriculture is the only way we can grow and support our health and our planet at the same time. Why just feed, when you can nourish?
Report: Nature Conservancy, Provide Food and Water Sustainably[285]

SOLUTIONS
- Filter your water.
- DON'T USE SYNTHETIC FERTILIZER IN YOUR GARDEN or YARD, or ON YOUR FARM PLEASE
- IF YOU'RE A FARMER and you want to switch to organic growing, we'll help you! Free yourselves from the chemical grip of poisons and get toxin free. Your best health awaits!
- The planet thanks you for choosing earth friendly fertilizer.
- Entrepreneurs and engineers are currently working on a way to replace synthetic nitrogen fertilizer with natural bacteria and probiotics. This is brilliant! Let's hope this gets to market sooner than later and synthetic fertilizer can be a thing of the past.

45. Nitrous Oxide

The overlooked factor in warming temperatures.
Where is it coming from? Synthetic nitrogen fertilizer on land
Yep, the same stuff destroying our water is destroying the air.

Synthetic fertilizer:
One of the most used substances on earth
Market Size: $169 Billion

The Problem: Nitrogen in fertilizer mixes with soil microorganisms releasing significant amount of nitrous oxide (and ammonia).

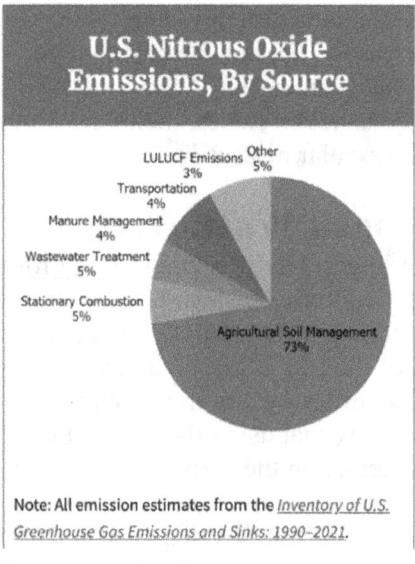

Note: All emission estimates from the *Inventory of U.S. Greenhouse Gas Emissions and Sinks: 1990-2021*.

Graph Source: EPA[286]

Nitrous Oxide Harms the Planet

- One pound is 265 times worse than 1 lb of CO2
- It lasts for 100 years
- Traps heat within the atmosphere
- causing warmer temperatures
- "Five key greenhouse gases are carbon dioxide, nitrous oxide, methane, chlorofluorocarbons, and water vapor.
- While the Sun has played a role in past climate changes, the evidence shows the current warming cannot be explained by the Sun." [287]

Government: The government says they want to end Climate Change, but Government allows and promotes widespread use of synthetic fertilizer and toxic pesticides.

Industry and Government Vs **Human Health and Planet:**
The synthetic fertilizer industry will do everything possible to make sure the world keeps using their products despite the harm.

What can you do? Avoid using their products, protect your family, help the earth, Be your healthiest by eating foods grown more in tune with nature. Support organic and biodynamic farmers. Help ban nitrogen synthetic fertilizers and save the planet. And of course, filter your water.

46. Nutrient Pollution

Nutrient Pollution in water refers to excess phosphorous and nitrogen pollution from agriculture and fertilizer runoff. The runoff goes into streams, rivers, and lakes where it proceeds to cause great damage and imbalance in the aquatic ecosystem.

"Nutrient pollution, caused by excess nitrogen and phosphorus in water or air, is the number-one threat to water quality worldwide and can cause algal blooms, a toxic soup of blue-green algae that can be harmful to people and wildlife. Around the world, agriculture is the leading cause of water degradation."

"In the United States, agricultural pollution is the top source of contamination in rivers and streams, the second-biggest source in wetlands, and the third main source in lakes. It's also a major contributor of contamination to estuaries and groundwater. Every time it rains, fertilizers, pesticides, and animal waste from farms and livestock operations wash nutrients and pathogens—such bacteria and viruses—into our waterways." Source: NRDC[288]

SOLUTIONS

- **Farmers**: switch to natural fertilizers and improve your soil health so your land absorbs carbon dioxide and embraces rain.

- **Gardeners:** Switch to natural fertilizers.

- **Swimmers and boaters and outdoor bathers**: don't use shampoo or soaps outdoors in the lake, ponds, streams or rivers, or the ocean. The suds contribute to toxic nutrient load & cause algae blooms & harm to wildlife.

- **Filter Your Water**

47. OIL DRILLING

Drilling Sites: Establishing and operating drilling sites involves roadways, trucking, and the hauling of heavy equipment, or constructing ocean rigs, all which wreak havoc on native habitats and ecosystems. Whether its drilling or fracking, both energy seeking processes have a negative impact on wilderness and wildlife; and often these disturbances are occurring on our public lands.

Wastewater: Extremely toxic wastewater from oil and gas drilling is disposed, dumped, and otherwise flowing freely without regulation into our waterways. For some ludicrous reason the EPA exempts this wastewater from monitoring. This is probably the most toxic destructive harmful waste that could be added to our water and what we most need to be protected from! Theoretically the wastewater is disposed underground into wells constructed under the aquifer, but how do we know if indeed this is where the water is going or if these wells are seeping or leaking into groundwater? For now we must look beyond why or how this came to be and focus on correcting this immediately.

"The key issue is that wastewater from oil and gas, regardless if it's originating from unconventional shale gas or conventional oil and gas wells, is not regulated by the federal Clean Water Act," Avner Vengosh, professor of geochemistry and water quality at Duke's Nicholas School of the Environment[289]

Let's get this industry regulated. No more Pollution! No more toxins in our water!

48. Oil Refineries

January 26, 2023: Washington, D.C. – "A national study of water pollution from oil refineries reveals that EPA is failing in its legal responsibilities to regulate the half billion gallons of wastewater a day that pours out of U.S. refineries, loaded with nitrogen, industrial salts, cyanide, arsenic, chromium, selenium, and other pollutants."[290] What more can be said. The EPA is failing to uphold the law and hold the petroleum and oil industry accountable. This is a horrible crime against our health, our families, our pursuit of a good life.

81 Refineries in the U.S. release:
- 1.6 billion pounds of chlorides, sulfates, and other dissolved solids (harmful to aquatic life)
- 60,000 pounds of selenium (can cause mutations in fish),
- 15.7 million pounds of nitrogen (as much as from 128 municipal sewage plants) *(Data: Oil's Unchecked Outfalls*[291]

> **Petroleum:** rock oil or oil from the earth. www.eia.gov

Refineries convert petroleum (crude oil) into three categories:[292]
- Fuels: gasoline, jet fuel, kerosene, refinery fuel
- Solvents, nonfuels: greases, wax, petroleum jelly, asphalt, lubricants
- Petrochemicals and Feedstocks for: BTEX, benzene, ethylene

"The federal Clean Water Act requires EPA to set limits for pollutants from industrial sources and update them at least every five years as treatment technologies improve. But EPA has never set any limits for refinery discharges of many pollutants, including selenium, benzene, cyanide, mercury, and many others. And EPA has also failed to update the few limits that were established nearly four decades ago, in 1985."[293]

From drilling to transport, manufacturing to fuel, carcinogens to lack of pollution control, oil contributes one hell of a lot of carcinogenic substances into the air we breathe and the water we drink. This isn't right, just, or necessary. Certainly not acceptable! Pollution control mechanisms exist, didn't they get the memo? Considering the industry receives trillions in subsidies yearly, why are they behaving so badly and why isn't the EPA protecting the health of the American people?

Carcinogens and man-made toxic substances emitted by Refineries include: Benzene, Toulene, Xylene, Ethylene

SPECIAL REPORT
CANCER ALLEY, LOUISIANA

Down in Louisiana, sits a stretch of land that's home to local residents. This area along the banks of the Mississippi River is close to the port and the Gulf. As such, in the 1980s it became the hub for oil refineries. Today this quaint area has been converted into a wasteland by the 200 oil and petrochemical facilities that set up shop. The majority of the residents have no option but to stay, for they can't afford to leave. Yet the water and the air quality make the area unfit for residence. Because of the extent of pollution, residents have "a 95% greater chance of developing cancer than the average American."[294]

Human Rights Watch, January, 2024: "Residents of Cancer Alley suffer the effects of extreme pollution from the fossil fuel and petrochemical industry, facing elevated rates and risks of maternal, reproductive, and newborn health harms, cancer, and respiratory ailments. Parts of Cancer Alley have the highest risk of cancer from industrial air pollution in the U.S. These harms are disproportionately borne by the area's Black residents. The failure of state and federal authorities to properly regulate the industry has dire consequences for residents of Cancer Alley."[295]

Houston, we have a problem! Similar to Cancer Alley, hundreds of refineries line the Houston Ship Canal. According to Houston Public Media, "Six specific refineries dump 55 million gallons of wastewater into local waterways <u>everyday</u>."[296] This problem is nationwide, as the Environmental Integrity Project points out, "81 oil and gas refineries discharge nearly 500 million gallons of polluted wastewater daily!"[297]

SOLUTIONS

We must get control of the toxic pollution! Let's put attention where it's due—on the parties responsible for the Pollution including the Refineries, the Petrochemical facilities, and the government!
To bring back health and to help the planet, we must stop the pollution causing disease and warming. The Union of Concerned Scientists is on to something[298], but let's not hold just the industries accountable for climate change, but also the government agencies who've been complicit in allowing these harmful toxins to go on indefinitely. And while we're at it, let's redefine this so people understand these pollutants harm our health and increase disease, not just sway the climate. EPA, you have a lot of explaining to do!

49. Oil & Gas Pipelines

Water is Life, Mni Wiconi!
It seems our country just can't stop building pipelines. If they don't leak and break apart so often it might not be such a problem. But as they do leak and leak a lot, we're all in danger from contaminated water and harm that goes with it. Pipelines can either carry oil or natural gas.

Between pipelines, drilling sites, leaks, accidents, and sabotage, our environment is quite vulnerable. Liquified natural gas (NLG) is transported via pipeline over the Appalchians, tarsands oil is not just moving across the plains, Enbridge Line 5 pipeline[299] threatens Mackinac Island and the entire Great Lakes watershed. Much of the infrastructure and pipes themselves are aging and teetering towards corrosion. If and when leaks and spills come, the fallout is tragic—habitats damaged, sometimes beyond recoverability.

Saving the Great Lakes from Tar Sands Oil

At this time there is an aging pipeline running along the bottom of Lake Michigan as well as traversing illegallly on the native Reservation of the Bad River Band of Lake Superior Chippewa. Line 5 is nearly 60 years old, and it transports 23 million gallons of oil daily! It's time for citizens of the Lake Michigan and Great Lakes watershed (Illinois, Michigan, Wisconsin, Minnesota, Ohio, Indiana, Pennsylvania, New York, Canada) to start our own Standing Rock protest. We must shut this pipeline down. Everyday it remains in operation, our health and our water is at risk. A lawsuit brought forth from the Chippewa resulted in U.S. district courts order to shut down Line 5 by 2026. However, Enbridge in February of 2024 appealed that decision in the circuit courts of Chicago, and President Biden asked the courts for a reconsideration as well! [300]We Must work together to shut down and reroute this monster immediately.

Recent pipeline leaks include:

Date	Pipeline and Location	Gallons
12/7/2022	Keystone Pipeline[301], Kansas	600,000
11/16/2017	Keystone Pipeline	200,000
01/2015	ExxonMobil Yellowstone River	50,000
07/2011	ExxonMobil Yellowstone River	60,000
07/2010	Tarsands Oil Ln.78 Kalamazoo River[302]	1,000,000+

TARSANDS OIL, LINE 5

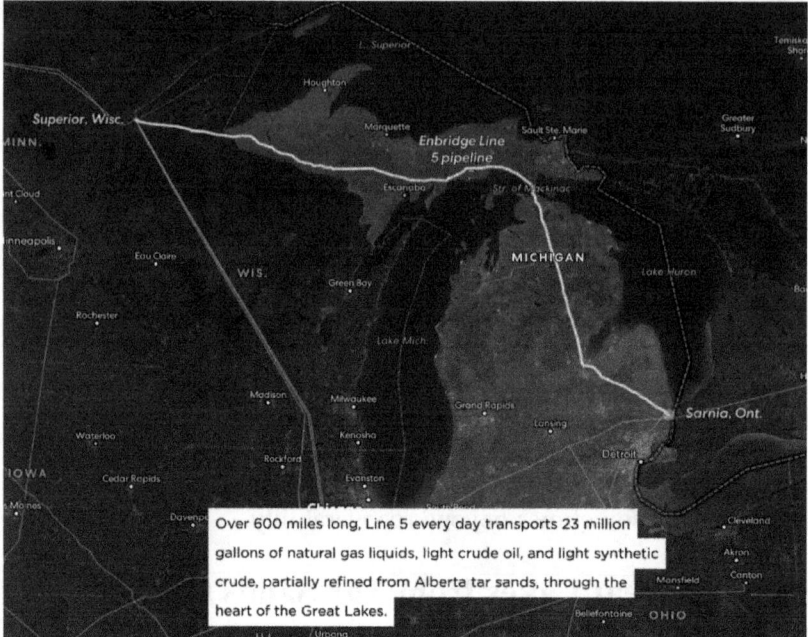

Over 600 miles long, Line 5 every day transports 23 million gallons of natural gas liquids, light crude oil, and light synthetic crude, partially refined from Alberta tar sands, through the heart of the Great Lakes.

Photo map Source: "A Battle for the Future of the Great Lakes"[303]

STANDING ROCK #NoDAPL

Now is the time for sound decision making and conservation. We can no longer jeopardize our fragile natural areas, waterways, rivers, or ground water. Until an accident proof vessel for transporting oil and gas is developed, pipelines shouldn't be built, especially not in or near fragile ecosystems and water sources. Fresh water is scarce on this earth, we must all act together to protect it! The fight over the Dakota Access Pipeline (DAPL) isn't over yet, the US Army Corps of Engineers will complete their study by the end of 2024. Continue to support the Sioux! We must continue urging Enbridge to avoid the Missouri River.[304]

SOLUTIONS

- Protect and defend our water. Pipeline safety is essential. Too many pipelines are threatening our water supplies and sensitive ecosystems. Help defend the Great Lakes before it's too late,
- Go to www.oilandwaterdontmix.org and sign the petition to stop tarsands oil flowing under Lake Michigan!

Let's all call the President, and ask him to stop Line 5 by revoking the presidential permit that allows it to operate![305]

DAKOTA ACCESS PIPELINE #NoDAPL

The fight over the DAPL Tarsands oil pipeline is not over! According to the NRDC, the pipeline is still tangled up in court, and the U.S Army Corps of Engineers is still preparing their environmental impact statement! The Corps regulates construction and infrastructure related to certain U.S. waters.[303]

Help Support the Sioux and residents along the Missouri River watershed protect their water. A simple negotiation could solve this dilemma. If the pipeline must be built, then let's ask the pipeline owner, Energy Transfer Partners, to find an alternate path for the pipeline—one that doesn't infringe on the Reservation or get too near the Missouri River where it threatens the drinking water. Then perhaps all parties can let this be built in peace.

Better still would be a wickedly new version of a pipeline that doesn't pose any risk whatsoever of breaking, leaking or spilling a single drop of oil. Now that would be worth celebrating!

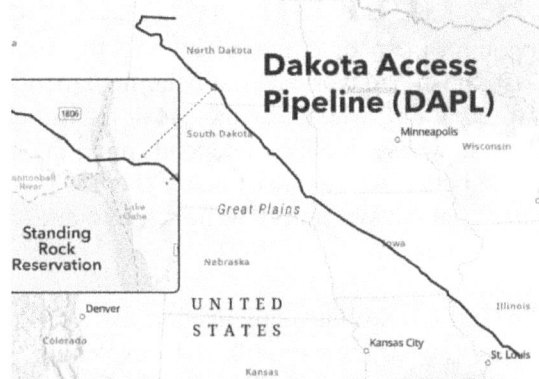

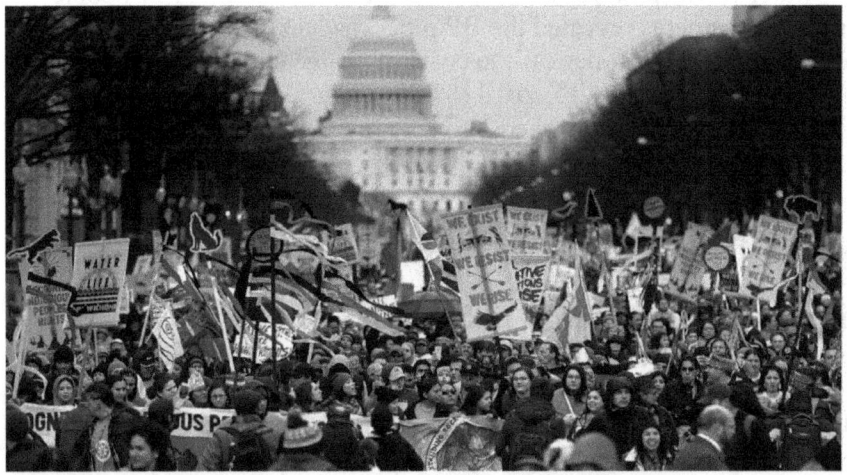

Protestors against the Dakota Access Pipeline in Washington, D.C., on March 10, 2017. NRDC, Photo *Credit: Justin Sullivan/Getty Images*[306]

50. Oil Spills

Despite repeated oil spills, accidents and tragic marine disasters, we still allow drilling anywhere permits are approved. Even worse, tankers and cargo ships, rail cars and pipelines continue transporting oil near and far. What can we do to prevent future accidents?
- BETTER TECHNOLOGY and DESIGN
- BETTER LEADERSHIP
- EARTH AND HEALTH BEFORE PROFITS

What toxins do oil spills add to the Water?
Benzene, toluene, ethylbenzene, xylene and more carcinogens[307]

THE GULF OIL SPILL, DEEPWATER
Tragic for the people, the marine life, the birds, the towns along the coast, the oil rig workers, the fishermen, people who enjoy eating seafood, for all who enjoy the ocean for its beauty and serenity and for all those whose livelihood depends upon the health of the ocean. We can do better, we can insist that if there is going to be drilling in ocean water, that the system has to be a sound one, one that will not ever result in this again.

The Gulf Oil Spill is recognized as the worst oil spill in U.S. history. Within days of the April 20, 2010 explosion and sinking of the Deepwater Horizon oil rig in the Gulf of Mexico that killed 11 people, underwater cameras revealed the BP pipe was leaking oil and gas on the ocean floor about 42 miles off the coast of Louisiana. By the time the well was capped on July 15, 2010 (87 days later), an estimated 4.9 million barrels of oil had leaked into the Gulf.[308]

What makes oil spills even worse is the chemicals used to clean up oil spills.

Dispersants: Making Oil Spills Worse!
Dispersants are a chemical soap designed, allegedly, to help clean up oil after a spill in a water body. Though they're used often now, they actually make the entire oil spill recovery nearly impossible☹ Like pesticides and personal care products, the dispersants have surfactants, which effectively carry the oil beyond the skin barrier. These cleaning dispersants in water carry the oil beyond the surface and comingle

within the water column and food chain. This makes it pretty (near) impossible for animals to avoid. Down the road, the chemicals in the dispersant formulas amplify health issues for people and marine life that have made contact with the water, the vapors, or sediment. Rather than making it easier to recapture the oil, dispersants break up the oil so finely that it becomes synonymous with the water, and it sinks to the bottom where
it degrades and releases toxins further. While the oil may look like it's gone, it hasn't actually disappeared—and the water will be compromised. Then, as the oil degrades further, the polyaromatic hydrocarbons (PAHs) from the oil bind with the dispersant particles, making them far more absorbable by people and animals alike.

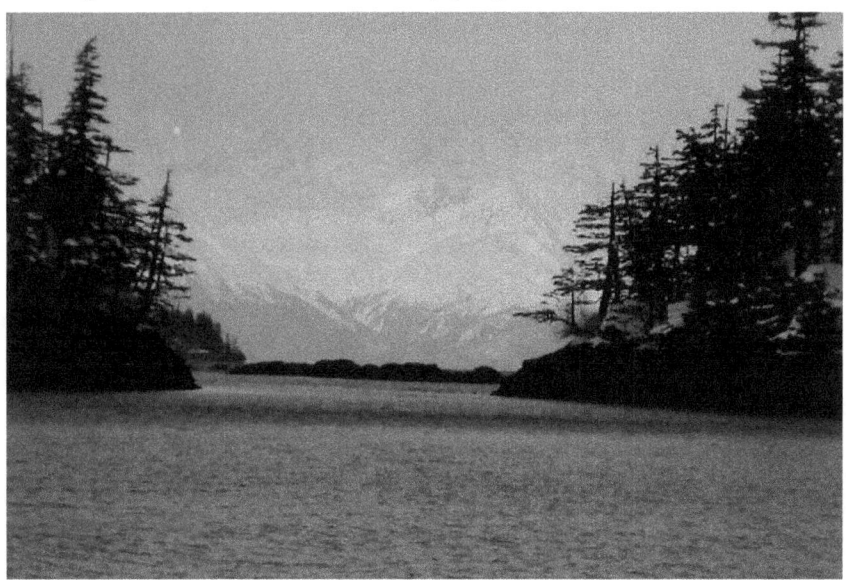

Prince William Sound, Photo Joanna Kappele

Remembering the Exxon Valdez Oil Spill

It was the early morning of March 24, 1989, and all the creatures in Prince William Sound were busy doing what creatures usually do. That was until the Exxon tanker ran aground and began gushing crude oil into what had been pristine waters. Quickly and without hesitation, nearly 30 million gallons of oil spread. Lacking oil-spill clean up knowledge, Exxon fumbled right out of the gate. Two days of calm weather provided clean-up workers with an ideal environment for recovery, yet the supplies were slow in coming. Booms weren't in place, and instead of full out effort, Exxon vied for chemical dispersants to make it look like far less of a disaster.

Of course, the marine mammals suffered immediate harm. Thousands of creatures—seals, birds, sea otters, porpoises, killer whales, sea lions, salmon, herring, ducks—lost their lives in the first couple of days. Stormy weather erupted on the third day and the whole project was up for grabs. Exxon supplied its own chemical stew to disburse the oil, products like Inipol (which has since been banned) and Simple Green. Rather than try to capture any more of the oil at sea, Exxon targeted the oily beaches. It was determined that hot, high-pressure washing would be necessary. In addition, the company added fertilizer in a process known as 'bioremediation.' This they thought would encourage healthy bacteria recovery on the shore. The fertilizer resulted in even worse deterioration of the ecosystem and further loss of critical habitat.

Through all of this, workers were not supplied with the protective clothing—necessary when working so closely with crude oil and the accompanying toxic chemicals. Exxon kept insisting that the chemicals being used were in small enough amounts so as not to present a health hazard. Yet, the workers would tell you another story. Many of them now have irreversible health problems. Their suffering reflects the true nature and harm of chemicals derived from petroleum, i.e. solvents, detergents, pesticides, etc.

DR. RIKKI OTT, OIL SPILL SPECIALIST
Perhaps better than anyone, Dr. Rikki Ott (Alaskan resident and Marine Toxicologist) explains the tragedy of oil spills and the mistake in using dispersants. She was there in Prince William Sound the day of the Exxon spill in 1989. She saw the same dispersant scenario occurring again in the Deep Water Gulf spill in 2010.

"The National Contingency Plan requires that as a priority, human health is protected... Second, is that the situation is stabilized, we don't do any more harm. And three, we are going to physically contain and remove the oil. That is a clean-up. Well, dispersants strike out on all three of those points," she expanded. "We know now that dispersants make it more toxic for people, they act like an oil delivery system. Strike out on stabilizing the situation, because oil plus dispersants make it worse for the ecosystem and people. Strike out on contain and remove the oil because once you add the dispersants, you push it into the water column – you emulsify it. It makes it impossible to remove the oil. So we have a law that conflicts with itself." Ott adds that the plan has not kept up with the times, noting no specific plans for tar sands or fracking chemical spills.[309] Her book is *Sound Truth and Corporate Myths*.

51. Packaging Waste

Food Waste, plastic waste, garbage, e-waste, and rubbish are huge problems mucking up water health everywhere. Individually and together, we can reduce our use of things that produce waste, especially plastic food packaging waste. Perhaps plastic of all kinds for food packaging must be banned. Until then, we can help by using less disposable plastic, avoiding plastic straws and utensils, water in plastic bottles.

Let's reduce use and eliminate waste. We can encourage companies to use biodegradable natural materials so we feel better buying their products. Through all of us working together, consumers, industry and government, we can help the planet in this way. If plastic could biodegrade it'd be different but it's here forever. The oceans of the world have no more tolerance for plastic.

Garbage and Recycling—Where does it Go?
It's debatable how and why so much plastic gets in the ocean. Is it because there's not enough garbage cans, or incentive to recycle? Or are the lids too flimsy and garbage blows away or falls out? Or is it that people are too careless and just throw their garbage any ol' place? (that is littering by the way). Or is it that we just don't have enough recycling centers? Or is it that garbage is taken out to the ocean and dumped carelessly? Or is it blowing off shipping vessels? Whatever the reason, humanity—that means All of Us—must be more conscientious and make less waste, and that which we make we must dispose of properly and recycle when we can. If we can all agree on that we can save the oceans and our planet.

Food Packaging Toxins— 3600 Chemicals!
Food packaging contains PFAS, neurotoxins, and carcinogens! More than 3600 toxic chemicals can leach into food from packaging![310] Where's the FDA? Single serve disposable plastic food packaging, utensils and straws makes up a giant mess worldwide. We must shift away from using such one trick plastic ponies. Plastic lasts forever, and we, nor the animals have forever to wait! Please do your part and avoid using plastic as much as you can. Avoid containers made of black plastic, as they're full of heavy metals from e-waste.[311] Use a paper or cloth bag, or piece of foil to wrap that filet instead of a styrofoam

container. Leftovers are a form of reusing, re-lifing, repurposing, and unused food is welcomed by those in need.

Food Waste: Food waste is a tremendous problem that each of us can shift. Some organizations like Food pantries can accept grocery and unprepared food.

Recycle, Reduce, Reuse—the 3 Rs: Recycling and reusing materials is a great way to keep garbage out of landfills and to conserve resources.

E-Waste: E-waste refers to electronic waste—computers, cell phones, calculators, radios, etc. Recycling has good intentions, but e-waste recycling could be causing more harm than good for the environment. E-waste is electronic, mechanical and technological waste. While containing minutiae-sized bits of metals and microchips that are of value, the main haul of these discarded devices go to a designated landfill awaiting reclamation that never comes. Sitting in perpetuity as they do, leakages and emissions of dioxins, toxins, heavy metals and hazardous substances become imminent. There has to be an entrepreneur out there who can figure out a solution to this one!

Hazardous Waste
- **Landfills**: release methane; ground seepage, climate crisis
- **Hazardous waste** contains toxins and heavy metals that contaminate groundwater and soil
- **Incinerating Garbage**: causes toxic air pollution, particulates; brings heightened levels of CO2, dioxin, VOCs, heavy metals, carcinogens and mercury in the air—all of which can cause diseases! This includes Biomass Power Plants.
- **E-Waste**: heavy metals, carcinogens, hazardous waste, flame-retardants and dioxins that seep into soil and groundwater.

SOLUTIONS
1. Use less, recycle more, save earth's resources
2. Buy goods in earth-friendly, health-friendly packaging.
3. Steer away from plastic, Styrofoam and unnatural materials
4. Compost food scraps and coffee grounds,
5. Help reduce garbage and pollution in your community.
6. Invent ways to convert waste into something useful☺
7. Avoid buying Tetra Packs, they're not recyclable.
8. Recycle your K cups or better yet, buy those that are reusable and save resources!

52. Paraquat & 2,4-D

This book would not be complete without including these popular herbicides found for growing grass and controlling weeds, and sprayed on a lot of crops! Paraquat, 2,4-D and Linurin are a mix of neurotoxins and carcinogens. Chances are something you eat today will bear with it the residue of one or all of them. Why in the world are such dangerous poisons used on food? There are plenty of farmers who prove we can grow abundantly without toxic chemicals. It's all in the methods and begins with the approach to soil.[312]

"About 1 billion pounds of conventional pesticides are used each year in the United States to control weeds, insects, and other pests."[313]

The main effects from overexposure include very serious harm to the brain and body. Exposure comes from drifting pesticides we breathe,[314] and in drinking water. The main culprits in this tale of neurotoxins includes 2,4-D, implicated in Lymphoma and Liver and Kidney Damage.[315] Paraquat, increase one's risk of developing Parkinson's.[316] Linuron,[317] which is banned in the EU is linked to MS[318], epilepsy, and Parkinson's! Paraquat, trade name Gramoxone, is used commercially to control weeds and grasses.[319]

EXPOSURE: Food and Water
Residues on food, in water, in the air, People and pets can be exposed to
- 2,4-D when walking on treated grass.[320] It's popular in weed and feed lawn products. 2,4-D is used on corn, soybean, sugarcane, wheat[321]
- Paraquat is used on lawns by commercial landscapers as well as on almonds, corn, grapes, soy, artichokes, pears, garlic, potatoes, wheat, strawberries and cotton.[322]
- Linurin is also used on grasses as well as these crops: soybean, cotton, potato, corn bean pea, winter wheat, asparagus, carrot and fruit crops[323]. Please rinse off your foods, better yet go organic and avoid these toxins (as long as they haven't drifted)! These manufacturers and the EPA have us in shackles. Enough! Reduce your exposure Stat! Cleanse these toxins out of your system with natural remedies.

53. Perchlorate

ROCKET FUEL: Perchlorate is the chemical name for rocket fuel. Vast amounts of this toxin leaked into the Colorado River from botched disposal at Lockheed Martin. Now it's severely spreading to water supplies across the country. Millions of people in at least 35 States drink water contaminated with it: Arizona, Nevada and Southern California water systems are all affected.

The Colorado River was hit hard. The river is the source from which hundreds of farmers derive water to irrigate crops. The impact on food irrigated with perchlorate have been found to contain **65 times** the amount of perchlorate originally found in the water itself![324] This is the sinister reality of bioaccumulation.

In 1997 authorities discovered groundwater contamination[325] was leaking into Lake Mead and ultimately the Colorado River. Manufacturing facilities in Nevada and Oklahoma City had been developing Perchlorate since the 1950s. Inadequate storage facilities at Lockheed Martin rocket and missile sites are also largely to blame. Because contamination occurred while working on behalf of the government, both the Henderson facility and Lockheed Martin avoided responsibility and removal costs.

HOW WE ARE EXPOSED
Contaminated water or eating food irrigated with perchlorate-tainted water, foods & bevs made with contaminated ingredients. Perchlorate is excreted by the body once exposure ceases.

HEALTH EFFECTS
Perchlorate is a thyroid toxin and hormone disruptor. It interferes with iodine absorption; causes hypothyroidism and scleroderma; impairs brain development; interferes with motor skill development; contributes to learning disabilities.

SOLUTIONS
- Filter your water. Reverse osmosis is best for perchlorate
- Avoid drinking contaminated water.
- Protect your health and thyroid with iodine rich foods like seaweed, switch from cooking with common table salt to a denser cleaner sea salt or Himalayan Salt.

54. PERC and TCE

Dry Cleaning Neurotoxins & Camp Lejeune

PERC, perchloroethylene is also referred to as Tetrachloroethylene is a colorless, nonflammable liquid used in dry cleaning. PERC is a toxic problem in that there are numerous sites where PERC has contaminated drinking water and caused cancer clusters.[326] Perc is one of the primary neurotoxins that's contaminated water at Marine Corps Base Camp Lejeune in North Carolina. **TCE, Trichloroethylene**[327] is the other culprit causing health problems for those at Camp Lejeune. It's used as a spot remover by dry cleaners, in solvents, degreasers and refrigerants.

HOW WE ARE EXPOSED
Contaminated drinking water, dry cleaned garments, correction fluid and shoe polish also contain PERC, contaminated air, contaminated food. "If your water source is contaminated with PERC, activities such as showering, doing dishes or running a dishwasher or laundry can cause PERC in the water to evaporate and contaminate your indoor air."[328]

The EPA, to their credit just in June of 2023 proposed a ban on all uses of PERC. This is exciting! However, it hasn't magically disappeared from the water its merged with. When the ban is implemented, it will surely help. While many cleaners have gone green or to other solvents, about 60% of drycleaners still use PERC and possibly Tri!

HEALTH EFFECTS
Chronic contact has been linked with neurological effects[329] including Multiple sclerosis, Parkinson's disease, ALS, Lou Gehrig's Disease, Depression, Fatigue, Behavior disorders, Concentration problems, kidney cancer, lung cancer, intestinal cancer, brain cancer, breast cancer, bladder cancer, neurological issues and birth defects, liver and kidney damage."[330] Cancer clusters and Parkinson's linked with perc[331]

SOLUTIONS

- Filter your water. "If your private well water is contaminated use an alternative source of water or a whole-house carbon filter and keep up with the filter maintenance." "[332]
- Use alternative methods to clean your clothes, wet cleaning.
- Ventilate: Take your clothes out of the dry cleaning bag and air them out in a well-ventilated area before hanging in closet.

55. PESTICIDES

Pesticides are a group of very harmful substances that include herbicides, weed killers, insecticides, and all the toxic agricultural products used to kill insects and plant life. They are bastards. They and their breakdown products end up in our drinking water. No one is safe, we are shackled whether we're in the city or the country, no place is safe unless it's a pesticide free zone--something we certainly need more of.

The companies manufacturing these killing substances are some of the most polluting and least concerned about our health.
2023: "**Pesticide manufacturing:** The EPA estimates that 31 pesticide chemical plants discharge pollution into U.S. waterways, including insect-killing ingredients, as well as nitrogen, benzene, cyanide and more. The EPA has not updated the guidelines for pesticide manufacturing since 1998!"[333] How strange that an agency dedicated to human health and the environment would let any company get away with such incredible harmful pollution. In what world are industry and corporate profits valued more than human health?

Manufacturing pollution combined with the excessive usage of pesticides in every town and parcel of land results in poison overload in our streams, rivers, and in our drinking water. Since these chemicals also reach the air and our food, we can—without realizing it—endure exposure from multiple routes. This takes a great toll on human and animal health.

One pesticide alone is trouble enough, but in water there are dozens, if not hundreds of toxic pesticides and other substances mingling together and traveling to the seas. They're also traveling right into our kitchens and into our bodies. Most filtration systems are incapable of fully filtering all these menacing toxins out. No one yet knows for certain what long term effects may be imposed from this array of chemical exposure. It's a bit like Russian Roulette.

Pesticides cover a wide range of products used for gardening, weeding, soil prep, farming, landscaping, fumigation, insect and pest control, even dog and cat flea collars contain them. They cause harm to all species who find themselves exposed. While the residues making contact with us personally may not be noticeable at the time, the damage to our bodies and our dear planet soon enough may be realized.

Pesticides, like other chemicals eventually breakdown to other substances. Once in the water, the pesticides degrade into transformation byproducts. It used to be thought that once a pesticide biodegrades the harm had vanished. Now scientists realize that after the pesticides deteriorate, the byproduct's endocrine-disrupting capacity can be significantly more dangerous than the parent pesticide.[334]

HISTORY OF PESTICIDES : CHEMICALS OF WAR

The dark reality about chemical pesticides and synthetic fertilizer is that their development sprung from the deadly poisons originally used in the World Wars. Fertilizer is made with former bomb-making materials. During WWII, BASF and Bayer were banded together as one deadly entity known as IG Farben, known then as the 'devil's chemist.'[335] The conglomeration taken to the Trials of Nuremberg for atrocities beyond comprehension. Fritz ter Mer, Bayer's Chairman, was found guilty of crimes against humanity and imprisoned for 12 years. Bayer, not only provided the Zyclon B Gas used to gas prisoners to death, they also performed gruesome experiments and unnecessary surgeries on unwilling victims.

These war chemicals—today's pesticides—were and still are designed to target the nervous system and brain[336]. They affect the endocrine system and thyroid, they can cause changes in our demeanor, and our sleep. They're implicated in Alzheimer's, ALS, Dementia, Epilepsy and Seizures, Multiple Sclerosis, Parkinson's, and all types of Neurological and Nervous System disturbances. They can trigger neural misfiring and mitochondria issues, affect digestion, weight, wound healing, memory. Pesticides are not good for us as you can see. They should not be in our water, in our air, or in our food. They should not be able to get into our body—that my friends is poisoning.

These anti-health corporations fathered the toxic pesticide industry and to this day, not only produce the most toxic and most sold herbicides, but also patent the seeds. They have quite the devilish grip on the global food supply and now under their umbrella, have come biotech and nanoparticles. I'm a little weary thinking of what harm may come from these newer substances ushered in by corporations who master poisons.

Today, we don't just have pesticides and herbicides to avoid, we have many wildly untested and questionable formulations of hormone-abducting and dangerous substances contaminating our water supply, food supply, and air supply. Our earth, our soil is harmed in such abundance by these products, it's a wonder anything can grow at all. The silent abduction is occuring every moment upon every person who walks the earth--the bees, the birds, the animals across the world are all victims in more ways than we can count.

How these products ever got approved for commercial use is a subject for an entire dissertation. The United States was not created for this level of deception and treachery. Who knew that one day our dinner table would be the gateway for such a breach of trust. The earth has been seiged by these dangerous entities imposing their injurious harmful goods all over us. This is not a simple time, health is indeed affected in countless ways from the intersections where random new particles and poisons collide. If only we could see all the toxins we face daily, then we'd understand all that confronts and hinders our health on both the physical and mental level. When one looks at the disease trends[337] rising since the 1990's, in tandem with GMO expansion and its pesticide usage, we must conclude that GMO farming is not improving global health, especially not for those who've been raised on them[338].

Herbicides and insecticides are nonselective, deadly substances that kill not just their target, but nontargeted species as well. If a flower is sprayed with an herbicide and a bee pollinates it, the bee will be poisoned. Pesticides drift in the wind, get carried away with runoff, and quietly make their way into our drinking water and our bodies.
All along these chemicals have done no favors for the planet, for ecosystems, for children, for peoples' health. They're making cancer more common, they're killing off pollinators—bees, bats, birds, butterflies-- animals of all kinds are disappearing from earth. Every person, every animal from the miniscule to the Keystone species is in danger.

Childhood Cancer: "Children are exposed to potentially carcinogenic pesticides from use in homes, schools, other buildings, lawns and gardens, through food and contaminated drinking water, from agricultural application drift, overspray, or off-gassing, and from carry-home exposure of parents occupationally exposed to pesticides. Malignancies linked to pesticides in case reports or case-control studies include leukemia, neuroblastoma, Wilms' tumor, soft-tissue sarcoma, Ewing's sarcoma, non-Hodgkin's lymphoma, and cancers of the brain, colorectum, and testes."[339]

TRANSFORMATION BYPRODUCTS

The transformation products resulting from pesticide degradation can surprisingly be more toxic than the original pesticide. Scientists are only beginning to discover how long these byproducts remain in the water and the environment and what further damage they may be causing. For instance, the insecticide Fipronil (commonly used in flea collars) and its transformation products have been identified in human blood and urine of 100% of people tested in China.[340]

In general, pesticides can be categorized as follows :

TYPE OF PESTICIDE	TARGETED ORGANISMS
Herbicides, Weedkillers	Herbs, Plants, Weeds, Invasive Species
Pesticides	Pests, Insects, Bugs
Insecticides Neonicotinoids Organophosphates,	Insects, Mosquito Spray, Fleas, OCPs, Organochlorine Insecticides
Fungicide	Fungus rot, Microbes
Fumigants	Soil organisms, Nematodes, indoor pests
Miticides, Acaracides	Mites, Ticks
Rodenticides	Rodents

Pesticides aren't just used to grow food, they can be found in many outdoor and indoor environments as they're marketed as products that make lawns beautiful, kill insects, get rid of weeds, grows your grass faster. When the exterminator comes, he brings neurotoxins capable of seriously harming you. When you need a hand with bugs or weeds, reach for a nontoxic solution to woo insects away and resolve the issue. Children are especially vulnerable to pesticides. "Pesticide use in homes may increase the risk of children developing leukemia or lymphoma."[341]

Common Pesticides Polluting our Drinking Water include:
1. **2,4-D:** Dow's 2,4-D works by attacking plants' roots and leaves by making the plant's cells grow out of control, like cancer. It's found in many Weed and Feed fertilizer combinations. It's used extensively on corn, soy, wheat, and sugarcane. Health effects include thyroid complication, hormone disruptions, Sarcoma, non-Hodgkin's Lymphoma, it damages human cells and causes cancer in laboratory animals. 2,4-D was created by Dow Chemical in the 1940s, until the 1990s it included dioxin.[342]
2. **Atrazine:** Widespread contamination, 60-80 million pounds used in United States yearly. Banned in the EU since 2004. Atrazine is an endocrine disruptor and reproductive toxin. Health effects include gender alteration, hormonal changes, reproductive disorders, Atrazine is made by ChemChina (formerly Syngenta).[343]
3. **Chlorpyrifos:** Neurotoxin, Organophosphate insecticide, miticide. Used to fight mosquitoes, termites, roundworms. On Feb 28, 2022 the EPA removed all allowable tolerances for Chlorpyrifos in food. That means it can no longer be used on food crops or to grow food. Chlorpyrifos patent, Dow1966.
4. **Enlist Duo:** Glyphosate mixed with 2,4-D. Used to control weeds; especially GMO corn, soybean, and cotton. In January, 2022 the EPA extended use of Enlist Duo. Made by Corteva Agriscience.
5. **Glyphosate:** Produced by Monsanto, now Bayer; glyphosate is the primary herbicide used to grow GMO crops, roughly 300 million pounds are used annually in the U.S. Since its development in 1974, over 18.9 billion pounds have been dispersed worldwide.
6. **Neonicotinoids:** Used e in U.S. Neonics kills bees and pollinators, threaten endangered animals. Used in flea collars☹ Bayer
7. **Paraquat:** Used extensively in U.S. Health Effects: Neurotoxin, Parkinson's. Made by Chem China. Banned in China and Germany where it was originally and currently manufactured.
8. **Surfactants:** Secret dangerous additives used in many pesticide and cleaning formulations. Surfactants increase ingredients ability to penetrate plant cells and human tissue. Mostly made by BASF.

LAWSUIT AGAINST THE EPA

"No one should get a free pass to pollute."
ENOUGH IS ENOUGH EPA, NO MORE TOXIC WASTE!
The EPA is being sued[344] by many environmental groups for failing to regulate wastewater from the most toxic industries ! How in the world did these clowns ever get a waiver ? Time for a big change!
The industries involved include the:

- Pesticide industry
- Plastics industry
- Fertilizer manufacturing
- Chemical manufacturing

Press Release, Center for Biological Diversity April 11, 2023:
"WASHINGTON— Environmental groups sued the Environmental Protection Agency today for failing to set limits on harmful chemicals like cyanide, benzene, mercury and chlorides in wastewater emitted by oil refineries and plants that produce chemicals, fertilizer, plastics, pesticides and nonferrous metals.

"The Clean Water Act requires the EPA to limit discharges of industrial pollutants based on the best available wastewater treatment methods, and to tighten those limits at least once every five years where data show treatment technologies have improved. But the agency has never set limits for many pollutants and has failed to update the few decades-old limits that exist — including limits set almost 40 years ago for oil refineries (1985), plastics manufacturers (1984) and fertilizer (1986).

"Outdated pollution-control technology standards meant that, for example, 81 oil refineries across the United States dumped 15.7 million pounds of nitrogen and 1.6 billion pounds of chlorides, sulfates and other dissolved solids (which can be harmful to aquatic life) into waterways in 2021.

"Twenty-one nitrogen fertilizer plants discharged 7.7 million pounds of total nitrogen, which causes algae blooms and fish-killing "dead-zones," and proposed new plants will add millions of additional pounds to that load. The EPA estimates that 229 inorganic chemical plants dumped over 2 billion pounds of pollution into waterways in 2019.

"No one should get a free pass to pollute. It's completely unacceptable that EPA has, for decades, ignored the law and failed to require modern wastewater pollution controls for oil refineries and petrochemical and plastics plants," said Jen Duggan, deputy director of the Environmental Integrity Project, which coordinated the action by the 13 environmental groups. "We expect EPA to do its job and protect America's waterways and public health as required by the Clean Water Act.

"For decades the EPA has let these dirty industries pollute our rivers and bays instead of making them keep pace with advances in technologies that tackle water pollution, as the Clean Water Act demands," said Hannah Connor, environmental health deputy director at the Center for Biological Diversity. "Forcing people and wildlife like endangered Atlantic sturgeon to bear the weight of toxic water pollution while industries rake in record profits isn't just morally wrong, it's also legally indefensible. The EPA needs to bring pollution standards into the 21st century.

"Despite the legal mandate for regular reviews and updates to keep pace with technology, the guidelines for 40 of 59 industries regulated by the EPA were last updated 30 or more years ago, with 17 of those dating back to the 1970s. Outdated standards mean more water pollution is pouring into U.S. waters than should be allowed because some plants are using technology standards from the Reagan era — before common use of the Internet, email or cell phones."[345]

WHAT CAN WE DO TO GET THE EPA ON POINT:
- Figure out how to get things done faster, expedite!
- Where are the weak links in the EPA? Replace them with people who care about human health and nature
Failing to regulate who's at fault? Leadership? EPA ? Lobbyists? Corporations? Pollution Waivers?
- Follow the Money and the EPA Waivers. End waivers
- Remove lobbyist influence and involvement in the EPA
- Fire Gov. employees paid by polluters, no conflicts of interest allowed. Time to get to work!

SOLUTIONS
- Protect yourself and your family by filtering your water
- Wash produce and vegetables, organic food reduces exposure
- Avoid antibacterial soaps, disinfectants, Quats, hand sanitizer

56. PFAS Forever Chemicals

A man-made compound that didn't exist a century ago, C8 (Teflon) is in the blood of 99.7 percent of Americans, according to the CDC, as well as in newborn human babies, breast milk, and umbilical cord blood.[346]

Besides harming our health, Production of PFAS cause Warming Temps and Climate Change! PFAS: Formerly known as PFCs (perfluoridated chemicals), PFAS are persistent organic chemicals. This means they don't break down or biodegrade but rather persist in the environment for years and years. PFAS include over 10,000 chemicals including PFOA, PFOS, Gen X, Teflon (C8). PFAS are rapidly and boldly dirtying our water supplies and migrating to our bodies. Due to the persistent life cycle of these compounds, there's no getting rid of them yet. They're in food packaging, stain resistant, water proof, nonstick, wrinkle resistant materials as well as firefighting chemicals.

Due to the toxicity of these substances, PFAS should not be consumed by any person or animal. Yet once in the water, they easily get in our drinking water. The EPA may set provisional health advisory (PHA) levels, but really we must ban their use altogether immediately. Children may be especially vulnerable to PFAS substances in the environment as thyroid carcinomas[347] are growing rapidly amongst this population.

HEALTH EFFECTS
Birth defects, thyroid cancer[348], thyroid carcinoma, cancer, learning and behavior challenges, endocrine disruptors, decreased fertility and hormone irregularity, weight gain and obesity, high cholesterol, irregular immune system, increases risk of cancer.

HOW WE ARE EXPOSED:
- Nonstick cookware (Teflon, Gen X)
- Food Packaging with grease-resistant coating (microwave popcorn, pizza boxes, fast food wrappers, straws),
- Stain resistant carpeting, clothing, furniture
- Wrinkle resistant clothing and materials
- Waterproof clothing and materials
- Some types of Dental Floss, tissue, toilet paper
- Drinking Straws, some dental floss brands
- Some Make up brands add PFAS
- Fertilizer containing Biosolids!

WATERWAYS COMPROMISED FOREVER
The most troubling water contamination problems to date include PFOA contamination from Dupont's Teflon facility. Under Chemours, Dupont created Gen X as a substitute that seems to be even worse. Today, regions of Delaware and West Virginia have super toxic levels of Gen X in their water supplies.

PFAS Can Be Found in Many Places[349]
PFAS can be present in our water, soil, air, and food as well as in materials found in our homes or workplaces, including:
- **Drinking water** – in public drinking water systems and wells
- **Soil, water, food**– from Biosolids sewage sludge fertilizer
- **Food packaging** – grease-resistant coatings, fast food containers, wrappers, microwave popcorn bags, pet food bags
- **Paper Tissues, Toilet Paper, Paper Straws sadly**
- Nonstick Cookware Wrinkle free, stain free, water-resistant
- **Pet Food Bags and Packaging can be coated with PFAS!**
- **Biosolids Fertilizer**—that's Human Sewage Sludge!
- **Fire extinguishing foam** - in aqueous film-forming foams
- **Manufacturing or chemical production facilities for** chrome plating, electronics, textile and paper facilities
- **Food** – when grown in soil fertilized with biosolids, food pkg
- **Household Products and Dust** –stain and water-repellent carpets, upholstery, clothing, and fabrics; cleaning products; non-stick cookware; paints, varnishes, and sealants.
- **Personal care products** – shampoos, floss, and cosmetics.
- **Protect yourself and your family**—Filter Your Water!

SOLUTIONS
- Filter your water, use filtered water for cooking
- Avoid food pkg, nonstick pans, food pkg, carpet, furn with PFAS.
- Tell the EPA to Ban PFAS in food packaging and products
- Reduce your exposure & replace items with nontoxic ones

> DuPont, 3M and other PFC manufacturers had ample indications decades ago that PFOA and other perfluorochemicals contaminate the blood of the general U.S. population. How and why they ignored the warning signs is one of the more disturbing chapters in the unfolding tragedy of PFC pollution.
> www.ewg.org/reports/pfcworld/part2.php

57. Pharmaceuticals

Pharmaceuticals and all types of drugs are infiltrating drinking water supplies. These substances are rarely filtered out with existing municipal filtering systems. Instead, they persist and mingle together causing a host of problems and challenges for animals and humans alike.

POLLUTION FROM PHARMACEUTICAL LABS
Pharmaceutical Manufacturing facilities are huge polluters! USGS scientists found that pharmaceutical manufacturing facilities are dumping waste into streams and rivers. Wastewater treatment facilities (WWTF) that receive discharge from pharmaceutical manufacturing facilities had 10 to 1,000 times higher concentrations of pharmaceuticals than effluents from waste water treatment facilities across the nation that do not receive pharmaceutical facility discharge. The release waters from these WWTFs were discharged to streams where the measured pharmaceuticals were traced downstream, and as far as 30 kilometers from one plant's outfall."[350]

DRUGS IN WATER CAUSING FEMINIZATION
Scientists are finding more and more troubling health effects from these peculiar mixtures. One particular study at the University of Wisconsin Milwaukee focused on the Type 2 Diabetes drug, Metformin.[351] Scientists have discovered that when in water, Metformin's effect is similar to the pesticide Atrazine, capable of feminizing male animals. Even though it's not a hormone drug, it's causing "reproductive and development problems in exposed fish. 84% of the young male minnows exposed to metformin levels commonly found in water developed feminized reproductive organs."

Where is the EPA? What is the answer to solving this crisis? None of us should be exposed to drugs from drinking water.

SOLUTIONS: FILTER YOUR WATER
- Surely facilities can install better pollution control. If these guys can't manage their toxic waste, they shouldn't be in business.
- EPA must regulate this waste as well as pesticide facility waste
- Time for a lawsuit to get them to stop this criminal activity

58. Phosphates

Phosphorous is an important mineral, but too much can get into water from fertilizer, detergents, dishwashing soap, and washing. Excess phosphates in water contribute to toxic algae growth and dead zones. The resulting low dissolved oxygen level triggers fish kills and harms aquatic animal life.

How Phosphorous gets in the Water
- From Agricultural Runoff
- From Chemical Fertilizer
- From Phosphate Mining and Fertilizer Facilities
- From Phosphates in soap, shampoo, detergents
- Don't use soap or shampoo outside in water sources

PHOSPHATES IN SHAMPOO HARM ANIMALS
Phosphates are added to many shampoos and soaps, detergents and cleaning products. These get into the water and contribute to toxic algae and other water diseases that harm animals in the water. This is the same problem with phosphate fertilizer. Now companies are adding surfactants to the potions which turns normal cleaners into power cleaners. This power boost comes at a cost to the animals and people who come across contaminated water or with the products themselves, perhaps even breathing the air near these manufacturing sites is damaging health. When rinsed down the drain, phosphates add to the nutrient load and trigger harmful ecological results.

Don't use Soap or Shampoo in any Lake, River, or Ocean
The next time you're camping and want to take a bath in the lake, please don't bring your soap or shampoo! Even the natural kind is bad for fish and birds. Such mixtures have long-term consequences for creatures that live in the water. Instead, use a bucket outside a good distance from the shore, or use a true shower with plumbing that takes the dirty water to a filtration center. Our filtration plants need some updating but for now it's the best we got.

SOLUTIONS
- Use soap and detergent products that have zero phosphates
- Don't use conventional fertilizer on your garden or farm.

59. Phosphate Fertilizer

RADIOACTIVE POLLUTION!
The US Produces 27 million metric tons of phosphate a year![352]

MANUFACTURING POLLUTION
Perhaps the worst synthetic fertilizer production problem comes from Phosphate mines. They are as bad for the earth and the water as you can imagine. These sites produce hazardous radioactive waste that is so toxic it's not allowed to be disposed anywhere but on site in open pits. Toxic gypsum stacks hover like mountains at these sites filled with millions of gallons of wastewater. When leaks occur, every aquatic organism in in its path dies. Red tides and toxic algae blooms follow.

PBS: "Phosphogypsum stacks, also known as gypsum stacks, are mountains of waste left over from fertilizer production. Some of that waste is radon and uranium. The EPA says that it's too radioactive to be buried, so it's piled in these stacks."

The Problem:
- Toxic Water Pollution, Hazardous Waste
- Gypsum mounds leak and spill, cause sinkholes
- Cause worsening Red Tides and Toxic Algae
- Fertilizer kills fish and animals
- Biohazard to People and Ecosystem
- Spills are frequent and deadly
- Contaminants cause human diseases
- Even after plants are closed, the toxic wastewater remains.

In 1997, "Fifty million gallons of wastewater from a phosphate fertilizer plant spilled into the Alafia River, and it killed almost everything, more than a million fish for 50 miles downstream."

SOLUTIONS: We must stop using and producing synthetic phosphate fertilizer. These corporations have to be more responsible or shut down. This toxins cause too much destruction to our health, to animals, to the waterways, to the atmosphere.
Filter your water.

NATURAL FERTILIZER

Soil quality can vary widely around the world. Soil gets depleted naturally overtime, and without anything added to it, either by nature or by humans, eventually nutrient levels will decrease.

As soil expert Dr. Charles Northern exclaimed in the 1930s, "Foods vary enormously in value, and some of them aren't worth eating as food. For example, vegetation grown in one part of the country may assay 1,100 parts per billion of iodine, as against 20 in that grown elsewhere. Processed milk has run anywhere from 362 parts per million of iodine and 127 of iron, down to nothing." Clearly vegetable quality depends on soil, and milk quality depends on the quality of the plants the cows are eating. Everything is so deeply intertwined.

So what can we do, what can farmers do? We must start with the soil. the soil, and nurture it. A few methods include:
- Local chicken manure has a high nitrogen content
- rock dust, or mineral manure—basically ground up rocks, granite in particular.
- Rudolph Steiner, the father of biodynamics developed soil amendments, replenishment methods using antlers and herbal preparations
- A simple way to restore soil between plantings and over winter is to plant cover crops like legumes or sweet clover, these plants magically convert nitrogen in the soil
- Instead of raking up your leaves and throwing them away put the leaves remain on your garden. Fallen leaves and plants naturally decompose and feed your soil.
- If you burn wood or plants, don't throw the ashes away but use these as fertilizer too! Lastly, don't forget the compost.
- Use worm casings, compost tea, natural things available from your local garden center
- Avoid BioSolids, Biosolids are full of PFAS and hazardous waste! Make sure fertilizer you buy doesn't contain biosolids.

60. PLASTIC

Microplastics, PVC, Styrofoam, Microbeads:

What do all these plastics have in common? They are derived from petroleum, they cause damaging health effects to people and animals, and they do not biodegrade.

PLASTIC: First developed in 1862, plastic is cherished by chemical companies for its versatility and durability. Plastic's usefulness, however, is offset by the amount of harm and pollution it causes throughout its lifespan. Once created, this nonbiodegradable material has an eternal lifespan. Thankfully, many people are starting to choose natural materials over plastic, and some methods of recycling plastic have been developed. While we continue to have plastics around us, it's important to use them less to lessen their impact on our health.

PVC, POLYVINYL CHLORIDE: Perhaps the worst of all plastics, polyvinyl chloride (PVC), or vinyl, is everywhere. Comprised mostly of chlorine, PVC is toxic from the moment it's produced—contributing dioxins, toxins, and a host of carcinogenic compounds into the air and water around us. PVC products, like shower curtains, off-gas toxic compounds like toluene, ethylbenzene and DEHP. These compounds are identified respectively as carcinogenic, developmental and reproductive toxins. Due to its high toxicity, PVC is not recyclable. In fact, tragically just one PVC container (identified by #3 or the letter "V") in a recycling load will render the entire batch unrecyclable.

PHTHALATES: Phthalates are a group of widely used compounds that are responsible for softening plastic. Found primarily in PVC products, phthalates also serve as an additive in perfume, lotions, nail polish, hair products and wood finishing products. Nearly 1 billion pounds of phthalates are produced throughout the world each year. The EPA has classified DEHP, an abbreviated name for *di(2-ethylhexyl) phthalate,* as a probable human carcinogen. It is often masked under trade names like Bisoflex 81, Eviplast 80, Octoil, Platinol DOP and Silicol 150. It may soon be added to the list of **P**ersistent **O**rganic **P**ollutants, as it demonstrates POP behavior.

Both Japan and the European Union have banned certain phthalates after overwhelming scientific evidence proved the harm they cause. Yet, the American Chemistry Council, which is comprised of and funded by many of the biggest corporate polluters, continues to deny the harm and danger phthalates and other petroleum-derived toxins cause. Furthermore, U.S. industrial lobbyists have been working overtime trying to persuade European companies to ease phthalate concern. Thankfully, some U.S. companies have expressed interest in limiting their use of phthalates.

POLYCARBONATE and BPA: Used to make many things like eyeglass lenses, roofing materials and hard plastic water bottles. Though a favorite among many manufacturers, PC contains the plasticizer bisphenol-A (BPA), a known endocrine disruptor. Beware the BPA alternatives, BPS and BADGE—which are equally if not more dangerous to health.

STYROFOAM is made of styrene, otherwise chemically known as **vinyl benzene.** The world must ban this hideous substance for eternity!

MARINE DEBRIS "Marine debris is any solid, manufactured material that is disposed of or abandoned into the marine environment. It may consist of plastic, glass, metals, polystyrene, rubber, derelict fishing gear and derelict vessels. **Plastics are estimated to represent between 60% and 80% of the total marine debris floating in the world's oceans.** Almost all of the plastic debris in the North Pacific consists of very small pieces of plastic floating at or slightly below the water surface. Such debris is composed of fragments of manufactured plastic products and also preproduction plastic pellets that were spilled at some point during shipping☹

MICROBEADS are sinister teeny tiny pieces of plastic that have been intentionally added to hundreds of personal care products. These may boost your cleaning regimen but at what cost to the planet? All of these particles once washed off your face go down the drain and eventually to the ocean where they are unwittingly swallowed by whales, dolphins, turtles, birds, and every marine creature imaginable.

PLASTIC WASTE: Plastic waste is a big problem. Plastic doesn't biodegrade and instead accumulates wherever it's tossed. Please be mindful and caring and either recycle plastic garbage or dispose of it properly. Litter only ends up hurting all of us in one way or another.

HEALTH EFFECTS
PVC Plastic chemicals cause cancer, harm the nervous system and contribute to birth defects. Phthalates are endocrine disruptors, and they

may cause DNA damage in sperm, affect semen quality, and cause kidney disease. Microbeads attract toxins and plastic and easily get eaten when marine mammals feed in the water. Every whale studied over the past 20 years has had microplastics embedded in all tissues sampled from lung and other areas.[353]

HOW WE ARE EXPOSED
Drinking water, consuming foods or warming foods and storing foods in plastic may cause plastic to leach into the foods. From cradle to grave the process of making Plastic to disposing of plastic is cursed.

Microbeads
It's estimated that 8 trillion beads wash down drains everyday! Across the world nations are scurrying to address microbeads, but with so many products still out there we're clearly not doing enough. Even though the US implemented a ban, they're still hidden in some products. For a full list of products see here

Microbeads are disguised under these words on the label: polyethylene, poly-ethylene glycol, polyacrylate, polyactic acid, acrylate. **Microbeads and plastic pellets are** teeny tiny pieces of plastic that easily pollute our waterways and oceans and cause immense harm to animals and to us. Lotions, skin cleansers, exfoliants and the like used to contain natural exfoliating agents like coconut shell or apricot kernel. Somewhere along the way many companies swapped out the natural stuff for these cheaper plastic imitations. This has contributed to devastating health consequences for countless aquatic animals who mistake them for food. The microplastics draw PCBs and other harmful pollutants with them, which then bioaccumulate in creatures that suffer the fate of swallowing them. The companies who manufacture microbeads should have their business licenses withdrawn. Thanks to pressure from GreenPeace and environmentalists worldwide, the UK in 2017 passed the most comprehensive ban yet![354]

> **"Research shows for the first time that persistent organic pollutants accumulate in the tissue of fish.**

Micro Plastics in Water
Plastic breaks down into tinier and tinier shreds of plastic. Products made of plastic, styrene, plastic polymers or plastic derivatives of any kind have become especially problematic for waterways, animal and human health.

Disposable Masks and Wipes
Disposable masks may have become useful and popular during Covid, but now they're a curse on the planet contributing to water pollution and wildlife distress. Like disposable wipes and all things plastic, masks have the tendency to block drains as well as interfere with wildlife well-being. Disposable masks: are made with plastic polymers "such as polypropylene, polyurethane, polyacrylonitrile, polystyrene, polycarbonate, polyethylene, or polyester."[355] Nanoparticles too! They do not biodegrade and take over 400 years to decompose,[356] all the while releasing microplastics into the environment. All ecosystems, animals, and humans are affected by the rising levels of plastic and microplastic contamination accumulating all over the world.

Microfibers
Microfibers are accumulating madly in the waterways and threatening animal survival. These microfibers are tiny pieces of micro filaments sloughing off nearly all materials in the wash cycle. All types of materials shed microfibers, but some of the fleece and synthetic fibers derived from petrochemicals may release more. These fibers do not biodegrade either unlike natural fibers. Ecologist Mark Browne discovered microfibers in sea trash[357] He discovered they comprise nearly 85% of all human-caused garbage washing up on shorelines! It's not just oceans that are affected, these fibers are turning up in the Great Lakes, in rivers, streams, and water bodies everywhere. Anywhere a sewer pipe leads, you'll find microfibers. If you can, install a filter on your washing machine. Wexco in Minnesota makes a filter called Filtrol that prevents the little microfibers from escaping. **Or go old school and make** your own with a pantyhose. That's what my mom used to do. ☺

SOLUTIONS: Avoid using Plastic
- Help clean up plastic pollution anywhere you see it
- Pressure your City and State Reps to ban Stryrofoam and plastic in your State,
- Filter your water and Go plastic free as much as you can
- Read more on Oceans and a Ban on Plastic pages 217-224

61. Plastic Pellets
Horrible Water Pollutant

Plastic pellets, otherwise called Nurdles are polluting and threatening oceans, waterways, fish and aquatic life everywhere!

Greatest Ship Wreck Containing Plastic, May 20, 2021, Sri Lanka: "The M/V X-Press Pearl caught fire while anchored off the coast of Sri Lanka, near the capital city of Colombo. According to news reports, the container ship was carrying nitric acid, urea fertilizer, sulphuric acid, ethanol, sodium hydroxide, lubricants and other chemicals, along with 78 metric tons (170,000 pounds) of a material known as plastic nurdles."[358]

"The tiny beads can be made of polyethylene, polypropylene, polystyrene, polyvinyl chloride and other plastics. Released into the environment from plastic plants or when shipped around the world as raw material to factories, they will sink or float, depending on the density of the pellets and if they are in freshwater or saltwater. Yet nurdles, unlike substances such as kerosene, diesel and petrol, are not deemed hazardous under the International Maritime Organization's (IMO's) dangerous goods code for safe handling and storage. This is despite the threat to the environment from plastic pellets being known about for three decades, as detailed in a 1993 report from the US government's EPA on how the plastics industry could reduce spillages. **An astounding 230,000 tons of nurdles end up in oceans every year.**"[359]

Where Do Plastic Pellets Come From? Natural Gas
"The roughly $6 billion Shell Monaca plant transforms a product of natural gas (ethane), extracted through hydraulic fracturing in the region's shale formations, into tiny plastic pellets used to manufacture single-use plastic goods like soda bottles and plastic packaging[360]

SOLUTIONS

We must hold the petrochemical and plastic industry accountable. Should they be allowed to make such toxic products that pollute our earth so? Shipping nurdles overseas must require better pollution prevention methods. In everything we do--industry and corporations especially this applies to you-we must be more earth minded and act with the precautionary principle in mind. Before profits, comes health.

PLASTIC RECYCLING

Red = Unsafe, Green = Safer

Most plastic is not recyclable, save for the kind labeled as #1 and #2. This is due to the fact that plastic melts at a very low temperature. It is difficult to properly remove the previous contents at this low temperature. If heated high enough to sanitize, toxic chemicals are released. This is why most plastic ends up in landfills. In one plastic recycling program, plastic is broken down into miniscule pellets and shipped overseas. This is leading to widespread plastic drift in the ocean.

NOT SAFE, NOT RECYCLABLE

3 **PVC, Polyvinyl Chloride. don't microwave!**
   NOT recyclable, Toxic, not safe, used in plastic wrap, teething rings, piping, baby and pet toys, shower curtains,

6 **PS, Polystyrene**
   NOT Recyclable *but can be reused*, Toxic, chemical leaching, major oceanic pollutant, used in carry out food & drink containers, packaging, egg cartons, **don't microwave!**

7 **Other: BPA, Polycarbonate,**
   NOT Recyclable, Toxic, chemical leaching, may contain BPA, Found in water bottles, sippy cups, **Don't microwave, Don't Reuse**

DEVASTATING OCEAN LIFE

1 **PET, Polyethylene Terephthalate**
   Recyclable, considered safe, used in water bottles

2 **HDPE, High-Density Polyethylene**
   Recyclable, considered safe, used in milk and laundry jugs

4 **LDPE, Low-Density Polyethylene**
   Borderline Recyclable (increasing) relatively safe, used in squeeze bottles, shrink wraps, dry cleaner, bread bags

5 **PP, Polypropylene**
   Recyclable, considered relatively safe, used in food packaging, yogurt containers, cereal bags. Bags for chips and pet food bags can contain PFAS coatings!

CONSIDERED SAFE, Not RECYCLABLE

PLA (corn-based) **Not Recyclable**, Compostable
Plastic Bags: reusable but plastic bags are **Not Recyclable**
Pizza boxes, greasy containers, used tissue= Not Recyclable

62. POPs

Persistent Organic Pollutants

Persistent Organic Pollutants are the most harmful chemicals on earth. They can be found in our water and in our food. According to the EPA, POPs are linked with disease, declines, and abnormalities in wildlife. In people, reproductive, developmental, behavioral, neurologic, endocrine, and immunologic adverse health effects have been linked to POPs.[361]

Similar to the EU's Substances of Very High Concern (SVHCs), these chemicals cause so much harm that in 2001 scientists from around the world began working together towards banishing them from the universe. Known as the Stockholm Convention, the aim was to protect people and the earth by banning these chemicals out of existence.

The original dirty dozen were chosen due to toxicity, persistence, and bioaccumulation, as well as capacity to travel vast distances via water and air. Because POPs stay in the environment for so long, they can still be found in waterways and the environment decades after use. The Stockholm Convention of 2001 bans the manufacturing and distribution of POPs in all countries who signed on. While the U.S. restricts use and manufacturing of POPs, the U.S. has not yet joined (or ratified) the Stockholm Convention.

Pesticides
Aldrin
Chlodane
Lindan
DDT, dichloro diphenyl trichloroethylene
Dieldran
Endrin
Heptachlor
HBC, hexachlorobenzene
Mirex
Toxaphene
Chlordecone
Alpha Hexachlorochyclohexane
Beta Hexachlorocyclohexane
Endosulphan
HCB, hexachlorobenzene (fungicide)

Industrial Chemicals
PCBs
PFOS
HBC, Hexachlorobenzene
PAHs
HBB, Hexabromobiphenyl
Perfluorooctane sulfonic salt
Perfluorooctane sulf. fluoride
Pentachlorobenzene

Byproducts
Dioxins
Furans

Flame Retardants
(PDBE)

63. PPCPs

PHARMACEUTICALS and PERSONAL CARE PRODUCTS

PPCPs, Pharmaceuticals and Personal Care Products, are an emerging group of pollutants found in drinking water. Scientists worldwide have only just begun to study PPCPs and the extent of their action, health effects, accumulation and interaction with other compounds. Because of the resilient nature of the many of the ingredients, they are found in both untreated and *treated* water. Our existing water treatment facilities are simply incapable of filtering out these types of mixtures.

Beware! These products act like micro terrorists in the environment, capable of harming every animal and human cell they touch. Reduce your exposure by filtering your water. Most common PPCPs: anti-inflammatory drugs, oral contraceptives, sun screen products, anticonvulsants, beta-blockers, antidepressants, bronchodilators, antibiotics, hypnotics, and synthetic fragrance. Because these things are normally not administered or ingested in combinations like these, scientists are testing aquatic creatures to determine long-term effects. Even more reason to avoid unfiltered tap water.

"When discharged into wastewater, pharmaceuticals and personal care products (PPCPs) become microorganic contaminants and are among the largest groups of emerging pollutants. Human, animal, and aquatic organisms' exposures to PPCPs have linked them to an array of carcinogenic, mutagenic, and reproductive toxicity risks. For this reason, various methods are being implemented to remove them from water bodies."[362]

SOLUTIONS

- Filter your water
- Avoid using anything with plastic microbeads.
- Don't flush unused drugs down the toilet.
- For body washes and foaming products, think soap, shampoo, laundry and dish detergent--avoid those containing toxins such as sodium lauryl/laureth sulfates, parabens, ammonium, phosphates, nanoparticles, antibacterial, deodorizer, synthetics
- When in doubt about a product, choose natural.

64. Power Plants

While much is said about air pollution resulting from Power plants, they're also notorious water polluters. In fact, "Discharges from power plants alone contribute a third of all the toxic pollution in our environment." Power plants create more point source water pollution than any other industry. A quick snapshot comparison:

Power Plant Type	Water Pollution	Air Pollution
Biomass - wood	Yes + Deforestation	CO_2, PM, Dioxin, CO, NO_2, SO_2, Ammonia
Coal	Heavy Metals, SO_2, Mercury +	Yes, PM, CO_2, SO_2, PM
Natural Gas	Mercury, Nitrate, Ammonia	Methane, NO_2, CO_2 NOx, PM
Nuclear	Yes, radioactive	none

BIOMASS: Worse for the Planet than Coal or Natural Gas!
Biomass using whole trees is a greenwash coup—cutting down forests and producing more CO_2 and Hazardous Air Pollutants (HAP) than coal or natural gas power plants! "Biomass power plants are California's dirtiest electricity source—releasing more carbon at the smokestack than coal. Adding to these harms, cutting trees for biomass energy reduces the forest's ability to sequester and store carbon."[363]

Why is our government subsidizing Biomass? "Because the government considers all forms of biomass energy as renewable, it qualifies for tax credits, subsidies and incentives in the U.S. These include:
- Renewable Electricity Production Tax Credit; and Renewable Energy Certificates: every mwh earns a credit that can be sold, traded or bartered, giving its owner the right to claim to have purchased renewable energy.
- The Investment Tax Credit reimburses 30% of biomass plant development if operation begins by 2024.
- Biomass is eligible for subsidies from the U.S.D.A.

Thermoelectric Power Plants (coal, biomass and nuclear plants) use water to produce steam which generates the electricity. It's estimated these facilities draw collectively over 136 billion gallons of freshwater daily. If you operate a facility that emits toxins of any kind, please install pollution control devices ASAP. Thank you.

65. RADIATION

RADIOACTIVE WATER
Spills and leaks aside, peculiar policies allow nuclear power facilities to discharge wastewater into nearby waterways. According to the Hudson River based Riverkeeper, "Government regulations allow radioactive water to be released from Indian Point nuclear power plant to the environment containing "permissible" levels of contamination. However, since there is no safe threshold to exposure to radiation, permissible does not mean safe."[364]

The Nuclear Regulatory Commission uses 50 miles as their standard for measuring risk to food and water supplies. Rather than monitoring closely, the NRC relies on facilities reporting discharge numbers themselves. In addition, nuclear plants are allowed to use local lakes and waterbodies for cooling purposes, which raises the potential for contamination and harm to ecosystems!

There are 99 nuclear reactors and 61 nuclear power plants operating throughout the U.S providing roughly one fifth of the nation's electricity. The Exelon Corporation is the country's largest producer of nuclear power with 14 plants nationwide. "Government regulators concede they have to balance the safety needs of aging plants, which require more maintenance, versus ordering cost-prohibitive upgrades at facilities that inherently are just a slip up away from catastrophe."[365]

FUKUSHIMA August 24, 2023: Despite objections from local fishermen and surrounding countries, Tokyo Electric announced it will soon begin dumping wastewater from the 2011 Fukushima disaster into the ocean. The water is tainted with tritium and has been stored at the nuclear plant since the accident. This is no small amount—"more than 1 million metric tons of treated radioactive water."[366] Apparently, "Tritium typically poses little risk to human health unless ingested in high amounts, and ocean discharges of diluted volumes of tritium-tainted water are a routine part of nuclear power plant operations. This is because it is a byproduct of nuclear operations but cannot be filtered out of water. Toxic water at the plant is being treated by a complex water-processing system that can remove 62 different types of radioactive materials except tritium.[367]

TRITIUM
"After a radioactive leak or spill, tritium is generally the first

radionuclide to be identified in groundwater. This is because tritium travels through the soil faster than other radionuclides. Leaks and spills at some sites (e.g., Indian Point, Braidwood) involved nuclides other than tritium (e.g., Cobalt-60, Cobalt-58, Cesium-134, Cesium-137, Strontium-90, Nickel-63), but those radionuclides are not included in this list."[368] nrc.gov

RADIOACTIVE SPILLS and LEAKS:
Exelon Power Stations, Illinois November 17, 2017
Radioactive waste continues to pour from Exelon's Illinois nuclear power plants more than a decade after the discovery of chronic leaks led to national outrage, a $1.2 million government settlement and a company vow to guard against future accidents, an investigation by a government watchdog group found. Since 2007, there have been at least 35 reported leaks, spills or other accidental releases in Illinois of water contaminated with radioactive tritium, a byproduct of nuclear power production and a carcinogen at high levels, a Better Government Association review of federal and state records shows. [369]

Palisades Nuclear Station, Michigan May 8, 2013
Nearly 80 gallons of water containing small amounts of radioactive tritium and possibly trace amounts of cobalt and cesium spewed into Lake Michigan, the Nuclear Regulatory Commission told the AP. Early Sunday morning, the tank was ruled inoperable and the nuclear power plant began powering down. This is reportedly the ninth time that the facility has been shut down since 2011.[370]

Three Mile Island, Harrisburg, Pennsylvania March 28, 1979
Three Mile Island shut down in 2019. The accident in 1979 was the most serious accident in U.S. nuclear power plant history.[371]

Naturally Occurring Radium Of course, some radiation occurs naturally in our water. As noted by the EPA, "Many of the contaminants found in public drinking water sources occur naturally. For example, radioactive radium and uranium are found in small amounts in almost all rock and soil, and can dissolve in water. Radon, a radioactive gas, created through the decay of radium, can also naturally occur in groundwater. If it is not removed, radon can be released into the air as you shower or wash dishes or do laundry."[372]

SOLUTIONS
- Filter your water
- Better pollution control methods must be installed at facilities

66. ROAD SALT

While it may seem harmless it is anything but! As with most things put outside on our sidewalks, lawn or on the roads, road salt runs off into streams and waterways causing massive contamination. Most road salt is comprised of Sodium and Chloride and as it runs off and accumulates in streams, rivers and lakes, it accumulates. This concentration of chloride is ruining ecosystems and killing wildlife. It's also harming us and making drinking water very toxic.

ROAD SALT & FLINT'S DRINKING WATER

Everyone by now has heard about the increased levels of lead in Flint's drinking water, but did you know it's related to road salt?[373] The Flint River has been severely polluted for years from industrial and automotive manufacturing. Also, over the years road salt run off has been increasing in concentrations in the river; this is the water drawn for tap water. The road salt made the water extremely corrosive. When corrosive water is drawn through water pipes, it will cause the metal in water pipes to leach into the water. The aging lead pipes throughout most of the homes in Flint were no match for the Flint River water.

Canada declared road salt a toxin in 2004 and restricted its use. Back in the United States meanwhile, an estimated 140 pounds of salt per person are distributed onto snowy roads each year! In some states like Minnesota that gets more snow and ice, that amount rises to over 200 pounds of salt per person per year! The time has come for the U.S. to implement better methods that eliminate ice without destroying the planet.

SOLUTIONS
- Filter your water
- Avoid using salt on your sidewalks and driveway. Instead: Try out *Ecotraction*, made from Volcanic Ash
- Sand or Old fashioned shoveling and non-clumping cat litter
- If you suspect your water is contaminated with lead, please filter, or find a source of clean water. You may have to purchase bottled water or have water delivered until your tap water is ok.

67. SEWAGE

Both untreated human waste and animal waste can pollute water. Untreated sewage is referred to as raw sewage. Certain cities are known to open storm sewers during intense storms to avoid overflow, but in turn raw sewage flows into nearby lakes, rivers, and oceans. In some parts of the world, it may occur more frequently. Private septic systems overflow as well, contaminating well water.

Biosolids is a fertilizer product many municipalities are making from sewage. It's a very toxic form of fertilizer that's being utilized on farm fields across the world, especially in America. From the PFAS contamination and other toxic hazards, it's no wonder disease is spiking in America. The biosolids assault on soil & health must end.

Exempt from Regulation: CAFO Animal Waste

Recently Indiana[374] earned the crown for most polluted lakes and rivers in the US, not swimmable or fishable! This it turns out is all due to factory farm runoff. In the summer of 2024, though Iowa became the Cancer Capital of America. In addition to all the pesticides pouring into Iowa's waterways, this could very well be related to the numerous CAFOs in Iowa spewing raw animal waste into the streams and rivers. Iowa has more CAFOs than any other State. [375]

What Makes Untreated Wastewater So Dangerous?
Information source: Springwelllwater.com
"Besides having a gross appearance and unbearable smell, wastewater typically contains harmful chemicals, heavy metals, and microbes known to cause various health problems. For instance, human and animal waste carries many disease-causing organisms, also known as pathogens. These pathogens can enter wastewater from human waste discharged from homes, businesses, and hospitals and animal waste from farms, meat processing facilities, rats, and other animals found in and around sewage. Similarly, toxic chemicals and heavy metals can leach into surface water from runoff from crop fields, industrial processes, mining, quarrying, and specific items put down the drain.

"Much of the wastewater – treated or untreated – eventually reaches our rivers, lakes, streams, reservoirs, oceans, and sometimes groundwater that serves well water systems. While municipal utilities that get water from surface water sources typically treat the water to ensure it is safe for consumption, the opposite is true for private wells.

"We assume that groundwater is pure – and sometimes it is. But well water contaminated by sewage is a common cause of wastewater-related disease outbreaks. This has much to do with the Environmental Protection Agency (EPA) and other federal bodies not regulating private wells.

"Due to the lack of regulation, well water tends to be more susceptible to contamination since people relying on private wells are usually responsible for ensuring the safety of their drinking water. In most cases, private well users are unaware of the dangers of drinking untreated groundwater. They also may not have adequate, modern systems installed in their homes to protect against potentially dangerous waterborne contaminants.

"When raw sewage reaches a drinking water source, the health risks can be plenty. Drinking sewage-polluted water can cause you to develop various diseases and illnesses or even die. In fact, one hundred years ago, epidemics of these sewage-related diseases helped limit the life expectancy of a U.S. citizen to about 50 years. Estimates vary for how many people sewage still sickens or kills each year, but they are all large.

Diseases linked with Sewage-Tainted Water include":[376]
- Diarrhea
- Typhoid, (Salmonella Typhi)
- Hepatitis A
- Cholera
- Parasitic Infection
- Salmonellosis
- Cryptosporidiosis
- Polio
- Dysentery

SOLUTIONS:
- Tell your officials, no raw sewage in the water! Keep our beaches open, and keep biosolids off our soil!
- Filter Your Water! Boiling & UV will kill most microorganisms. If you swim in tainted water, shower after. Install a shower filter.

68. STORMWATER

Stormwater Runoff is a very easy way for pollutants to bypass filtration and get directly into waterways. Paved roads, streets, sidewalks and any impervious pavements don't allow rain to be absorbed, but rather flow faster downhill. There are many things we can do to at home or business to lessen stormwater runoff. These include:
- Plant a rain garden or mini wetland between your yard and waterways
- Create a bioswale to capture runoff near roads
- Put rain barrels out to capture rain
- Make your soil healthier so it will absorb rain
- Use less pesticides and harmful chemicals on your yard and garden
- Clean up animal waste and keep yard clippings and leaves out of the street
- Don't dump cleaning rinse water, soapy car wash water, or paint rinse water in the street (these all contain chemicals that need to be filtered before entering waterways).

To help your town avoid excess water flows, reduce water usage during storms.

Help reduce overflowing sewage systems: resist doing laundry, running the dishwasher, and taking long showers on rainy days.

Bioswale

A bioswale is created to collect excess rainwater, filter it and help it soak into the ground. Bioswales are a more complex rain garden with layers and drain pipes underground.

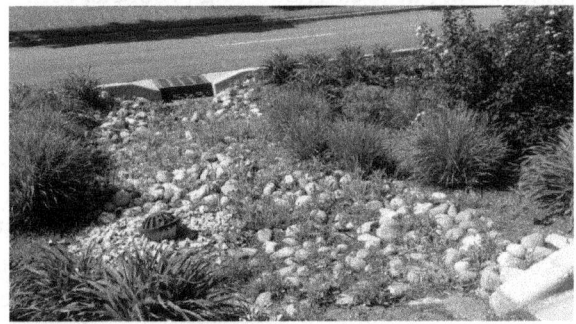

Image: Milwaukee Metropolitan Sewerage District[377]

69. STYROFOAM

POLYSTYRENE, STYROFOAM: While convenient and cheap, this plastic easily leaches into the product contained within its walls. It's a neurotoxin and causes cancer in animals. Do not heat or microwave any foods or beverages in Styrofoam.

The 2 most abundant Plastics found inside People: Polyethylene (plastic water bottles) and Polystyrene (styrofoam).[378] **Stryofoam is made from Styrene, which is Vinyl Benzene.**

When a Styrofoam cup is filled with a cold or hot beverage, the chemicals in the styrofoam break down and seep into your drink. These are not ordinary chemicals, these are benzene and vinyl styrene-- potent carcinogenic chemicals that should never enter your body. Anytime a food or beverage is in contact with polystyrene, seepage occurs-increasingly so the warmer the said food or drink is. Making matters worse, polystyrene contributes to the hole in the ozone layer! It doesn't biodegrade, nor is it recyclable, so anything made from this Styrofoam will still be here 500 years from now. That's sad.

HEALTH EFFECTS
Polystyrene is an endocrine disruptor (mimics and adversely affects hormonal balance), it's carcinogenic, it's bioaccumulative (gets stored and increases in fatty tissues in our bodies), causes neurological changes, fatigue, depletes ozone layer, harms animals and wildlife.

HOW YOU ARE EXPOSED
Styrofoam packaging, dishes, containers, food wrapped on Styrofoam trays, take-out packaging, building products, ceiling tiles, foam boards

SOLUTIONS
- Filter your water.
- Don't buy, eat, drink or reheat anything in a Styrofoam
- Help ban Styrofoam in your city and state
- Avoid using or purchasing anything in plastic, plastic bags.
- Use cloth or canvas and reusable bags when shopping
- Reduce, reuse and recycle any plastic you can. Currently, only two types of plastic are recyclable; the rest end up in landfills.

70. SUNSCREEN

While intended to protect our skin and prevent burning, sunscreen substances easily get in the water too. soak into our skin and on our health. They also can kill coral reefs and harm animals in the environment. Using natural mineral sunscreens is the best choice.

SUNCREEN SPRAYS CONTAIN BENZENE!
The problems with sunscreen sprays is they don't just land on our skin but thanks to wind and weather, mostly land everywhere around us. In so doing the spray contaminates everything nearby, sand, people, and water. Making matters worse, scientists have just discovered most sprays contain benzene![379] Benzene causes cancer and belongs nowhere near our bodies.

NANOPARTICLES HARM DOLPHINS and CORAL
According to Surfrider, you want to avoid nanoparticles in sunscreen. Both zinc oxide nanoparticles and titanium dioxide nanoparticles as these are bioaccumulative and ridiculously harmful for aquatic species in that they: reduce reproduction, accumulate in gills, cause behavior changes, bleaches coral, causes mortality in brine shrimp, reduces fecundity of crustaceans, increases uptake of heavy metals, reduces birth rates and impairs growth of zebrafish, reduces immunity of carp, causes respiratory and oxidative stress, damages intestines and gills of rainbow trout. These poor animals are guinea pigs for the industry as nanoparticles are not regulated or monitored by any government agency. But don't think the industry would not invite us.

Human health effects include: bioaccumulation of course, and: penetration of epidermal cells, stimulating release of free radicals, cross blood brain barrier. Nanos may come coated by the manufacturer with aluminum oxide nanos or other materials intended to block undesirable interactions with water and oxygen (air). Go figure. Sounds perfectly safe to put in countless products, doesn't it? Titanium dioxide nanos cause cancer for rodents when inhaled, thus take heed and avoid sprays containing titanium dioxide nanoparticles.[380] Nanoparticles, incidentally are not regulated or monitoring by the U.S. government.

Avoid These Most Dreaded Sunscreen Ingredients:
- **Benzene:** carcinogenic

Avoid These Most Dreaded Sunscreen Ingredients:
- **Benzene:** carcinogenic
- **Oxybenzone:** gets into bloodstream, breast tissue, endocrine disruptor (ED), toxic to sperm, pro-carcinogenic, contributes to coral bleaching and fish mortality, reacts with chlorine to create hazardous byproducts, banned in Hawaii
- **Octinoxate**: harms thyroid, hormones, affects behavior
- **Avobenzone**: on the FDA watch list for further testing
- **Homosalate:** Banned in EU limit 1.4%, US allows 15%!
- **Octocrylene**: breaks down to Benzophenone, carcinogen
- **Dioxybenzone:** Endocrine disruptor, harms marine life
- **Padimate O:** damages DNA, allergic reactions
- **Sulisobenzone:** Endocrine Disruptor

The National Ocean Service says bad ingredients:[381]:
- Impair the growth and photosynthesis of green algae
- Accumulate in coral, inducing bleaching, damaging their DNA, deforming their young, and even killing them
- Induce defects in young mussels
- Damage the immune and reproductive systems of sea urchins
- Decrease fertility and reproduction in fish
- Accumulate in the tissues of dolphins, which can be transferred to their young

SOLUTIONS
- Use natural mineral sunscreen that does not contain nanoparticles.
- Practice Sun Smarts: Wear sunscreen on exposed areas, Wear hat, sunglasses, protective clothing during peak hours..
- Avoid sunscreens that have health harming ingredients-nanos
- Surfrider's list of Reef Friendly: REN, Avasol, Manda
- Help reduce smog and air pollution that traps heat. If we can ban substances that deplete the ozone layer, we seriously imrove our chances for reducing skin cancer and relieving the planet of air pollution that traps heat. This means less crazy heat waves and such. We need sun for our health, plants need sun, animals and life needs the sunlight.

BEST SUNSCREENS

Reef Friendly, Mineral Based, Broad Spectrum, Non Nano

BRAND	REEF Safe	NO Nanos	NO Parabens	NO OCTINOXATE NO OXYBENZENE	Plastic Free	SPF
Reef Repair	yes	yes	yes	yes	no	30
Blue Lizard	yes	yes	yes	yes	no	50
Isdin Eryfotona	yes	yes	yes	yes	no	50
Hawaiian Tropic Mineral	yes	yes	yes	yes	no	50
Thrive Regenerative Skincare	yes	yes	yes	yes	no	50
SurfDurt	yes	yes	yes	yes	yes	30
Raw Elements Mineral	yes	yes	yes	yes	no	50
Babo Super Shield Mineral	yes	yes	yes	yes	no	50
Sports and Waterproof						
Think Sport Clear Zinc	yes	yes	yes	yes	no	50
Verta	yes	yes	yes	yes	no	45
Maui Naturals Surfer Honey	yes	yes	yes	yes	no	30
Badger Sport Mineral	yes	yes	yes	yes	no	40
Stream to Sea	yes	yes	yes	yes	no	30
Gentle, safe for Sensitive Skin						
Tatcha	yes	yes	yes	yes	no	50
MDSolarSciences	yes	yes	yes	yes	no	50
Pipette Mineral	yes	yes	yes	yes	no	50
Blue Lizard Sensitive	yes	yes	yes	yes	no	50
Sun Bum Mineral	yes	yes	yes	yes	no	50
Raw Elements Face	yes	yes	yes	yes	no	30
Kids Formulas						
Thinkkids	yes	yes	yes	yes	no	50
Thinkbaby	yes	yes	yes	yes	no	50
Blue Lizard Kids	yes	yes	yes	yes	no	50
Blue Lizard Baby	yes	yes	yes	yes	no	50

www.Adoreyourplanet.com

Information gathered from labels, National Geographic, Travel and Leisure, and from personal experience.

71. SURFACTANTS

Surfactants are an emerging contaminant of great concern with a history of secrecy. Nonylphenol Ethoxylates (NP/NPEs) are perhaps the most used surfactants added to detergents and soaps, personal care and cleaning products, washing agents, pesticides, hand sanitizers, Round up, latex paint, automotive products and such. They've largely gone undisclosed on labels under the umbrella of 'trade secrets.' Facilities that produce surfactants emit tons of air and water pollution yearly. Wastewater treatment facilities expel surfactants back into the water. Surfactants are a 40 billion industry, projected to grow

Surfactants are included in formulations to increase a products absorbability within numerous surfaces including human skin and plant tissue. Under the TSCA, the EPA is rethinking NPs. This is in line with the 2000 EU ban on surfactants. Surfactants can be found in:
- Cleaning Products
- Detergents and Soaps
- Hand Sanitizers
- Pesticide Formulation

HEALTH EFFECTS
Highly toxic to aquatic life, causes blindness in fish,
NP has been detected in human breast milk, blood, and urine and is associated with reproductive and developmental effects in rodents.[382]

HOW WE ARE EXPOSED
Contaminated Water, using products containing NP and other surfactants.

SOLUTIONS
Consumers can avoid products with NP/NPEs by looking for products with EPA's Safer Choice Label on the shelves of major retailers. When you see the safer product label on a product it means that EPA scientists have evaluated every ingredient in the product to ensure it meets stringent human health and environmental criteria. Learn more about consumer products that carry the safer product label.

72. TCP 1,2,3

Dow's Telone and the Shell Corporation's D-D were once the most used fumigants in the State of California and Hawaii. However, the companies knew one of the ingredients in their toxic blends was not capable of dissolving in soil and knew it would contaminate ground water. Both companies knew how dangerous it was, yet to save disposal costs they secretly reused it. This is so often the case with large corporations—more concerned about profits and saving money when not harming people should've been their main concern. Now millions of Americans are drinking water contaminated with TCP 123.

TCP should have been disposed of as hazardous waste. This is a perfect example of why Superfund matters, and corporations must be accountable for cleanup costs. Several cities are now suing both companies for cleanup costs. "[383] TCP is a known carcinogen. Shell discontinued producing DD and TCP was removed from Telone in the 90s, yet the contaminant remains in water. California authorities suggest a threshold no greater than 1 part per trillion, while the EPA has a reporting requirement at 30 parts per trillion. TCP has been found in drinking water and wells throughout California but also in Hawaii and in 20 other states.

The EPA has let TCP go unregulated for years but is currently reevaluating. California does regulate it as a water contaminant.

Health Effects

It's a manmade chemical that's not meant for ingestion. The EPA classified TCP as likely to be carcinogenic to humans based on the formation of multiple tumors in animals.[384]

SOLUTIONS

- Filter your water. Activated carbon or better filters it.[385]
- Protect yourself and avoid products containing TCP: metal degreasing agents, toxic cleaning supplies, varnish removers

73. TEFLON + GEN X

Teflon contains perfluorooctanoic acid (PFOA), also referred to as C-8. Dupont has been making Teflon and telomers (form of PFOA) since the early 1950's, and was aware of the danger since the early 1980's. DuPont recently paid over $300 million for withholding that information. These chemicals are persistent organic pollutants. Blood tests of people all around the globe show very high levels of PFOA. Gen X was created as a substitute for Teflon, but now is found to be 10x worse than Teflon.

As reported by *Democracy Now*, PFOA is so prominent in our environment that it's been detected in 99 percent of Americans who've been tested, including newborn babies. These substances simply do not go away nor breakdown, but remain in our bodies. PFOA and PFOS were originally produced by 3M, but as the EPA started becoming concerned with these chemicals circa 1999, 3M discontinued production and Dupont took over. After being sued, Dupont sold off this division to Chemours who in recent years created Gen X to replace PFOA. Gen X is currently causing great concern in North Carolina where it's been detected in the drinking water. There are no regulations yet for Gen X nor have health risks been exactly determined. [386]

HEALTH EFFECTS: During the lawsuit against Dupont in 2011, it was determined conclusively that overexposure to perfluorinated compounds can cause testicular and kidney cancer, liver tumors, ulcerative colitis, pre-eclampsia, and thyroid disease. It's suspected of contributing to birth defects also, but findings were inconclusive.

HOW WE ARE EXPOSED TO PFAS and PFOA:
PFOA and GEN X can be found in contaminated water, nonstick cookware, fast food packaging (coating on Styrofoam and other plastics).

SOLUTIONS
- Filter your water, avoid nonstick pans and other PFAS
- We have a right to know if our water is contaminated.
- Contact the EPA: PFASs must be banned

74. TEXTILES

Many clothes and fabrics are made with dyes and toxic chemicals. These chemicals are some o the worst contaminants in our waterways. They can harm our bodies and the ecosystems surrounding clothing factories worldwide. Many brownfield sites today are former leather tannery locations; eather dying uses harsh toxins like Chromium. During laundry, textile toxins and microfibers wash into water ways and the planet's drinking water sources. Green Peace published a great report on the issue, <u>Toxic Threads</u>, that's well worth a read. Toxins used by many clothing manufacturers, especially the cheaper brands, sorry to say, include substances that gravely harm animals and people, water and ecosystems everywhere.

What's Used in Clothes Making?
- **Alkylphenols**: endocrine disruptors, cleaning, dying
- **Chromium 6**: Leather Tanneries
- **Flame Retardants** are applied to fireproof clothing and materials, endocrine disruptors, harm thyroid health, mood and sleep, can cause cancer
- **PFAS**: waterproof materials like Goretex, wrinkle proof items, as well as anything stain resistant, grease resistant, nonstick
- **Formaldehyde**: wrinkle free, static-free, stain free.
- **Chlorinated paraffins** fire retardants, leather and textiles.
- **Anti-fungal agents** known as Organotin Compounds are used in socks, shoes and sports gear treated to prevent odor.
- **Chlorobenzenes** harm thyroid, liver, and nervous system.
- **Azo dyes**: main types of dye used by the textile industry. Some break down into aromatic amines and can cause cancer.
- **Chlorinated solvents**: used to dissolve substances and clean fabrics, they harm the nervous system, liver and kidneys.
- **Phthalates**: reproductive toxins used in fake leather, vinyl
- **Heavy Metals**: neurotoxins found in dyes and pigments,
- Adidas, Nike and Patagonia have pledged to keep PFAS out of their clothing.

Brands who do good and treat animals nicely
There's a new rating system. Check it out here: www.goodonyou.eco

SOLUTIONS: wash clothes with phosphtate free detergent

75. Train Derailments

TRANSPORTING TOXINS BY TRAIN

Train cars often carry hazardous materials, known as hazmat cargo. In February, 2023 the awful accident in East Palestine, Ohio reminded us of the danger when these trains derail.

Train cars full of Vinyl Chloride, Benzene, Ethylene Glycol and other dangerous poisons were set on fire to prevent an even more catastrophic explosion. How can the companies transporting these hazardous materials do so without an emergency barrier and devices in place to prevent the spilling or threat of fire should these train cars fall off the track? The methods and safety guards currently being used clearly are not enough.

Can't shipping be made accident proof? If not why don't we ban companies from using and distributing these substances? Or at least not ship them! It's time the U.S. join the Stockholm Convention. Clearly, we don't have the technology to safely transport these wretched substances, so why are they being transported? Why are they even being used at all? Vinyl Chloride is harmful from cradle to grave, used to make plastic, flooring and PVC pipes. Benzene has no safety limit, any contact can cause cancer. (It's in styrofoam!)

Major Train Accidents and Fires in the last 20 Years

Year	Location	Toxins
9/15/2023	Nebraska	Perchlorate acid Explosion
2/3/2023	East Palestine, OH	Vinyl Chloride, Benzene
2020	Bellingham, WA	Crude Oil
2012	Paulsboro, NJ	Vinyl Chloride
2005	South Carolina	Chlorine Gas

Note: Burning Vinyl Chloride converts it into **Phosgene gas**[387] a highly toxic warfare gas used in WWI! Not good! No bueno.

76. Vinyl Chloride

Vinyl chloride is a manmade chemical that is not found in nature. Almost all vinyl chloride is used to make a type of plastic called PVC, which is used in pipes, wire and cable coatings, car parts, housewares, and packing materials.[388] PVC is made from Petroleum at Petrochemical Facilities.

Vinyl chloride will travel through your body in your blood. Your liver will break it down into other chemicals, some of which can be more harmful than the vinyl chloride itself. Some of these new chemicals can be stored in your body for a long time.

TRADE NAMES
Vinyl chloride can go by many names on labels including: Chloroethene, Chloroethylene, Ethylene monochloride, Monochloroethene, Monochloroethylene, VC, VCM, Vinyl chloride monomer (VCM)

TARGET ORGANS
Liver, central nervous system, blood, respiratory system, lymphatic system

HEALTH EFFECTS
Liver Cancer, brain cancer, blood cancer, lung cancer, weakness, Rare form of liver cancer, Hepatic Angiosarcoma, leukemia

HOW WE ARE EXPOSED
Contaminated water, Vinyl window coverings, flooring, shower curtains, clothing, epoxy resin pipes, PVC, in dining ware, medical equipment, decorations, tobacco smoke, plastic kitchen and household wares

PVC: "Like most plastics, PVC is made with fossil fuel feedstocks. Unlike other plastics, PVC/vinyl also contains substantial amounts of chlorine, upwards of 40%."[389]

SOLUTIONS
- Filer your water for drinking and cooking.
- Avoid vinyl chloride materials

77. WASTE Plastic & Paper

PLASTIC and FOOD PACKAGING: Plastic is a huge problem, especially when it doesn't get thrown away or recycled. Plastic packaging leads pollution in the oceans. Once in the water, plastic gets swallowed by whales, turtles, dolphins, fish, birds, every creature is exposed. There's so much plastic in the oceans from people and commerce, that all these animals are likely eating plastic every time they open their mouths to feed.

If enough plastic is consumed, animals get sick and unable to digest food. If plastic is small enough it can penetrate animal tissues and organs causing who knows what to their amazing selves. Plastic essentially causes animals to starve before we can find out what else may come for them. We must absolutely must, cease the use of disposable plastic and plastic packaging. Please avoid these at home and when dining out:

> Thank you Las Vegas MGM Hotels for banning plastic straws!!

- Straws
- plastic cups
- plastic lids, caps
- plastic water bottles
- plastic bags
- Styrofoam (vinyl benzene)
- plastic utensils: fork, knife,
- plastic cups
- six pack rings
- single use plastic

PAPER PRODUCTS: Paper products are derived from trees, and often, endangered forests! This is a planetary problem for us all. Trees and forests provide us with oxygen that we need to breathe and live. Trees also filter the air pollution and make air cleaner for us to breathe. At this time in the world we need trees more than ever for these two reasons alone.

> **New York City and Maine: Thank you for banning Styrofoam in 2019!**

Trees absorb CO2 (Carbon Dioxide) much like a sink that holds water. When trees and forests are removed to make paper products, we've lost what the planet needs most. Pollution control and clean air. Right now, the majestic Boreal Forest in northern Canada is being decimated to make toilet paper.[390] This is the world's largest intact forest. What a misuse, a sad plan for such beneficial essential natural resources.

Bleached paper products create yet another problem—dioxin pollution in our waterways. When I worked for Greenpeace in 1989 this was my first campaign —ending chlorine bleaching at the paper mills. Since then paper mills have cleaned up their act somewhat, yet dioxin is a persistent pollutant and remains a big problem. Today you can find advisories against eating fish in many rivers and lakes throughout the country due to dioxin & other persistent pollutants.

PAPER PRODUCTS TO AVOID
- Avoid paper from endangered forests
- Avoid paper products that are chlorine bleached
Paper napkins, Paper towel, paper plates, toilet paper
Tissue, writing paper, copy paper, wrapping paper

SUSTAINABLE PAPER PRODUCTS INCLUDE:
- Recycled paper products
- Bamboo and Hemp derived paper materials

SOLUTIONS
- Avoid single use plastic food utensils, bags, containers
- Avoid plastic straws
- Avoid chlorine bleached paper products, or
- Avoid paper products from endangered forests
- Use cloth napkins, handkerchiefs, dish towels, wash cloths
- Use earth friendly dishes, utensils, reusable cups
- Avoid using Styrofoam
- Be sure to throw garbage away in the bin, recycle it, or reuse.
- Help clean up litter even if you didn't put it there, Planet thanks u. Don't be a litterbug.
- Let's go big and encourage all companies to reduce their plastic packaging, and Urge the Government to Ban Styrofoam in all things, especially packaging.
- Avoid bleached paper products. Be part of the solution and reduce your own personal use of harmful plastic materials and bleached paper goods.
- It's going to take practice, one day at a time. We're so used to getting a straw in our drinks, for instance. We have to start somewhere. Next time you're out, just say no straw please, *unless* it's paper from an *un*endangered forest and has 0 PFAS.
- Save Trees, don't cut them down for paper or tissue or Biomass! Use Bamboo paper products instead!
- Save the Oceans, help get the plastic out of our seas please.

78. Window Cleaner

2-BUTOXYETHANOL: This window-cleaning toxic chemical is found in many cleaning and car products. It goes by many names: ethylene glycol monobutyl ether, ethylene glycol butyl ether, ethylene glycol n-butyl ether, Butyl Cellosolve, butyl glycol, butyl Oxitol, glycol butyl ether, Dowanol EB, Gafcol EB, Polysolv EB, and Ektasolve EB. Common abbreviations for 2-butoxyethanol include BE and EGBE.

"Ethylene glycol is a clear, colorless liquid with a sweet smell—but its effects are anything but sweet. One might think the government regulates it, but that is not so. Instead, this and other toxic chemicals are often found in home cleaning products and can be toxifying your house without your knowledge. While the EPA may be soft, The New Jersey Department of Health declares, "2-Butoxyethanol should be handled as a carcinogen—with extreme caution. It can damage the liver and kidneys. There may be no safe level of exposure to a carcinogen so all contact should be reduced to the lowest possible level."[391]

HEALTH EFFECTS
2-Butoxyethanol can lead to headaches; a depressed nervous system; and irritated eyes, nose, and throat. It targets the kidneys, liver, lymphatic system, blood, respiratory system and nervous system.

HOW WE ARE EXPOSED
Contaminated water, toxic emissions found near the manufacturing facilities, using toxic cleaning products. Most of the popular ones all contain ethylene glycol.

SOLUTIONS
- Buy a nontoxic kind or make your own window cleaner. Mix 1 cup water with 1 cup white vinegar, add a teaspoon of dishwashing liquid if desired and mix. Pour into a spray bottle and start cleaning. Make other cleaning products with safe ingredients like vinegar, baking soda and essential oils.
- Write to your senators & representatives. We need to fix the Toxic Substances Control Act (TSCA) and regulate toxins better.

79. XENOBIOTICS

Xeno = foreign, biotics = of or pertaining to life. According to the Merriam Webster Dictionary, Xenobiotics are defined as: a chemical compound (such as a drug, pesticide, or carcinogen) that is foreign to a living organism.[392] Once ingested, xenobiotics are absorbed, transformed, digested by our gut flora. Some are synthesized, excreted, or reabsorbed, some cause no problems, some do.

"Humans ingest a multitude of small molecules that are foreign to the body (xenobiotics), including dietary components, environmental chemicals, and pharmaceuticals. The trillions of microorganisms that inhabit our gastrointestinal tract (the human gut microbiota) can directly alter the chemical structures of such compounds, thus modifying their lifetimes, bioavailabilities, and biological effects. Our knowledge of how gut microbial transformations of xenobiotics affect human health is in its infancy, which is surprising given the importance of the gut microbiota. We currently lack an understanding of the extent to which this metabolism varies between individuals, the mechanisms by which these microbial activities influence human biology, and how we might rationally manipulate these reactions."[393]

HEALTH EFFECTS
Depending on type of toxin or xenobiotic, health effects can include: Nerve and memory impairment, peripheral neuropathies,[394] numbness, pain or tingling in extremities, diabetes, gut and digestive disorders, anxiety, depression, sleep disorders, behavior changes, cancer, autism, dementia, muscle weakness, weakness, lack of energy, slow healing, complications with lungs, kidneys, internal wiring and systems.

SOLUTIONS
- Filter your water
- Reduce exposure to toxins and xenobiotics
- The FDA and EPA must stop being so lenient with toxins in products, manufacturing, and industrial unregulated pollution!
- Help Stop the Flow of health-harming substances entering our waterways. Join the crusade to wake up the EPA and FDA and take back our health! Find out more at www.adoreyourplanet.com.

TOXIC SUBSTANCE CONTROL ACT
TSCA[395]

Established 1974
Updated in 2016: Frank R. Lautenberg Act

Scope of TSCA
Applies to the full lifecycle of chemicals:
- Manufacturing
- Processing
- Distribution and Use
- Waste management

"Certain chronic diseases and disorders are on the rise in the human population, in a manner that can only be explained by environmental factors. Second, studies in laboratory animals as well as human epidemiological studies link exposures to certain chemicals to those same chronic diseases."[396]

TSCA is regulated by the EPA.

Toxic Substances Not Controlled by TSCA:
- Pesticides (EPA)
- Personal Care Products, Cosmetics (FDA)
- Pharmaceuticals (FDA)
- Food and Food Packaging (FDA)

SECTION THREE
IN DANGER:
Human Health & Planet
- **Animals**
- **Ecosystems**
- **Waterways**
- **People**

> The nation behaves well if it treats the natural resources as assets, which it must turn over to the next generation increased, and not impaired, in value.
> **President Theodore Roosevelt**

Water's effect on wildlife

Poor water quality can harm species and habitats, and must be assessed in activities such as wastewater discharge. Many factors are known to cause poor water quality: temperature, sedimentation, runoff, erosion, dissolved oxygen, pH, decayed organic materials, pesticides, and an array of other toxic and hazardous substances.

The poor quality of irrigation drainage water and discharges from collecting systems are known to cause the accumulation of toxic substances as well as reproductive and developmental problems in shorebirds, waterfowl, and fish.
U.S. Fish and Wildlife Service

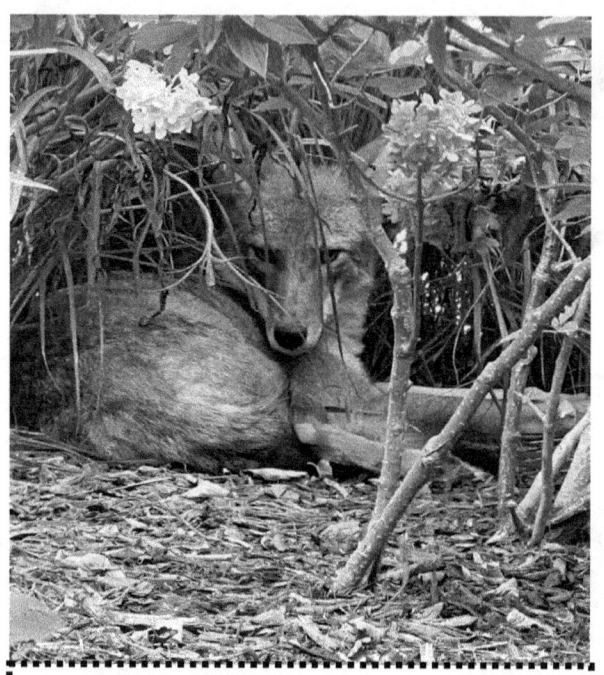

I am in favor of animal rights as well as human rights. That is the way of a whole human being.
President Abraham Lincoln

1. Animals in Danger

The greatness of a nation and its moral progress can be judged by the way its animals are treated, Gandhi

The plight of wild animals around the world is not great. While many are adapting to loss of habitat from human activity and development, they're also forced to endure human made pollution. Especially for animals who live in water this is such an unfair burden. Yet all animals and people alike are harmed when water they drink is corrupted by toxic substances. By polluting water, industries and people cause animal disease and extinction.

ANIMAL WELFARE ACT

The Animal Welfare Act (AWA) requires that minimum standards of care and treatment be provided for certain animals bred for commercial sale, used in research, transported commercially or exhibited to the public. Let's get all animals including farm animals and all animals trapped or held in captivity included in the Animal Welfare Act.

MARINE MAMMALS PROTECTION ACT

The Marine Mammal Protection Act (MMPA) was enacted on October 21, 1972. All marine mammals are protected under the MMPA. The MMPA prohibits, with certain exceptions, the "take" of marine mammals in U.S. waters and by U.S. citizens on the high seas, and the importation of marine mammals and marine mammal products into the U.S.

Congress passed the Marine Mammal Protection Act of 1972 based on the following findings and policies:
- Some marine mammal species or stocks may be in danger of extinction or depletion as a result of human activities;
- These species or stocks must not be permitted to fall below their optimum sustainable population level ("depleted");
- Measures should be taken to replenish these species or stocks;
- There is inadequate knowledge of the ecology and population dynamics; and Marine mammals have proven to be resources of great international significance.[397]

Captivity: Captivity is yet another tragic imposition affecting animals the world over. Factory farms, fur farms, zoos, aquariums and other unfortunate environments that provide far too little space for wild animals to be healthy. Wild Horses are captured and held hostage by mean people at facilities where they are no longer allowed to run, be with family, to be themselves, wild and free. Whales and Dolphins are stolen from the wild seas and sent to aquariums to entertain for the rest of their lives. These are small pools for them, hardly adequate living situations.

Sonar: Sonar in water is killing numerous whale species and dolphins. The animals ear drums are damaged so badly they can't prevent beaching themselves. Currently, there are no laws or regulations protecting animals from water pollution, or sonar, or ensuring that they're treated humanely while held captive at farms or facilities. Animals of all kinds are inquisitive and playful. They feel pain when injured, and feel scared when treated cruelly.

WHALES: 2023's failure to get Toki back to the sea in time, and her tragic instead of magic ending is so telling of the times we're in. How wrong it is to keep these incredible creatures in captivity. We must free all Orcas and Dolphins and let them be free as they're meant to be. If we must observe them and be entertained, let us go to them and watch them play in the sea. What kind of industry is this that robs whales of their freedom and family?

WILDHORSES: Wild horses in America are fighting for their lives. Why? Because people are mismanaging our Public Lands. The US Department of the Interior's Bureau of Land Management (BLM) is making a mess of Public Lands. These horses-- symbols of freedom and America are being bullied and harassed by obnoxious helicopters. Forced into tiny corrals, the horses are harassed and treated very poorly.

These incredible majestic horses are Keystone Species for their habitat and the Public Lands ecosystem. They have a right to live on Public Lands forever. They are not harming anyone. Yet due to leases for mining, drilling, and cattle, the government somehow determined that the horses have to go. This is so wrong! Most of the horses are sold at auction, and many of them end up in slaughterhouses in Mexico.
We must help these horses remain free on our Public Lands where they belong. It's outrageous that the Department of the Interior authorizes the Bureau of Land Management to capture them. BARBARIC! This is a violation of the Law established to protect them, the Free Roaming Wildhorse and Burro Act of 1971. America, America, God shed his grace on thee.

Endangered Species Act

When Congress passed the Endangered Species Act (ESA) in 1973, it recognized that our rich natural heritage is of "esthetic, ecological, educational, recreational, and scientific value to our Nation and its people." It further expressed concern that many of our nation's native plants and animals were in danger of becoming extinct.

The purpose of the ESA is to protect and recover imperiled species and the ecosystems upon which they depend. It is administered by the U.S. Fish and Wildlife Service and the Commerce Department's National Marine Fisheries Service (NMFS). The FWS has primary responsibility for terrestrial and freshwater organisms, while the responsibilities of NMFS are mainly marine wildlife such as whales and anadromous fish such as salmon.

Some of the Species listed:

Aspen Tree	Foxes	Rattlesnake
Bats	Fir Tree	Sage Grouse
Bears	Frogs	Salamanders
Beetle	Garter snake	Sea Turtles
Bison	Gecko	Seals
Butterfly	Grasshopper	Snails
Cactus	Iguana	Sparrow
Caribou	Jaguar	Spruce Tree
Condor	Kingfisher	Sumac
Coral	Lynx	Tern
Crayfish	Milkweed	Toad
Cypress Trees	Monkeyflower	Tortoise
Dolphins	Mussels	Warbler
Fairy Shrimp	Oak Tree	Whales
Falcons	Owl	Alligator
Fern	Panthers	Whooping Crane
Finch	Pine Tree	Wolf
	Mountain Lion	Woodpeckers
	Puma	Yellow Billed Cukoo
		Wild Horses

WHAT CAN WE DO TO HELP:

- Take care of the earth, help animals
- Take personal responsibility for keeping your garbage and toxins out of waterways,
- Organize a neighborhood clean-up, beach clean ups
- HELP SAVE BIODIVERSITY and KEYSTONE SPECIES
- **Write to your Senators and Reps and insist that we protect Wild Horses and Burros. We must enforce the protections established under 1971's Free Roaming Wildhorse and Burro Act. for wild horses out west**
- Don't use soap or shampoo in lakes, rivers, or oceans
- Help keep water ways and oceans clean
- Conserve water use
- Be part of the solution, help end pollution
- Help reduce dead zones and toxic algae by curbing pesticide and fertilizer runoff,
- Avoid plastic & toxins
- Leave places better than when you found them

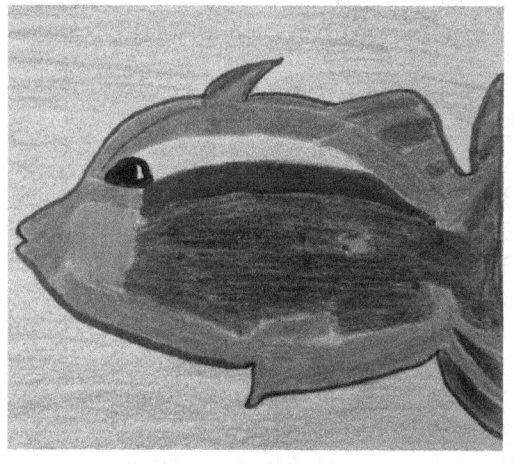

- Take care of the wild places you go and respect the wild animals

> "Water is uniquely vulnerable to pollution. Known as a "universal solvent," water is able to dissolve more substances than any other liquid on earth and mix with it, causing water pollution."

- Do the right thing. Be nice to animals

2. Ecosystems in Danger

Visible evidence of toxic wrongdoing can be witnessed everyday throughout all the world's ecosystems. Wildlife, flora, and fauna in all its majesty is sorely injured by humanity's discourteous behavior. Pollution assaults, be it toxic pesticides, overuse and misuse of unnatural substances, or wrongful waste management—it all results in vast amounts harm to our natural resources. Animals and ecosystems depend on water and air just as we do. Their health, like ours, depends on a clean and safe environment. Pollution affects ecosystems in every corner of the world. The big and the little creatures alike are all impacted. How it effects every creature varies by species and exposure level as well as duration.

Being citizens of the earth bears a responsibility to care for our co-inhabitants to some degree, the least of which is to keep our surroundings, our environment clean and free of harmful substances. While as individuals we can make some impact, it's going to require industrial and government participation to achieve success. Has not the time come for this collaboration? Disease and Cancer rates do not have to keep driving upwards for humanity, nor does toxic pollution have to continue. We are sensible beings, so let's act sensibly and stop the toxic pollution. It's not that difficult. Step one, any industry causing water or air pollution must cease doing so immediately.

ECOSYSTEMS

Ecosystems are habitats, home for a diverse collection of animals and plant life. Ecosystems vary by location and natural elements. Some are woodlands, forests, treetops, mountaintops, deserts, prairies, grasslands, savannah, in the soil. Ecosystems are in the water also—oceans, lakes, wetlands, creeks. Ecosystems can be viewed from many vantage points, with a big picture lens, or smaller like a tide pool or even tinier as in a drop of water if you're looking under a microscope. Life comes in all sizes and types in this amazing world we live in. Nature is full of living creatures adapted to their surroundings, their habitat. These are natural communities of animal and plants and insects in balance, keystone species holding neighborhoods together, symbiotic relationships between creatures helping each other survive.

Balance is the key to the health of an ecosystem. Nature has established ecosystems that we are fortunate to share this beautiful planet with.

Delicate they are even when teeming with strong beasts weighing two tons. Left alone, ecosystems do wildly well and generally recover from adversity and afflictions that may come their way. Unfortunately for many animals and ecosystems, mankind's interference has led to loss and instability. From managing wolves in Yellowstone, to frogs and amphibians bathed in endocrine disruptors, to the wild horses stolen from their land and corralled for auction, to oil spills in the most pristine waters in the world--we continually demonstrate our disregard for the planet and all its ecosystems. I do believe though that on this blue planet there are more of us who care about helping the planet than there are who want to cause harm. So, Humanity, let's get to work.

What's Harming Animals and Ecosystems:
- Toxic pollution released into the waterways
- Monocropping farming & rampant use of insecticides
- Agricultural Runoff & Untreated sewage going in water
- Excessive use of pesticides
- More Roundup used in desiccating crops
- Biosolids used as Fertilizer!!!!
- Oil spills, Pipeline spills, Shipping disasters
- Plastic Pellets, Microbeads, Plastic garbage, packaging waste
- Factory Farm Confinement, GMO Animal Feed, Traps and inhumane people
- Toxic industrial pollution & chemicals in water and in the air
- Poaching, big game hunting, trapping, USDA's Wildlife Services

Pollution, especially toxic wastewater and agricultural pollutants harm ecosystems and all life forms—human beings, animals, trees, plants, soil, wildlife, virtually every aspect of the natural world. Is this something we must endure? Can't we do better than to allow irresponsible industries to destroy our planet with their destructive methods and chemicals? This is our home they're destroying. Without the planet we have nothing. Together we can and must change this. Just think, imagine, without all these chemicals, the world may become not just healthier but happier and more peaceful too! Maybe people would have an easier time getting along and resolving their differences. Certain pollutants are known for causing aggression and depression. Rather than close or end all these businesses, there must be a way to innovate and be resourceful. It's not as if toxic substances add a degree of usefulness to any product. If industries want to keep operating, they need to use safe substances not toxic ones. Is that too much to ask?

We have one world, we all have one body, shouldn't the companies we buy products from be taking care of this world also? Shouldn't their products support and bring us health? Any pollutants emitted by industry impact us all— either now, or eventually contributing to the planet's toxic load. Alternatives must exist or can be invented that will be safe and nontoxic from start to finish. There are ways to capture emissions before they leak and escape. Emissions can be turned into fuel and energy somehow. Pipelines and boats can certainly be made to be leakproof without chance of mishap.

For those corporations who can't or won't, or don't want to, close them down until they decide to be health friendly. We don't need to instill taxes on all, when we could just change the way things are being done. That's how to clean up the environment and put climate change in reverse. The corporations and industries must cease polluting the water and the air. Period. We can't just let them trade carbon credits and continue polluting. Trading credits for pollution is nothing, no winners-- a no win game for the Planet. Let the polluters suffer the consequences for what harm they commit, hefty fees and higher taxes. Why exempt any polluting industry or pay them tax dollar subsidies when they don't need it? Right now, we need their help not vice versa.

We live in such careless times, but it does not need to remain that way. I'm tired of all the entitled corporations harming our world, aren't you?

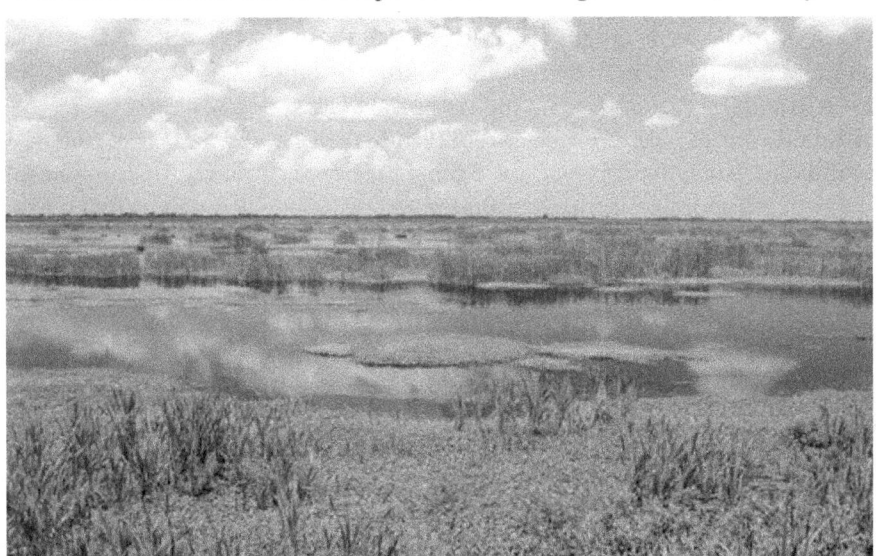

Source: USDA[398] Wetland's Conservation Program

3. Groundwater in Danger

Aquifers, Rivers, Streams, Lakes, and Wetlands throughout this country sustain us and provide our most essential resource for life: water. The magnificent waterways are all interconnected within the earth's water cycle. There's scientific consensus that the water on earth remains constant and has since the beginning of time. What falls from the sky becomes the lake and the groundwater, and that water eventually evaporates one day to return once again somewhere as condensation falling from the clouds. This is why keeping water clean is so important. The new level of toxic contaminants mankind has created will continue causing harm for all species, mankind included. It's vital we replace the most toxic amongst them and let health rule.

Aquifers & Groundwater

While many of our water sources can be seen from above, many of us obtain our drinking water from the vast water located beneath the surface of the earth. Ground water is comprised of water that makes its way through the soil and cracks in the earth to the bedrock below. Underground aquifers, rivers, streams, and caves lie beneath us almost everywhere. Residential wells draw from this water as do industries and municipalities.

When more water is drawn and pumped out than what is replaced by rain and precipitation, the water levels fall. In some places, water levels have shrunk considerably and the risk of water shortages abound. Through careful, considerate, and mindful use of water we can maintain healthy and sustainable levels. We must take care of these gifts of water and prevent spoilage through pollution. As we gather ourselves together to end corporate pollution of all kinds, we will indeed save our waterways.

Groundwater Pollution Goes Undetected

According to the USGS (US Geological Survey), "Contaminants can be natural or human-induced. Groundwater will normally look clear and clean because the ground naturally filters out particulate matter. But, natural and manmade chemicals can be in groundwater.

THE WATER CYCLE

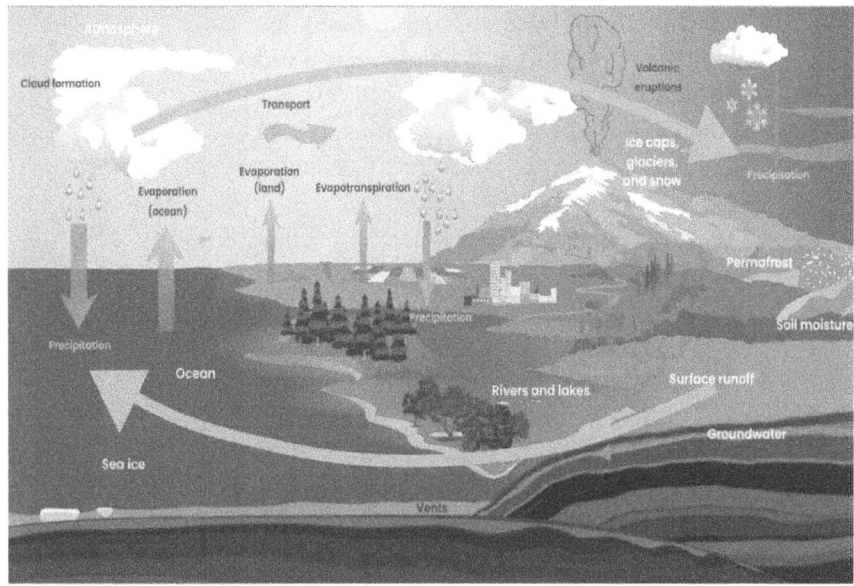

The Water Cycle, Source: PBS[399]

As groundwater flows through the ground, metals such as iron and manganese are dissolved and may later be found in high concentrations in the water. Industrial discharges, urban activities, agriculture, and disposal of waste--all can undermine groundwater quality.
Contaminants can be human-induced, as from leaking fuel tanks or toxic chemical spills. Pesticides and fertilizers applied to lawns and crops accumulate and migrate to the water table. Leakage from septic tanks and/or waste-disposal sites also can introduce bacteria to the water; and pesticides and fertilizers that seep into farmed soil can eventually end up in water drawn from a well. Or, a well might have been placed in land that was once used for something like a garbage or chemical dumpsite. In any case, if you have your own well supplying drinking water to your home, it is wise to have your well water tested."[400]

Threats to Aquifers and Groundwater:
- Agriculture Runoff, Pesticides, Factory Farm Waste (not regulated), Toxic Pesticides: herbicides and insecticides
- Phosphate Mining slurry and sink holes
- Unregulated waste from pesticide manufacturing
- Unregulated waste from pharmaceutical manufacturing

Threats to Aquifers and Groundwater *(cont.)*:
- Lawn Chemicals, Weedkillers, Insecticides
- Chemicals applied to golf courses and fields
- Pollution from petrochemical facilities
- Unregulated waste from the Plastics industry
- Unregulated waste from the Fertilizer industry
- PFAS pollution
- Unregulated Pharmaceutical and Biotech pollution[401]
- Nanoparticle pollution
- Fracking, drilling, mining, wastewater and underground injections (not regulated)
- Nitrate from fertilizer Runoff
- Synthetic fertilizer
- Unregulated industrial pollution
- Arsenic, manganese and heavy metals
- Dicamba, Glyphosate, Chloryrifos and all toxic pesticides

So far in this book, we reviewed many different contaminants that are mucking up are precious water sources. For far too long, governments have sacrificed the integrity of our planet's water resources in exchange for corporate and industry growth. As a result, bodies of water the world over are tainted with toxins. We also have allowed construction of pipelines to carry fossil fuels over and under fragile water sources. Will we ever learn? If industries discontinued releases of harmful pollutants and responsibly cleaned up their waste, we can decelerate and reverse this damage. Unfortunately, most industries are not yet reducing their toxic chemical wastewater emissions and many have avoided regulations. Population growth and pollution have drastically increased the need for people, government, and industry to quickly act responsibly in matters concerning water.

SOLUTIONS

Let's put pressure on the EPA and our State Officials to end water pollution. All toxic pollution must be regulated and must be stopped. We have no time to waste! Help get your elected officials on board and your Mayor involved, especially if you have serious water pollution and related health issues in your town.

4. Lakes in Danger

Lakes are wondrous ecosystems teeming with life. The animals that live in and depend upon lakes for survival include countless species of birds and water fowl as well as amphibious creatures and fish and scores of other animals that use the lakes for hydration, bathing, hunting and lodging. The importance of lakes big and small around the world cannot be overstated. Local animals as well as migratory animals of every kind have a relationship with these magical bodies of water.

Besides providing life and sustenance, lakes can also be abused and ill conserved. When pollutants and degradation enter these waterways, the results are ever not enchanting or life giving. Larger lakes may have the advantage of dilution—meaning when assaulted by pollutants, the vast size can help dilute the offensive agent. Smaller lakes and ponds sadly don't have that ability. In either case, only so much of any pollutant can be absorbed by lakes before effects begin to show.

One of the most harmful additions to lakes at this time falls within the agricultural runoff category. Fertilizer, pesticides, and agricultural waste can convert a lake brimming with life to a graveyard quickly if too much nitrate and phosphorous enter bringing toxic algae to life.

THE GREAT LAKES

The Great Lakes are considered the most significant bodies of fresh water in the world. While vast in size, these lakes are not immune to health issues and water loss. Five lakes all interconnected hold over 20% of the world's fresh surface water.

In recent studies, the Great Lakes are identified as especially polluted. This disturbs not only the quality of the drinking water in towns that rely on them, but also the health of the marine and aquatic life as well as the lake ecosystem at large. Lake Michigan has been identified as heavily polluted with mercury, which in turn affects everyone living near the lake and drinking water derived from it. Besides mercury pollution in the lakes, one of the greatest crimes is the dumping of raw sewage. Cities like Milwaukee have chosen this as a way to combat flooding during heavy rainstorms. In May of 2004, for instance, Milwaukee dumped 4.6 billion gallons of raw sewage in the lake.[402] In so doing the entire aquaculture ecosystem was bombarded with parasites, bacteria, and viruses. This is not a reasonable solution to prevent flooding. Such actions violate the Clean Water Act, result in beach closings, and cause undue harm to the lake and the species residing within it. The government and the EPA must uphold the laws that protect our resources and penalize those who violate such laws

TAR SANDS OIL THREATENS GREAT LAKES!

Right now, a Tar Sands oil pipeline, Line 5, crosses under lake Michigan. We must get this pipeline shut down! See Pipelines, pages 132-133!

Risks to all lakes and bodies of water include:
- Toxic Pollutants, industrial discharges, and bad manufacturing
- Agricultural runoff and Toxic Algae
- Sewer and stormwater runoff
- Plastic, Microbeads, Microfibers
- Cargo ship discharges, Invasive Species
- Toxic products that get washed down drains, quats
- PCBs, DDT, flame retardants, toxic chemicals, heavy metals

Pollution impacts not just wildlife in the lakes but everyone living near the lakes and drinking water derived from them.

Plastic: Plastic litter, garbage and products containing plastic microbeads are devastating all water bodies worldwide. Lakes, streams, beaches, oceans, wetlands are all affected and all creatures living in or dependent on these waters are suffering. This is tragic and completely preventable. Humans create the plastic waste, litter and garbage. Through mindful action we can stop the pollution.

Toxins: Toxins from industry, cleaning chemicals, personal care products, agricultural run off, and garbage hurt the lakes. These substances migrate to the water from discharge pipes, they settle from air pollution, from ships, from nearby drilling and fracking sites, they get washed down drains and toilets, they come from pharmaceuticals and they inevitably cause great harm. Debris on shores as well as on the lake bottoms add to this toxic load. The majority of these pollutants are endocrine disruptors, reproductive toxins and carcinogens.

Even the best water purification facilities at this time can't remove them all, so drinking water derived from the lakes can have residues of these substances. Animals living in the water have no escape or filter to protect them or the food they eat.

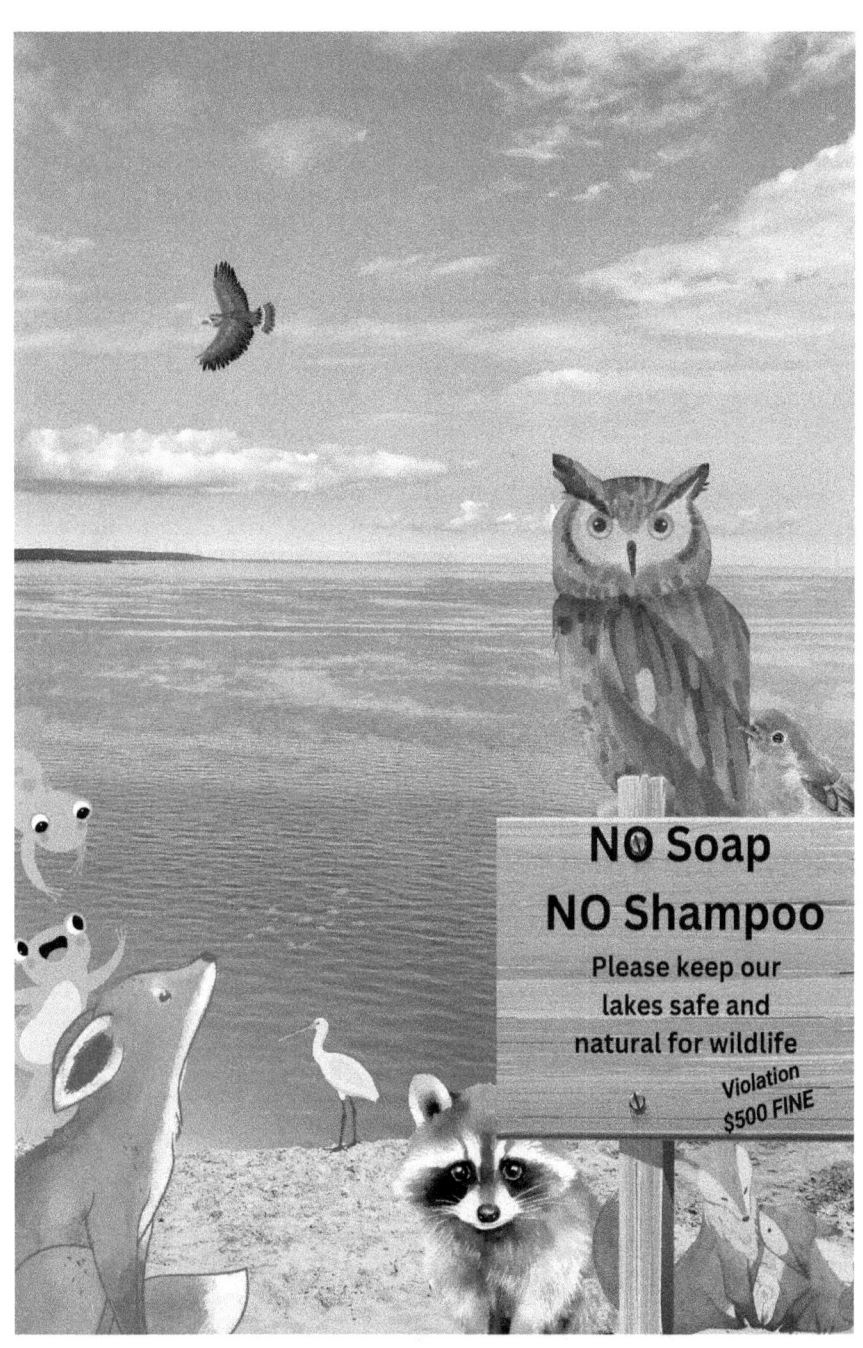

Raw Sewage: Besides industrial pollution in the lakes, one of the dangerous discharges is raw sewage. Sewage itself contains not just what is expelled but anything poured down the drain; so essentially, it's household cleaners, pharmaceuticals, personal care products, you name it. Dumping raw sewage into the lakes is typically chosen as a way to combat flooding during heavy rainstorms. For instance, in May of 2004, Milwaukee dumped 4.6 billion gallons of raw sewage into lake Michigan. In so doing, the entire aquaculture ecosystem was bombarded with parasites, bacteria and viruses. Is this a reasonable method to prevent flooding? Such actions violate the Clean Water Act, result in beach closings, and cause undue harm to the species residing within the water.

Water Loss: Water loss can be natural or spurred by climate change, or it can be from bottling water or from dredging. "The historic changes and dredging of the St. Clair River over the years has resulted in changes to the riverbed that has increased the amount of water going down the river, carrying more and more water out of Michigan and Huron, through the lower Lakes, and out to the ocean. This water is irreplaceable," explains Roger Gauthier, Lead Hydrologist for the Great Lakes Commission. "It has reached a point where the damage is profound. It is now threatening the hydrological integrity of the entire upper Lakes. Since 1970, the drainage hole, which continues to grow larger, has resulted in an overall water level decline of nearly two feet, or 60 centimeters, in Lakes Michigan and Huron and Georgian Bay. If put together in one place, that two-foot loss would be the size of a block of water one mile high and four miles long by four miles wide. Georgian Bay Association[403]

Microfibers: Microfibers are a rather new discovery bringing harm to fish and water life. The culprit seems to be washing clothes. These tiny fibers wash off synthetics, fleece, and most fibers in the laundry and go with the rinse water down the drain and eventually into the waterways.

BAN PLASTIC
BAN STYROFOAM
BAN PLASTIC PELLETS
SAVE THE GREAT LAKES!

Call the President and ask him to stop Line 5 by revoking the presidential permit that allows it to operate![404] (More information available on pages 132-133). Thank you.

Review: Agricultural Operations and Water Quality

"Agricultural operations can have significant effects on water quality, due to the extent of farm activities on the landscape, the soil-disturbing nature of those activities, and associated impacts from sediment, nutrients, pesticides, and herbicides. The National Water Quality Assessment shows that agricultural runoff is the leading cause of water quality impacts to rivers and streams, the third leading source for lakes, and the second largest source of impairments to wetlands. **About a half million tons of pesticides, 12 million tons of nitrogen, and 4 million tons of phosphorus fertilizer are applied annually to crops in the continental United States.** Soil erosion, nutrient loss, bacteria from livestock manure, and pesticides constitute the primary stressors to water quality.

"Why? Nutrients in fertilizer and livestock manure, pesticides, and other substances don't always remain stationary on the landscape where they are applied. Runoff, infiltration, and irrigation return flows can move these contaminants into local streams, rivers, and groundwater. Rainfall and snowmelt transport the majority of these pollutants to surface waters, but other factors (e.g., cattle loafing in stream corridors, stream channel erosion) can also degrade water quality.

"The effects of this runoff vary widely, depending on the type of operation, landscape conditions, soils, climate, and farm management practices. Increased levels of nitrogen and phosphorus from fertilizer and manure can stimulate algal blooms in lakes and rivers, which can lead to the development of hypoxic (low oxygen) conditions that are harmful to aquatic life. Algae can also affect recreational uses of local streams, downstream reservoirs, and estuaries. Excessive sedimentation from erosion can overwhelm aquatic ecosystems, smother breeding areas, and degrade coastal and marine ecosystems—including coral reefs. **Bacteria and nutrients from livestock and poultry manure can cause beach and shellfish bed closures and affect drinking water supplies. Pesticide runoff to streams can pose risks to aquatic life, fish-eating wildlife, and drinking water supplies.**

"Pollutants from agricultural operations can also enter groundwater and degrade sources of drinking water. **Human health impacts might occur as a result. More than 13 million U.S. households obtain their drinking water from private wells.** Pollution from pesticides, fertilizers, and animal manure can enter groundwater depending upon local land use and geologic conditions."[405] *SOURCE: EPA*

SAVING WHALES

Threats to Whales, Dolphins, Porpoises and Marine Animals

THREAT	SOLUTION
Fishing nets and gear	Ropeless fishing gear[406]
Ship Strikes, Collisions	NOAA lower speed limit please
Plastic Pollution	Clean up Ocean, don't litter
Sonar	Reduce use of Sonar

Whales are a Planetary Keystone Species whose relationship with phytoplankton supplies the oxygen we need for survival.[407]

NOAA: Please fast track lowering the speed limit for ships and sea vessels

"One way to lessen the number of ship strikes is by imposing lower speed limits for vessels. In 2022, NOAA proposed changes to the speed rules they implemented in 2008 for vessels longer than 65 feet to protect critically endangered North Atlantic right whales."[408]

SOLUTIONS

- Contact your elected officials and ask them to support and fast track NOAA implementing slower speed rules for ships, ban plastic, and organize beach and sea trash clean ups.
- Help clean up plastic pollution. Plastic is killing countless animals in the seas and on land.
- Help keep toxins and plastic out of the waterways. Toxins are a burden to waterways and influence warming temperatures
- Help commercial fishermen transition to ropeless fishing technology to save dolphins, whales, turtles and other animals.

5. Oceans in Danger

The world's oceans are in a very fragile state. Some people are under the impression that oceans have the capacity to purify and rebalance themselves under any condition. This is simply not true. Excessive amounts of pollution, plastic, oil drilling, carbonic acid, and overfishing are destroying the oceans.

> Future generations would not forgive us for having deliberately spoiled their last opportunity and the last opportunity is today.
> **Jacques Cousteau**

Oil spills alone cause extensive and irretrievable harm. Because of rising fungus and virus infections, coral reefs are dying, starfish are dying and many marine species are in danger. This further adds to the desecration of what once was a balanced, sustainable ecosystem.

HARMS TO OCEANS INCLUDE:
- **PLASTIC** does not biodegrade. Microbeads, Microfibers and plastic of all kinds result in ocean garbage patches,
- **OIL DRILLING** and **OIL SPILLS:** releases vast amounts of heavy metals and methane into the marine environment. How about we make pipelines and ships that won't leak and are crash- and explosion-proof?
- **FERTILIZER, PESTICIDES, FARM RUNOFF**
- **NANOPARTICLES in SUNSCREEN**
- **BRINE FROM DESALINIZATION**
- **SHIPS COLLIDING WITH ANIMALS**
- **OVERFISHING** due to modernized fishing techniques—such as long-lining, oversized nets and bottom trawling—a wide variety of ocean life is harmed. Sea turtles, starfish, seabirds, dolphins and countless other species (often referred to as *bycatch*) are constantly caught in nets and left for dead.
- **PERSISTENT ORGANIC POLLUTANTS** Whales and seals contain a very high amount of bioaccumulative toxins like dioxin and PCBs in their bodies.
- **SONAR** can kill whales, dolphins and porpoises

Oceans & Plastic

The Plastic Graveyard

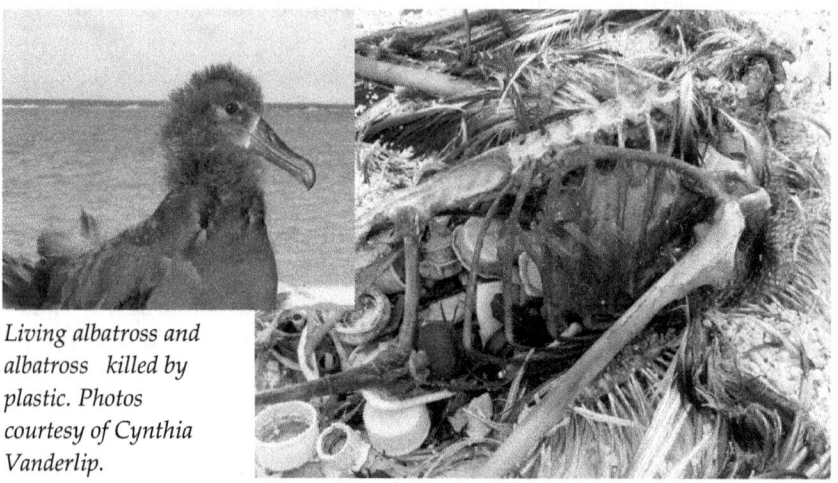

Living albatross and albatross killed by plastic. Photos courtesy of Cynthia Vanderlip.

The oceans are in a dire state. From plastic pollution and garbage patches to drilling, oil spills, and excess pollution emissions the Oceans need our help! We have a responsibility as citizens of the earth to do what we can to preserve and care for our oceans. Keeping our impact to a minimum is crucial. Imagine if each of us, every citizen on earth took responsibility for the plastic they used and kept our use of plastic to null. If each industry became more earth friendly and refused to sell or use substances that caused harm to oceans or people! Then we just might turn the tide and save our wonderful oceans.

CAUSES OF OCEAN DEGRADATION
- POLLUTION, SPILLS, OLD FISHING GEAR,
- PLASTIC, WASTE, TOXINS, PELLETS, WARMING
- IRRESPONSIBLE PEOPLE & INDUSTRIES

DEAD ZONES

When agricultural runoff loaded with fertilizer enters water systems, the high phosphorous and nitrogen levels cut off oxygen. This causes eutrophication, otherwise known as Dead Zones. Marine life cannot live in water without oxygen. Pesticides worsen Dead Zones.

World's Largest Dead Zone in Gulf of Mexico

"This large dead zone size shows that nutrient pollution, primarily from agriculture and developed land runoff in the Mississippi River watershed is continuing to affect the nation's coastal resources and habitats in the Gulf. These nutrients stimulate massive algal growth that eventually decomposes, which uses up the oxygen needed to support life in the Gulf. This loss of oxygen can cause the loss of fish habitat or force them to move to other areas to survive, decreased reproductive capabilities in fish species and a reduction in the average size of shrimp caught."[409]

RED TIDE: Red Tides occur mainly in the Gulf of Mexico. This is where phosphate mining/fertilizer facility waste combines with agricultural runoff. The result is extensive bacterial infestation and fish kills, otherwise known as Red Tides. Sugarcane farming runoff may be increasing the frequency.

STARFISH: Scientists have determined that a virus is behind the massive starfish die-off in the Pacific Ocean. Could ocean acidification also be to blame? What is it that's making their immune systems so weak that they are not able to fight this off and survive? Perhaps it's natural and has no chemical or radiation precursor, but considering all the toxic pollution dumped in the ocean one must wonder.

OCEAN ACIDIFICATION

The oceans are a carbon sink absorbing carbon dioxide. Scientists estimate the oceans are capturing roughly 22 million tons daily, and this is causing increased acidity levels. Not all sea animals can or will be able to adapt. Eventually the oceans will reach a saturation point and no longer be able to absorb CO_2 but will instead release it.

BAN PLASTICS
BAN SYNTHETIC FERTILIZER
BAN TOXIC PESTICIDES
FINE POLLUTERS
EPA PLEASE
REGULATE ALL INDUSTRIES

PLASTICS in the OCEAN

Top 3 Plastics found most on the Ocean Floor:
1. **POLYPROPOLENE**
2. **POLYETHYLENE**
3. **POLYESTER**

The total amount of microplastics deposited on the bottom of oceans has tripled in the past two decades with a progression that correlates with the use and production of plastics since the 1960s. Researchers explain that the sediments analyzed have remained unaltered on the seafloor since they were deposited decades ago. "This has allowed us to see how, since the 1980s, but especially in the past two decades, the accumulation of polyethylene and polypropylene particles from packaging, bottles and food films has increased, as well as polyester from synthetic fibers in clothing fabrics," explains Michael Grelaud, ICTA-UAB researcher. The amount of these three types of particles reaches 1.5mg per kilogram of sediment collected, with polypropylene being the most abundant, followed by polyethylene and polyester. Despite awareness campaigns on the need to reduce single-use plastic, data from annual marine sediment records show that we are still far from achieving this. Policies at the global level in this regard could contribute to improving this serious problem.[410]

POLYESTER: #1 PET, Polyethylene Terephthalate
- plastic bottles

POLYETHYLENE: #2 HDPE, High-Density
- milk and laundry detergent jugs, disposable utensils

POLYETHYLENE: #4 LDPE, Low-Density Polyethylene:
- squeeze bottles, shrink wraps, drycleaner and bread bags

POLYPROPYLENE: #5 PP,
- food packaging, yogurt containers, chip bags, cereal

PLASTIC PELLETS

Yet another type of microplastic harming wildlife and accumulating in fish are plastic pellets. Petrochemical companies must stop making plastic.

SOLUTIONS

- Don't Litter or be a litterbug, put trash in garbage can or recycle it
- Please Don't use products with microbeads
- Install a filter on your washing machine to capture microfibers
- Keep plastic and all garbage out of waterways
- If you see plastic debris in the street, please get it in the trash.
- Avoid using or buying plastic, biodegradable natural materials are best for planet and for us.
- Ask K Cup makers to use biodegradable materials, not plastic
- Don't use toxic fertilizer and pesticides that get in run off.
- Please all construction, cosmetic and consumer product manufacturing companies, please cease adding plastic microbeads to products you produce.
- BE A WATER PROTECTOR.
- HELP TEACH OTHERS NOT TO LITTER, AVOID PLASTIC, KEEP OUR OCEANS AND WATERWAYS CLEAN.

THE OCEAN CLEAN UP MODEL

An entrepreneur, Boyan Slat, has designed one of the most intriguing pollution filtering mechanisms that could potentially remove all the litter currently recking havoc in the oceans. Let's hope this works! www.theoceancleanup.com.

BE A PLASTIC HUNTER

If you see it pick it up to keep it out of the oceans. Then put it in the trash or the recycling bin. Thank you! Please wash your hands after.

- Six Pack Rings, Plastic Bottles and Bottle Caps
- Plastic Bags, Straws, and Styrofoam
- Plastic utensils, Plastic packages and containers
- Any and all things made of plastic

Worldwide Plastic Treaty

Plastic is all around us, in countless products and containers, things we use everyday. While plastic containers and all can be useful, plastic doesn't biodegrade. As a result, it is the most abundant toxin spewing uncontrollably across the surface of the earth- from oceans and lakes, to cities and towns. Now it's making its ways inside of our bodies! Plastic harms all animals and plants and everybody in its path. Reduce, reuse, recycle, and repurpose plastic when possible. Get creative!

End Plastic Pollution
Today there is hope plastics will be banned in the near future! In March 2022, A Resolution to end plastic pollution was adopted by the United Nations Environment Assembly.[411] The goal is by the end of 2024 a framework that can be used internationally for governments to work together in banning plastic pollution.

Many hotels and restaurants and Cities (NYC) and Maine have banned single use plastics and plastic straws, and styrofoam containers, and plastic bags, but more involvement is needed.

This is going to take all of us, persons and companies, governments and cities, and industries at all levels including transport and manufacturing, the supply chain. Transocean vessels carrying plastic pellets and recycling debris need a fool proof system of non-spillage, or we just can't ship such things any more. The ocean cannot tolerate any more abuse, and neither can our health absorb any more exposure.

Thank you to to those who care about tackling the plastic issue. We are making strides toward reducing toxic substances. Let's continue the work and use our momentum to diminish all the hazardous toxins harming our planet and our bodies. The impacts of plastic production and pollution on the triple planetary crisis of climate change, nature loss and pollution are a catastrophe in the making. Reported by Pew Trusts: Plastic production soared from 2 million tons in 1950 to 348 million tons in 2017. The industry is valued at $522.6 billion (US) and is expected to double by 2040!!![412] Could our world endure such a doubling of that magnitude! I think not. Thank God for this Treaty! Just in time! Exposure to plastics can harm health, have a negative effect on fertility, hormonal, metabolic and neurological activity.[413]

SPECIAL REPORT
RED TIDES

Red tides have been occurring for hundreds, perhaps thousands of years. Yet today's pollution stemming from agricultural runoff and fertilizer facilities is likely the reason they're worse and more frequent.[414] Like factory farms have manure ponds, phosphate fertilizer facilities stretching from the Louisiana Gulf Coast to Florida have radioactive gypsum ponds[415]. This stuff is so unsafe the EPA won't allow disposal anywhere![416] "Because the wastes are concentrated, phosphogypsum is more radioactive than the original phosphate rock."[417]

Add to that all the runoff from Florida's sugar cane and citrus farming. Much of this runoff is diverted away from the wetlands that would naturally filter out pollutants, and sent instead directly to the sea.[418] Toxic pollution from Florida's phosphate fertilizer facilities frequently escapes into waterways[419] and ocean water.[420] Is this mix of contaminants exacerbating the blooms? Bad storms and hurricanes cause more toxic water and dust from the radioactive gypsum mounds to get into the sea. National Geographic pointed out that the recent prolonged red tides of 2017 all followed massive hurricane seasons.[421]

Distinguished Mote Marine Laboratory can't state with certainty that there is a link between the red tide, "Karenia Brevis" and fertilizer pollution, but admits when the algae moves toward shore it feeds off the nutrients produced from human sources. "Florida red tides develop 10-40 miles offshore, away from human-contributed nutrient sources. Red tides occurred in Florida long before human settlement, and severe red tides were observed in the mid-1900s before the state's coastlines were heavily developed. However, once red tides are transported to shore, they use human-contributed nutrients for their growth."[422]

SOLUTIONS

- Reduce & avoid synthetic fertilizers and pesticide usage.
- Where's the EPA? No more radioactive gypsum mounds!
- Filter your water
- Help your community stop the use of synthetic fertilizer and pesticides
- Keep you kids and your pets out of stinky water with algae or red tide
- Stay away from these toxic waters

6. Rivers in Danger

Rivers, streams, and watersheds throughout the world are in danger from pollution, primarily toxic industrial pollution and agricultural runoff. For decades, corporations, industries, citizens and towns have used waterways for unwanted waste materials. There are also unintended leaks, spills, and accidents that cause further damage to these precious resources. As a result, rivers and other bodies of water are tainted with toxins like dioxin, mercury, PCBs, heavy metals, pesticides, phosphate fertilizer, oil spills, coal ash, motor oil and human sewage.

If industries discontinued the releases of harmful pollutants and responsibly cleaned up their waste, we might be able to reverse this damage. Unfortunately, most industries are not reducing their toxic emissions. Many have avoided restrictions and oversight, like those in the energy and fracking sector, where they're exempt and free to take advantage of loopholes in the nation's water protection laws.

> **SECTION 303 of the Clean Water Act, Total Pollution Loads**
> What does the Clean Water Act require? Section 303 of the Clean Water Act requires States to establish water quality standards for waterways and then to identify those streams failing to meet the standards. Streams failing to meet standards are identified as impaired and put on the State's 303(d) list of impaired waters. 303(d) listed waters then become the subject of "Total Maximum Daily Load" (TMDL) regulations. A TMDL calculates the maximum amount of an offending pollutant the stream can receive -- from all sources including from a pipe, off the land or from the air -- and still meet water quality standards. The allowable pollution load (TMDL) is then allocated amongst all pollution contributors -- point and non-point sources. If the state fails to carry out this mandate, the Environmental Protection Agency is supposed to do it.
> Source: www.waterkeeper.org

Water pollution not only harms our health in countless ways, but it also increases our dependency on bottled water. Although it may seem like an exaggeration, water that's clean enough for drinking is a limited resource. Population growth and pollution have drastically increased the need for people and industries to act responsibly in matters concerning water.

WHAT'S GETTING IN THE RIVER?
Rivers are heavily polluted with fertilizer nutrients, phosphorous, nitrates, dioxin, PCBs (even though these were phased out decades ago) and other compounds. In addition to agricultural waste, sewage, chemicals and heavy metals also pose a serious problem. As a result, aquatic life everywhere is suffering. We will not see our rivers recover unless we strengthen pollution regulations. This is critical as drinking water in many areas of the world comes from nearby rivers and lakes. It is in everyone's best interest to protect the world's water sources.

Pollutants entering Our Lakes and Rivers include:
Fertilizer Runoff, Atrazine and herbicides, pesticides, phosphate and nitrate pollution, Biosolids, Factory farm animal water, Fracking and oil wastewater discharge, wastewater, Pipeline spills, Oil spills, industrial drainage, toxic chemicals, hazardous waste, dioxin from paper mills and industry; Coal ash, drilling and mining waste, gypsum stacks, pharmaceuticals and personal care products, untreated sewage, logging and mining, mountaintop removal, perchlorate, pharmaceuticals, PFAS, Gen X, flame retardants, mercury, hazardous waste, AMPA, endocrine disruptors, carcinogens, neurotoxins, ...

THE PEOPLE WHO MAKE THINGS BETTER
The Fox was an activist and advocate for water health and nature. He fiercely opposed water pollution. He let companies know when they were doing something wrong. He spent all his time trying to clean up the Fox River near Batavia, Illinois. He was a real hero fighting pollution at the source. We can all be like the Fox and be caretakers of our planet and of each other.

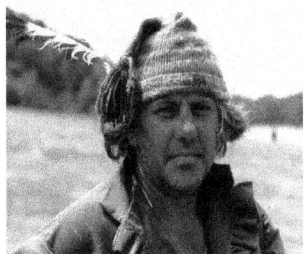

The Fox, James Phillips, 1930-2001, Hero of the Fox River

SPECIAL REPORT
TOXIC ALGAE
STAY OUT OF LAKES WITH TOXIC ALGAE!
PROTECT YOUR PETS FROM TOXIC ALGAE

Toxic Algae blooms can exist in freshwater or salt water. In recent years cases of Toxic Algae have become more threatening to us all. Due to fertilizer run off and toxic pesticide overloads in the water supply, toxic algae blooms are getting more and more serious. This has deadly effects on animals and marine life.

It's believed that agricultural runoff is the primary driver causing algae blooms. However, the increased presence of toxic pesticides like roundup in our waterways in conjunction with the fertilizer runoff is fueling the blooms and making them deadlier than ever.[423] Sustainable farming practices that grow food without harmful toxins is the fastest way to reduce this type of pollution from entering water.

SOLUTIONS
Do not swim or eat fish in lakes or waterways when you see or smell algae present. AVOID STINKY WATER AND LAKES!
- Protect your pets! Keep your dogs away from lakes and beaches contaminated with toxic algae, it is deadly to dogs and animals. If you dog or pet makes contact with toxic algae call the pet poison hotline (855) 764-7661, and seek veterinary assistance immediately!
- Filter your water
- Help Develop a solution to cleaning up toxic algae. The Everglades Foundation offered a $10 million prize to anyone who could develop a solution to remove phosphorous from water.
- The sugar producers in Florida use heavy amounts of fertilizer and pesticides resulting in some of the worst toxic algae cases seen in recent years.
- **We must protect Fresh Water Resources**

7. Wetlands in Danger

August 29, 2023: THE U.S. SUPREME COURT GREATLY REDUCED PROTECTIONS FOR WETLANDS! [424]

In a striking setback for saving the planet, The Supreme Court withdrew protections that prevented the filling in of wetlands. Wetlands have been protected from fill and development since the inception of the Clean Water Act. This ended on August 29, 2023.

The Symphony of the Wetlands

Wetlands are not just living works of art, but they're functional serving as barriers and purification centers. The dynamic architecture of a wetland ecosystem is extraordinary, and the fact that they absorb and filter pollution and keep water sources cleaner is desperately needed now. Wetlands with their tall grasses, marshes, and little critters provide a natural sanctuary and vital habitat for an amazing array of wildlife.

Any filling in or loss of wetlands, puts not just animals, but humans more at risk. Without wetlands, more people will be exposed to greater amounts of pollution and health harming substances. Communities will be at risk of greater destruction during storms. Drinking water systems will have to work harder to remove health-harming substances. Oceans will suffer more from the pollutants not filtered by the barrier wetlands.

PURIFYING WATER NATURALLY

Many wetland plant species absorb toxic heavy metals. Today, in many areas—water and sediment that would normally nourish and support the health of wetlands is redirected elsewhere. This has made it all the more urgent for us to do whatever is necessary to maintain these ecosystems. Simply put, restoring and preserving wetlands is vital for our health and the environment.

"The value of the purification function of wetlands is significant: New York City recently found that it could avoid spending US $3-8 billion on new waste water treatment plants by investing just $1.5 billion in buying land around the reservoirs upstate and protecting the watershed that will do the job of purifying the water supply for free." www.ramsar.org[425]

If you have the means or are Mayor or work in your city government, help push for more wetlands in your community. Wetlands can help keep your local watershed healthy for all.

Edge of Field Wetlands Protect Waterways

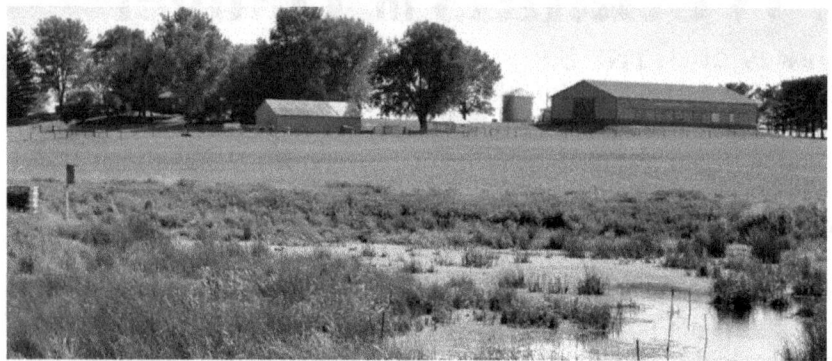

Source: Wetlands Initiative

"Constructed wetlands are a cost-efficient, long-term, highly effective tool to reduce nutrients exiting fields that could otherwise affect local waterways. A relatively small wetland, around 6% of the tile-drained agricultural area, can reduce nitrogen by nearly 50%. If applied at scale, this approach could help address excess nutrients from farms throughout the Midwest."[426]

Urban Wetlands, More Valuable than Ever!

"Half of humanity about 4 billion people live in urban areas today. By 2050 that proportion will reach 66% as people move to cities in search of jobs and a vibrant social life. Cities account for around 80% of global economic output. As cities expand and demand for land increases, the tendency is to encroach on wetlands, they are degraded, filled in and built upon. Yet when left intact or restored, urban wetlands make cities liveable:

- **Reduce flooding** : Wetlands act as giant sponges that absorb flood waters. Rivers, ponds, lakes and marshes soak up and store heavy rainfall. In coastal cities, saltmarshes and mangroves work as a buffer against storm surges.
- **Replenish drinking water**
  Groundwater aquifers, rainwater and rivers are the source of almost all drinking water. Wetlands filter the water that seeps into aquifers, helping to replenish this important water source. Protecting rivers and limiting harmful run-off also helps safeguard the water supply.
- **Filter waste and improve water quality**
  The silt-rich soil and abundant plants in wetlands function as water filters, which absorb some harmful toxins, agricultural pesticides and industrial waste. Urban wetlands also help treat sewage from households."[427] Convention on Wetlands www.Ramsar.org

WATER & HEALTH SOLUTIONS

- Wetlands take care of us. We must do our part to take care of them and keep them strong where they are.
- If you have a farm, add a growing barrier or edge of field wetland on the edge of your lot to filter out pollutants before they get to the water.
- Be a water protector. Help show and teach others not to litter as most litter ends up in waterways.
- Protect your local watershed.
- Don't use products containing microbeads or toxins
- Avoid using plastic disposable items, and help dispose of any plastic you do use into the recycling or rubbish bin.
- Opt for personal care products with natural ingredients
- Don't use toxic cleaning products
- Don't put toxic chemicals down the drain
- Help the lakes heal. Join Alliance for the Great Lakes.
- Together we can find better solutions than discharging toxins, and in so doing prevent contamination of the Lakes.
- If you can, add a filter to your washing machine drainpipe
- Industry on the shores of the lakes as well as cargo ships and tankers can do a better job keeping the lakes clean.
- If farms reduced synthetic fertilizer and pesticide use, it'd reduce harmful runoff, reduce toxic algae and dead zones.
- We have much work to do to protect and recover the polluted rivers and streams throughout the world.
- Do what you can to keep our water and waterways uncontaminated. Use more green and less toxic substances.
- Help clean and prevent water pollution in your community.
- Let's eliminate fracking's wastewater loophole
- Industry must keep their pipelines from harming our water
- Learn more about wetlands and peatlands from the Convention on Wetlands at http://www.ramsar.org/
- Current list of endangered rivers: www.americanrivers.org
- Help restore protections for Wetlands and if it takes going back to the Supreme Court that is what we must do!
- Encourage your community to restore native wetlands

SPECIAL REPORT
PEOPLE IN DANGER

2024 — "the First Year the US Expects More than 2 Million New Cases of Cancer. The American Cancer Society reports lower overall cancer death rates, yet incidence is increasing for many common cancers, including 6 of the top 10."[428]

> 2009--President's Cancer Panel Report:
>
> "Weak laws and regulations, inefficient enforcement, regulatory complexity, and fragmented authority allow avoidable exposures to known or suspected cancer-causing and cancer-promoting agents to continue and proliferate in the workplace and the community. Existing regulations, and the exposure assessments on which they are based, are outdated in most cases, and many known or suspected carcinogens are completely unregulated. Enforcement of most existing regulations is poor. In virtually all cases, regulations fail to take multiple exposures and exposure interactions into account. In addition, regulations for workplace environments are focused more on safety than on health. Industry has exploited regulatory weaknesses, such as government's reactionary (rather than precautionary) approach to regulation."
>
> [429]

WATER POLLUTION

Water pollution harms people as well as the environment. These contaminants can be natural or manmade. This book covers a wide variety of manmade contaminants and those resulting from inproper and antiquated methods of resource management.

Definition of Contaminant
The Safe Drinking Water Act (SDWA) defines "contaminant" as any physical, chemical, biological or radiological substance or matter in water. Drinking water can reasonably be expected to contain at least small amounts of some contaminants. Some contaminants may be harmful if consumed at or above certain levels in drinking water. The presence of contaminants does not necessarily mean that the water poses a risk. A wide array of contaminants mingled together can present different or an increased health risk.

Contaminant Types
Toxic Substances, Carcinogens, Heavy Metals, Neurotoxins, Reproductive Toxins, Endocrine Disruptors, and Microbes can all be seeping into our water night and day from many sources. Unfortunately, existing wastewater treatment facilities are largely unable to filter out all types of pollutants. And even more troubling, the EPA doesn't regulate all pollutants yet, so many slip by without public warning.

Point Source: from an exact location, identifiable like a discharge pipe from manufacturing facility or refinery, or an oil spill.

Nonpoint Source is difficult to pinpoint the source. Examples of nonpoint source include rain that washes runoff pollutants into waterways, or in the case of persistent organic pollutants that travel far and wide. The EPA categorizes factory farm pollution as non-point source, yet logically the polluting sites can be identified. Not all makes sense with the government's approach to controlling toxic pollution today. One of my heroes who used to lead the EPA is Eric Schaeffer. He got so fed up under the Bush Cheney presidency that he left to start his own firm, the Environmental Integrity Project. As he says, "The failure to confront agriculture is probably the biggest program failure of the Clean Water Act."[430]

Unregulated Pollution: There is a wide range of carcinogens and toxic substances getting into water because of outright negligence on the part of industry and government. The industries that don't have to follow pollution rules include the pesticide industry, the fertilizer industry, the plastics industry and the chemical industry. Chemical includes the fossil fuel industry, particularly petroleum refineries and LNG (liquified natural gas)—these are the substances turned into chemicals, plastic and feedstocks that different compounds are made from. US Oil Refineries are in complete violation of the Clean Water Act and may be causing the most obscene amount of damage to our waterways[431]—*reported* effluents in one year total 1.6 billion pounds of toxins, 16 million pounds of nitrogen, and 60,000 pounds of selenium. Rather than tell the truth, the American Fuel & Petroleum Manufacturers trade group told NPR, "We have made great progress in environmental stewardship under the Clean Air Act, the Clean Water Act and many other environmental regulations, and continue to innovate to evolve our operations and products."[432] This from the group behind lowering

Agricultural Pollutants are some of the most harmful toxins getting in our water. Today's modern farming methods are quite different and use far more dangerous substances than in our grandparents' day. This is a serious matter that needs attended to before we all see ourselves on our death beds. What's even more terrible is the excessive use and mingling of these toxins in the water. Excessive animal waste matter and the synthetic toxic substances used by conventional, GMO and especially, the large corporate factory farms do not belong in our drinking water.

Glyphosate is a severely harmful herbicide found in nearly every stream and waterway tested. It's used in hundreds of gardening products, all GMO crops, as well as other crops and grains to expedite harvest- a process known as desiccation. It's used by landscapers and gardeners and grounds keepers. The weedkiller is sprayed plentifully on genetically engineered crops such as corn and soybeans that have been modified to be tolerant 'roundup ready' as the term goes. Many farmers also use it on fields before the growing season, including spinach and almond producers. It is considered the most used herbicide in history."[433]

What can Farmers Do? *(Source EPA)*[434]
- **Ensuring Year-Round Ground Cover:** Farmers can plant cover crops or perennial species to prevent periods of bare ground on farm fields when the soil is most susceptible to erosion and loss
- **Planting Field Buffers:** Farmers can plant trees, shrubs and grasses along the edges of fields;
- **Implementing Conservation Tillage:** Farmers can reduce tilling..

MIDWEST FARMING

It's more important than ever to get contaminants out of our water supplies. Every state where chemical agriculture is plentiful may start seeing disease rates doubling. Adding to the problem is nanoparticle exposure, which causes cancer to spread faster within the body.

In Minnesota, Families blame farm nutrient contamination for heavy cancer toll. *"Every family along here was affected, Everyone."*[435]

FACTORY FARMS in Iowa: 4025[436]

"An ethanol-producing facility in northeast Iowa expelled excessive pollutants into the air for several years that can cause cancers and other health effects, according to the Iowa Department of Natural Resources." *Iowa Capital Dispatch*[437]

With more than 200 million pounds sprayed annually in the US alone, glyphosate is found in the urine of 93% of everyone tested, as well as 99% of the people in France![438] **It's not just America that has been betrayed, these chemicals are used around the world!**

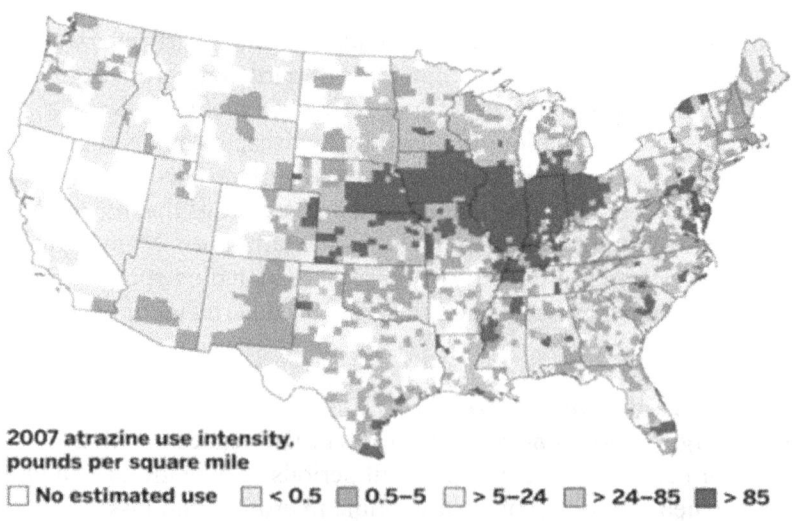

Human Health

All living creatures are influenced negatively by water pollution. Pollution in any form is detrimental, but that which compromises water or air quality has direct impacts on our well being. That's why it's so vital we end pollution. Disease risk is increased through exposure to pollution. Depending on the contaminant and duration, exposure can lead to dire health situations. Some of the diseases caused by pollutants in water and air include:

- Metabolic Disorders
- Cancer
- Neurotoxins and nervous system disorders
- Reproductive problems
- Thyroid problems
- Digestive system problems
- Learning disabilities, autism
- Birth Defects
- Lowered IQ
- Infertility and reproductive problems
- Stomach Cancer, Uterine Cancer, Prostate Cancer
- All types of Cancer!
- And on and on the list goes...

10 WORST POLLUTANTS
1. Oil Refineries Carcinogens, Reproductive Toxins
2. Pesticide Carcinogens and Neurotoxins weedkillers, herbicides, insecticides,
3. Raw Sewage Pathogens, Factory farm runoff
4. Nitrate pollution from synthetic fertilizer
5. PFAS Pollution
6. Heavy Metal Pollution and Neurotoxins
7. Chlorypyrifos, Dicamba, Atrazine & Glyphosate
8. Toxic dirty hazardous crap!
9. PLASTIC IN ALL FORMS
10. SYNTHETIC FERTILIZER (used on fields, yards, and in aerial fire extinguishing on forest fires)

SPECIAL REPORT
IOWA CANCER SURGE

Headlines recently report Iowa's new position: America's Cancer Capital.[439] Surely the extensive use of pesticides and toxic agricultural runoff has contributed to these results. After years of dominating GMO corn and ethanol farming, the condition of waterways and drinking water sources in Iowa is sub standard at best. It's just a fact, cancer-causing pesticides and other toxins flowing from factory farms do not encourage health.

Could these cancers have been avoided in a cleaner environment? GMO crops may sound fine and dandy, I'm sure the roundup ready salesman is a real nice guy! But when you realize this farming system uses millions of pounds of cancer-causing pesticides to grow food, you have to wonder. These pesticides end up in not just the drinking water and waterways, but everything else too: the food, the animals, the ethanol and alcohol produced, the private wells, the soil and air. Over exposure to carcinogenic neurotoxic substances increases risk of cancer and continued exposure interferes with healing.

It's not just Iowa, drinking water everywhere is contaminated with these pesticides and runoff compounds. Double the trouble when animals are fed GMO feed. If we have any sense at all, and truly want to reduce human and animal disease, this will serve as our wake up call. It's time for us to stand up and defend our families, defend our land, defend our friends. Cancer is increasing everywhere. When carcinogens get in the water, we must remove them. It's not healthy for humans or animals to consume toxic water. If we care at all, we must demand the government tighten its rules, push back on the Big Ag Chemical companies, and get the toxic crap out of farming. We must get back to using healthier more natural methods of growing food. We must resuscitate soil health and all else will follow. GMO farming only leads to disease for the soil and for us. Let's jump ship and return to natural organic and regenerative farming as fast as we can.

IOWA: CANCER CAPITAL OF THE U.S.

There are many contributing factors that can increase cancer rates including radon, which is particularly elevated in midwestern states. Data shows that in 2021, 14,500,000 pounds of pesticides were doused on corn grown in Iowa. Ethanol farming uses Atrazine, Roundup and ridiculous amounts of cancer-causing substances as seen below.

Pesticide Use on Corn - Iowa and Program States: 2021

Active ingredient	Iowa		
	Planted acres treated	Yearly rate	Total applied
	(percent)	(lbs per acre)	(1,000 lbs)
Fungicide			
Azoxystrobin	13	0.093	155
Propiconazole	13	0.100	166
Prothioconazole	9	0.115	138
Trifloxystrobin	9	0.101	121
Total [2]	26		786
Herbicide [3]			
Acetochlor	48	1.342	8,306
Atrazine	69	0.861	7,663
Clopyralid	14	0.078	143
Glyphosate	11	0.738	1,057
Glyphosate iso. salt	25	0.805	2,600
Glyphosate pot. salt	24	0.929	2,920
Mesotrione	47	0.114	699
S-Metolachlor	16	0.856	1,799
Total [2]	96		29,390
Insecticde			
Bifenthrin	7	0.065	58
Total [2]	13		175

Data (USDA)[440] Page 232, Corn Pesticide map (Chem & Eng News)[441]

Could the intense application of pesticides in Iowa for well over 20 years be causing Cancer uptick? Why do these crops need so much pesticide, if the corn is for ethanol, does it matter if its partially eaten by bugs? If the plants are so weak and can't defend themselves, something is not right with the soil. Remove the crappy fertilizers so the soil can improve. Healthy soil makes healthy, strong plants.

AGRICULTURAL RUNOFF EFFECTS

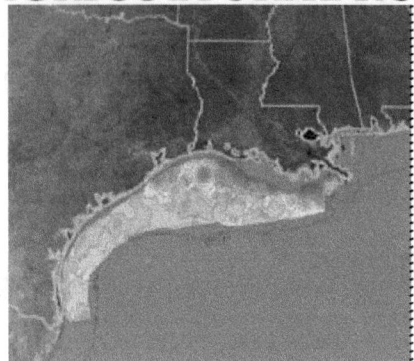

Map Source: NASA
According to National Geographic, there are over 415 Dead Zones worldwide.[442]

The Dead Zone
Fertilizer nutrients, notably phosphorous and excess nitrogen cause toxic algae blooms and dead zones. The largest dead zone in the world sits where the Mississippi River meets the Gulf of Mexico. "Scientists have determined this year's Gulf of Mexico "dead zone," an area of low oxygen that can kill fish and marine life, is 6,705 square miles, an area roughly about the size of New Jersey.
Source: USA Today Aug 1, 2024

Agricultural Effects on the Mississippi River
Toxic pollutants can affect human health either because they contaminate drinking water supplies or because they accumulate in the fat or tissue of fish, which are consumed by human populations. The primary toxic substances due to fish consumption are currently PCBs and chlordane. Although dieldrin is currently the basis for fish consumption advisories in Illinois, other states may follow suit.

The second category of toxic pollutants which is of concern to human health includes those substances that pose threats to drinking water. Based upon the fact that they have either shown exceedances of maximum contaminant levels (MCLs) or had a significant impact on water treatment needs, **Atrazine** and **Nitrate** are considered to be of top priority. Both produce localized and seasonal problems, but are of basin-wide concern. Nitrate is additionally of priority concern because recent research suggests that the Upper Mississippi River is a major source of nitrogen in the Gulf of Mexico. www.umrba.org

THE HEAVY HITTERS

- **Carcinogens**
- **Endocrine Disruptors**
- **Heavy Metals**
- **Neurotoxins**
- **Reproductive Toxins**
- **Proposition 65**
- **Toxic Substances**

Cancers Related to Toxins in Contaminated Water

Cancer Type	Pesticides: toxins used for killing insects, plants, all life	Other Toxins
Brain	Pesticides[443], sulfuryl fluoride	Microbes radiation
Breast	Atrazine, Chlorpyrifos, fungicides[444][445] Glyphosate, OP, OCPs[446], Dieldrin, Aldrin, DDT[447], Dichlorobenzene[448]	
Colon, Colorectal	Agricultural runoff, [449]Chlorpyrifos[450] Carbaryl, EPTC, Dicamba, Trifluralin, Imazethapry, Pendimethalin, Acetochlor, Nitrate in water[451]	Microbes, Protozoa P. Hominis[452],
Esophageal	Nitrate, OP, OCPs[453],	
Kidney	Nitrate in water[454], p-DCB[455], fungicides	Arsenic
Leukemia	(acute myeloid) glyphosate[456], p-DCB	Benzene
Liver	Neonics,[457] p-DCB[458], fungicides	Arsenic, parasites[459]
Lung	Dicamba, chlorpyrifos Carbofuran, diazinon, dieldrin, OCPs, Pendimethalin, metolaclor[460]	Arsenic, radon
Melanoma Skin cancer	Carbaryl, Parathion[461], Mancozeb pesticides, Organochlorine Pesticides (OCPs), , OP organophosphates	Arsenic
NHL (non-hodgkins-Lymphoma)	glyphosate[462], OP Diazinon[463], OCPs,	
Ovarian, uterine	OCPs, dichlorobenzene, neonics, carbamate	
Pancreas	Glyphosate, Mancozeb, Spray Sulfur[464]	Arsenic[465]
Prostate	Nitrate in water,[466] synthetic fertilizer	Arsenic
Stomach	Nitrate[467], Atrazine[468], OCPs	
Testicular	Early exposure to pesticides[469]	PFAS
Thyroid	Nitrate in water[470], Paraquat and Glyphosate[471], neonics, carbamates	perchlorate
Bladder, bile duct	Carbamates, Fungicides	Arsenic, liver flukes[472]
Bones	Carbamate fungicides	

1. Carcinogens

"Environment has the principal role in causing sporadic cancer."[473]

President's Cancer Panel Council

CARCINOGENS are toxins that cause Cancer. It's been realized that most cancers are caused by environmental factors, not genes. In fact, the good news is that through nutrients and epigenetics, many cancers can be reversed and prevented. "Compounds found in dietary phytochemical preparations such as teas, garlic, soy products, herbs, grapes and cruciferous vegetables are now generally accepted to defend against the development of many different types of tumors as well as acting as epigenetic modulators that impact not only the initiation, but also the progression of oncogenesis."[474]

What's in the products we buy today, the formulations? So many products today contain a secret new ingredient: nanoparticles. From sunscreen and after shave to candy and beverages, check your labels. Though not tested for safety, scientists have discovered, "Nanoparticles cause cancer to spread faster."[475]

SOLUTIONS

In order to prevent the many diseases and cancers caused by environmental factors and toxic substances the President's Cancer Panel[476] suggests these actions be undertaken:

- Exposure to pesticides can be decreased by choosing, to the extent possible, food grown without pesticides or chemical fertilizers and washing conventionally grown produce.
- Reduce exposure to antibiotics, growth hormones, and toxic run-off from livestock feed lots by choosing free-range meat
- Avoid consumption of processed, charred, and well-done meats to reduce exposure to carcinogenic heterocyclic amines and polyaromatic hydrocarbons.
- Properly dispose of pharmaceuticals, household chemicals, paints, and other materials to keep drinking water clean
- We can also choose products made with non-toxic substances
- Similarly, reducing or ceasing landscaping pesticide and fertilizer use will help keep these chemicals from contaminating drinking water supplies.

THE DANGERS OF INSECTICIDES

These chemicals are harming people and killing the environment. Many pesticides are cholinesterase inhibitors. "**Cholinesterase**, or **acetylcholine**, produced in the liver, is one of many important enzymes needed for the proper functioning of the nervous systems of humans, other vertebrates, and insects. Nerve impulses are transmitted across synapses through the release of a chemical called acetylcholine. After the stimulating signals are transferred, cholinesterase is released by the body and the acetylcholine is broken down into its acetyl and choline components and removed from the synapse, allowing other signals to pass through.

Cholinesterase inhibiting chemicals, notably organophosphates insecticides and carbamate pesticides do not allow cholinesterase to end the stimulating signal, which causes a build-up of stimulating signals in the nervous system. Because they cannot be removed, the stimulating signals continue firing in the body which results in the uncontrollable movements that are the sign of cholinesterase inhibition including rapid muscle twitching, convulsions, and others."[477]

Since the EPA approves pesticides based on safety studies provided by the manufacturer, of course we have to question the validity of any safety studies. Also, these safety studies typically only examine the main ingredient, not the full pesticide formulations!

We know we were lied to about the safety of PCBs for years, as well as dioxin, and Agent Orange only to finally have the truth revealed[478]. When it is found that manufacturers have deceived us and knowingly provided faulty safety studies, and harmed our health for years, what will be done? Perhaps it's in their best interest to reveal the truth about their products and start saving human lives. How swift will be the jury? These companies have the ability to reformulate their products into better, safe versions that harm none. God help them get to it!

2.Endocrine Disruptors

EDCs, Endocrine Disruptors are substances that interfere with our endocrine system. Many chemicals and substances in our everyday lives interfere with our health on such a subtle level that most people remain unaware they're affected. Health problems creep in but are attributed to getting older, aging when actually it may be the result of exposure to EDCs or another health harming substance.

What is the Endocrine System?

The endocrine system is that part of your body related to your hormones, and includes the Thyroid and Pineal glands. These glands control many bodily functions from how tall you will grow, when you will begin puberty, how you handle stress, to how tired or energetic you feel. For a full list of all the endocrine disrupting chemical check out the TEDX, an Endocrine Disruption Exchange created by the late Dr. Theo Colborn. She was dedicated to raising awareness about these issues and to helping people live in a nontoxic world. http://endocrinedisruption.org/.

WHAT ARE ENDOCRINE DISRUPTORS?

Endocrine disruptors are chemicals that may interfere with the body's endocrine system and produce adverse developmental, reproductive, neurological, and immune effects in both humans and wildlife. A wide range of substances, both natural and man-made, are thought to cause endocrine disruption, including pharmaceuticals, dioxin and dioxin-like compounds, polychlorinated biphenyls, DDT and other pesticides, and plasticizers such as bisphenol A. Endocrine disruptors may be found in many everyday products– including plastic bottles, metal food cans, detergents, flame retardants, food, toys, cosmetics, and pesticides. The NIEHS supports studies to determine whether exposure to endocrine disruptors may result in human health effects including lowered fertility and an increased incidence of endometriosis and some cancers. Research shows that endocrine disruptors may pose the greatest risk during prenatal and early postnatal development when organ and neural systems are forming. [479]

HORMONE ENDOCRINE SYSTEM INFORMATION

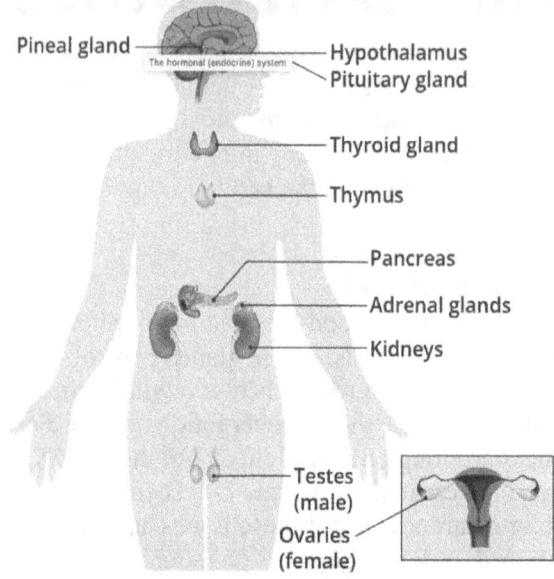

Image and Page Source: Health Direct[480]

Key facts
- The hormonal system, also called the endocrine system, is a network of glands and organs in the body that produce hormones.
- Hormones regulate all the cells in your body, controlling your body's metabolism, growth and many other functions.

3. Heavy Metals

Excess heavy metal exposure causes illness in a myriad of ways. Heavy metals contaminate water, dust, air and smoke. They can be particularly problematic in warfare zones, near drilling, mining, or manufacturing sites.

HEAVY METALS
Aluminum, Manganese, Nickle, Arsenic, Barium, Silver, Beryllium, Cadmium, Zinc, Chromium, Lead, Mercury, Tin, Vanadium, Molybdenum

HEALTH EFFECTS
Behavioral changes can result, as can learning disabilities; neurological disorders, memory disorders; autism; lowered IQs; confusion, mineral deficiency diseases; hormonal imbalances; chronic liver disease; respiratory issues; chronic bronchitis; inflammation in the lungs; kidney disease; organ malfunction; lethargy and weakness; muscle spasms and tremors; excessive sweating; irregular heart beat; headache; aches in the bones, weakened bones; aggressive tendencies and violence; nausea; chronic muscle pain; fatigue; insomnia; impaired immune function; numbness, tingling in hands and feet. Some heavy metals double as NEUROTOXINS damage the brain and nervous system: Lead, manganese, aluminum, fluoride, arsenic, barium, toluene, PCBs, methylmercury

HOW WE ARE EXPOSED
Contaminated water, toxic waste, dust, smoke, exhaust; pesticides and fertilizer; MMT, particulates and aerosols; cigarettes and e-cigarettes; oil refineries and petrochemical manufacturing, nanoparticles

SOLUTIONS
- Reduce exposure to carcinogens, toxins and heavy metals.
- Protect your health! Filter your water and eat lots of deep green leafy vegetables and foods rich in chlorophyll and silica, extra vitamin c, flax seeds, extra glasses of clean water.

4. Neurotoxins

NEUROTOXINS are substances that damage the brain and nervous system. Overexposure to neurotoxins can cause your brain and nervous system to malfunction. Neurotoxins are synthetic or natural substances that can be found in the air, in contaminated water, in contaminated soil, in food, in beverages, in personal care products, in microwave popcorn packaging, in products containing flame retardants, in dry cleaning chemicals, etc.

They are implicated in the development of many diseases of the brain and nervous system including: Memory disorders, Autism, ADHD, learning disorders, lowered IQ, behavioral development, brain disorders, abnormal brain development, epilepsy, dementia, Parkinson's, Alzheimer's, Senility, concentration disorders, neuropathy, numbness, tingling in extremities, pain in feet, impaired judgement, delayed response, memory loss, hyperactivity, aggressiveness, insomnia, anxiety disorder, mental retardation, inflammation of myelin sheath.

Exposure to a type of air pollution called fine particulate matter, or $PM_{2.5}$, has been identified as a risk factor for dementia.[481]

SOLUTIONS

- Filter your water. Wash hands with soap and water.
- Avoid neurotoxins in food by eating organically
- Avoid exposure to pesticides, herbicides, fungicides and chemical fertilizer. These substances can be found in water and food as well as near facilities using them, parks, outdoor mosquito spraying, etc.
- One of the keys to brain health is keeping your inner body in balance, particularly your gut biome. Have you taken lots of antibiotics in your life, do you consume sweets or alcohol? You may have yeast overgrowth in your gut that can compromise brain health. Getting the gut microbiome back to balance helps prevent disease in the brain.
- Reduce your exposure to disease-causing substances.
- **Sulfur Dioxide (SO2):** inhalation causes memory impairment.
- SO2 is found in polluted air, acid rain, exhaust, smoke. SO2 is also used in solar radiation management (SRM) experiments in the atmosphere. We must stop the advancement of the SRM aerosol program before SO2 levels cause further harm to the air we breathe.

Nervous System Afflictions

Nervous System Disease	Pesticides associated with Nervous System and Mitochondria disfunction	Other Toxins Associated
Alzheimer's/ Memory Loss Dementia	2,4-D,[482] Dieldrin, Rotenone, Paraquat[483] Chlorpyrifos, DDT	SO2, Microbes, fungus, Candida[484], Heavy metals, Air pollution
MS	Agricultural runoff, nitrate in water[485]	Bacteria, Clostridium perfringen[486]
Parkinson's Epilepsy	Paraquat[487] Chlorpyrifos	Perc, heavy metals, aluminum Nanoparticles, Nutritional deficiency
Depression	Glyphosate[488], dicamba	Perchlorate in drinking water
Learning Disabilities/ Lower IQ/	Chlorpyrifos,[489] 2,4-D	Lead, heavy metals
ADHD	Chlorpyrifos, Glyphosate, 2,4-D	
Stroke	High levels of Pesticides[490]	Mineral deficiency
Aggression	2,4-D[491], High levels of pesticides	Manganese Heavy metals
Schizophrenia	Organophosphate pesticides[492]	Heavy metals
Autism	Organophosphates,[493] insecticides, glyphosate[494]	
Neuropathy neurotoxicity	Exposure to microplastics[495] and nanoparticles, neurotoxins and xenobiotics, carbamates, organophosphate insecticides[496]	Toxins, injury, bacteria, heavy metals, Chemotherapy

5. Reproductive Toxins

Reproductive toxins impact us in many ways. Essentially, they can be harmful to all the organs and cells involved with our sexual expression and function. They act like endocrine disruptors, disturbing hormones involved with everything from ability to get pregnant to low sperm count, pregnancy health, endocrine system health, reproductive system health. More than anyone else, Theo Colburn (1927-2014) championed this subject matter. To delve more into how these toxins interfere with your health, and your family's health, please visit the Endocrine Disruption Exhange.

Reproductive toxins can cause: low birth weight, spontaneous abortion, development challenges, birth defects, erectile dysfunction, menstrual issues, tumors, PCOS (polycystic ovary syndrome), fibroids, uterine and ovarian cancer, testicular cancer, endometriosis, prostate cancer, kidney cancer, breast cancer and everything in between. The State of California's Proposition 65 stands as one of the most respected and thorough roundup of reproductive toxins. Carcinogens are also included. The list is updated yearly.

PROPOSITION 65[497]

California's Proposition 65, also called the Safe Drinking Water and Toxic Enforcement Act, first became law in the state in 1986. It is intended to help Californians make informed decisions about protecting themselves from chemicals that could cause cancer, birth defects, or other reproductive harm.

Proposition 65, the Safe Drinking Water and Toxic Enforcement Act of 1986, was enacted as a ballot initiative in November 1986. The Proposition was intended by its authors to protect California citizens and the State's drinking water sources from chemicals known to cause cancer, birth defects or other reproductive harm, and to inform citizens about exposures to such chemicals. Proposition 65 requires the state to maintain and update a list of chemicals known to the state to cause cancer or reproductive toxicity. http://www.oehha.ca.gov/prop65.htm

6. Respiratory & Digestive

Respiratory toxins can damage the lungs and airways, restrict breathing capabilities and stress the heart and cardiovascular system, triggering dysbiosis in the whole body system. Avoid using products that harm your lungs.

Respiratory Toxins include:
- Carbon Monoxide (CO)
- Sewer Gas, Hydrogen Sulfide (H2S)
- Ammonia
- Smoke, cigarette smoke, air pollution, forest fire smoke
- Aerial spraying of herbicides, insecticides, bug killers
- Glyphosate[498], 2,4-D
- Nanoparticles
- VOCs
- Heavy metals, toxic gases,

Digestive toxins (DT) harm the stomach and intestines as well as the liver, pancreas and gallbladder. DTs can trigger chronic inflammation, metabolic disorders, upset microbiome causing an imbalance of hostile gut bacteria. DTs can prevent absorption of nutrients, and breach the gut brain barrier leaching beyond the intestinal wall into the bloodstream, which affects the nervous system as well as the endocrine system, hormones and behavior. DTs cause a host of systemic diseases including IBD, Colitis, Crohn's Disease.[499]

Digestive toxins include:
- Contaminated food and water
- Salmonella, E.Coli, protozoa, cysts, microbes, parasites
- Glyphosate[500]
- Gluten (for those who are sensitive)
- Refined sugar in excess, High Fructose Corn Syrup
- High sugar processed foods
- Genetically modified proteins
- Alcohol

7. Toxic Substances

President's Cancer Panel Report [501]

"The true burden of environmentally induced cancer has been grossly underestimated. With nearly 80,000 chemicals on the market in the United States, many of which are used by millions of Americans in their daily lives, are understudied and largely unregulated, exposure to potential environmental carcinogens is widespread."

Toxic Substances are toxins that harm all. Most of these toxins are in use throughout the world, unless they're banned in a particular country. These toxins generally harm all life, on land, in the water, or through the air. This includes all people and animals and plants. These substances cause serious water pollution, and are interconnected with most of our diseases and cancers They affect well-being, behavior, and overall health in many ways. The toxins can be grouped as:

- **Neurotoxins**: harm brain and nervous system,
- **Carcinogens**: cause cancer, weaken immune system
- **Endocrine Disruptors**: harm thyroid, endocrine, reproduction
- **Heavy Metals:** neurotoxins, accumulate in body, affect brain
- **Reproductive Toxins**: disease, infertility, birth defects, cancer
- **Respiratory and Digestive Toxins** trigger disease, weaken gut-brain axis, the nervous system, and epithelial network
- **Fungal, bacterial, viral** cause a wide range of diseases
- **Nanoparticles**: combination of Neurotoxins, Heavy Metals

EFFECTS TOXINS HAVE ON US
- Harm physical health, cause disease, cause cancer
- Harm mental health, cause behavioral changes, increase risk to brain
- Contribute to environmental degradation, biodiversity loss

SOLUTIONS:
- Avoid toxic substances and carcinogens
- Filter your water & wash your hands with soapy water
- Choose food grown without toxins and products made naturally
- We must get the EPA to enforce rules for industries that have <u>no</u> pollution rules, especially those that outright contaminate water daily such as oil refineries and petrochemical facilities, pesticides manufacturers, fertilizer facilities, plastics and PFAS facilities, ethanol facilities, and factory farms amongst others.

SPECIAL REPORT
PESTICIDE CATEGORIES

Herbicides (Weedkillers)
These are used abundantly on farm fields, growing GMO crops, for lawn care, landscapers, golf courses, parks, athletic fields, gardens. These are carcinogens and endocrine disruptors mostly. Examples: Glyphosate (Roundup), Atrazine, 2,4-D, Dicamba, Paraquat, Glufonisate, etc.

Insecticides (the most harmful to humans)
These are deadly carcinogens and neurotoxins that target the nervous system and cross the blood brain barrier. They not only target insects, but also animals and humans' nervous system. Insecticides inhibit essential nerve synapses and enzymes resulting in impairment, mitochondrial dysfunction, or death. These kill pollinators and beneficial insects and cause chronic neurodegenerative conditions—like Parkinson's in people. Insecticides include: Organophosphate (OP) insecticides, Organochlorine pesticides (OCPs), Carbamates, Neonicotinoids, Pyrethroids, Mitochondrial Complex I Inhibitors, Miticides, and Acaracides. Commonly used insecticides in the U.S. include: Chlorpyrifos, Clothianidin, Thiacloprid, Imidacloprid, Thimethoxam, Endosulphan, Pyridaben, Pirimicarb, DDT, Dieldrin, Aldrin, Hexachlorocyclohexane (HCH), etc. [502]

Formulations Increase Pesticide Danger
Formulations of products are proving to be more toxic than individual chemicals. These formulas contain adjuvants, inert substances, and surfactants that increase absorbilty, "Roundup was found in this experiment to be 125 times more toxic than glyphosate. Moreover, despite its reputation, Roundup was by far the most toxic among the herbicides and insecticides tested. This inconsistency between scientific fact and industrial claim may be attributed to huge economic interests, which have been found to falsify health risk assessments and delay health policy decisions." [503]

SECTION FOUR

SOLUTiONS DEPARTMENT
WATER

"Our lives begin to end the day we become silent about things that matter."
Martin Luther King, Jr

SOLUTiONS WATER
PROTECT YOUR FAMILY
KEEP WATER CLEAN

The importance of clean water cannot be overstated. The luxuries of today's modern world cause water sources to be contaminated. Tap water may appear clean but it contains disinfection byproducts and other unmentionables that you really want to filter out. If your water is discolored or has a funny smell you especially need a filter.

To know what contaminants are present, you can check the EWG.org database, or the consumer confidence report (CCR) that comes with your water bill. You can also call the water department for the most recent water quality report for your area. If you have your own well, you are responsible for getting the water tested. If you like, you can get your own test kit at www.mytapscore.com.

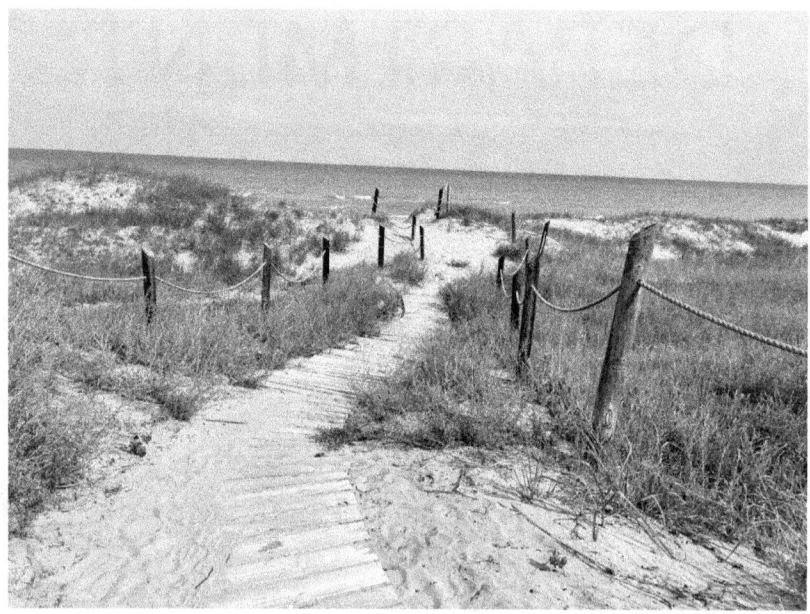

- Filter your water
- Make art that raises awareness and inspires light and love
- Care for each other and for the earth.
- Don't litter! Take personal responsibility!
- Communicate, talk, write, call, post, tag us #filteryourwaternow

SOLUTiONS WATER

FILTER YOUR WATER

The most effective water filters can either be installed at your sink, or a gravity filter that sits on your countertop. There are also whole home filters, refrigerators filters, and pitcher filters but these are somewhat limited in what they remove. The most effective filters are:
- Reverse osmosis
- Carbon block filtration or activated charcoal
- Reverse osmosis with carbon filtration and ultraviolet light

A filter system requires regular maintenance. Depending on the type of system you install and how much water you use, filters need to be changed regularly—usually every 3-6 months. Use filtered water for drinking, for making beverages, coffee, tea, baby food, and for all your cooking needs.

Take care of your health and your family with filtered water.

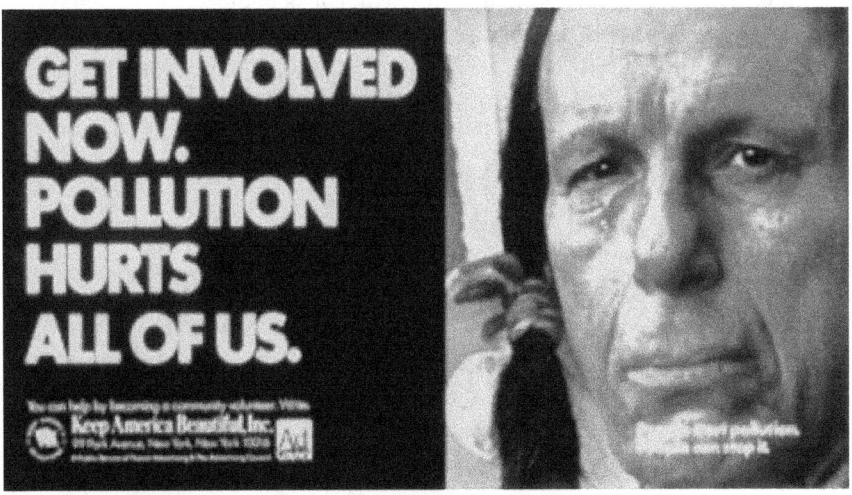

What happened to the PSAs?
From the Public Service Campaign, Keep America Beautiful

SOLUTiONS WATER

Be a Water Guardian
From The President's Cancer Panel Report, 2009
"Filtering home tap or well water can decrease exposure to numerous known or suspected carcinogens and endocrine-disrupting chemicals. Unless the home water source is known to be contaminated, it is preferable to use filtered tap water instead of commercially bottled water.

Storing and carrying water in stainless steel, glass, or BPA- and phthalate-free containers will reduce exposure to endocrine-disrupting and other chemicals that may leach into water from plastics. This action also will decrease the need for plastic bottles, the manufacture of which produces toxic by-products, and reduce the need to dispose of and recycle plastic bottles."

CONSERVE WATER
Be mindful when using water. We can conserve water by installing more efficient faucets in our home and kitchen. Take shorter showers, install high efficiency dishwasher, turn off water while brushing your teeth, limit and combine laundry loads to run washer less each week, replace toilets with newer models that use less water per flush, repair leaky faucets and appliances, fill your garden and yard with native plants that thrive in your climate under existing weather conditions

WHAT WE CAN DO:
- As much as we can, let's keep water clean.
- Drink and cook only with clean filtered water
- Avoid plastic, phthalates, BPA, and all endocrine disruptors
- Keep chemicals, plastic, and microbeads out of the water.
- Clear out PFCs, PFAS, as well as fire retardants from your home. Avoid nonstick cookware and check labels
- Don't use any herbicides or toxic fertilizer on your lawn or garden
- Don't use Road Salt to deice driveways, use volcanic ash
- Keep toxic chemicals out of your home and your cleaning supplies
- Avoid using plastic straws and disposable plastic as much as possible

SOLUTiONS WATER
PROTECT THE GREAT LAKES

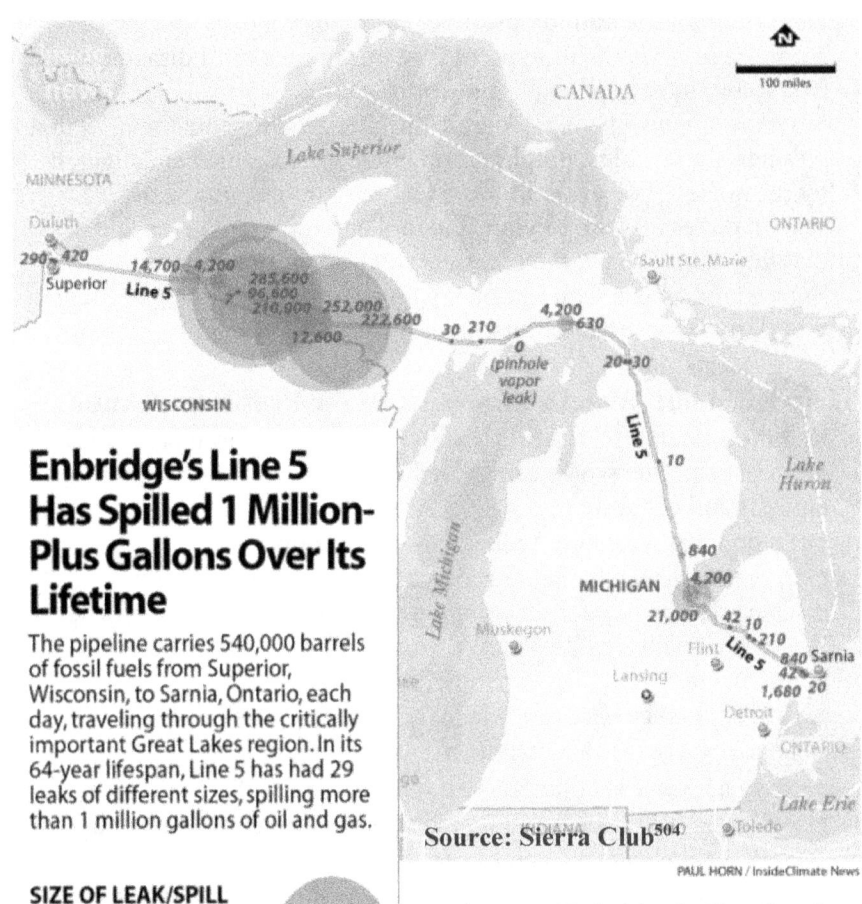

Enbridge's Line 5 Has Spilled 1 Million-Plus Gallons Over Its Lifetime

The pipeline carries 540,000 barrels of fossil fuels from Superior, Wisconsin, to Sarnia, Ontario, each day, traveling through the critically important Great Lakes region. In its 64-year lifespan, Line 5 has had 29 leaks of different sizes, spilling more than 1 million gallons of oil and gas.

Source: Sierra Club[504]

PAUL HORN / InsideClimate News

SIZE OF LEAK/SPILL in gallons
<500   1,000   10,000   100,000

Help stop Enbridge's Tar Sands Oil Line 5 that threatens the Great Lakes watershed! See more on pages 132-133. Until pipelines are built with 110% accident-proof technology, they must not be located in sensitive habits, or in places that threaten our fresh water resources. Let's keep supporting the Sioux and protect the Missouri River. #NoDAPL. We must protect America and end the insanity! Protect your health, filter your water, protect the earth and all of God's creatures.

SOLUTiONS WATER

PROTECT THE OCEANS
- Help keep plastic and toxins out of the waterways
- No more offshore drilling permits in our oceans until disaster proof technology is created. No more spills!
- No more Sonar. The Navy agreed in 2015 to limit sonar testing that was harming whales, dolphins and other sea creatures endangered by the noise. They can still use sonar but not in ecologically sensitive areas. Write to your senators and representatives and ask that they help expand the areas in which sonar use is banned.
- Support the Ocean Conservancy www.oceanconservancy.org and the Marine Conservation Institute, www.marine-conservation.org

Help Keep our Water Sources clean for People and Animals
- End the assault on the world's water sources: no more pesticides, no more plastic. The world can't tolerate anymore, it's sickening us, animals and ecosystems.
- Let's do what we can to reduce plastic pollution
- Corporations must be held accountable for their waste water and discharges, and pay for cleaning up any damage they have caused. Water treatment facilities aren't capable of purifying all of the pollutants now entering our water.
- As sad as it is, beware of toxins when choosing fish to consume.

Our bodies are 70% water
- As long as water is contaminated, protect yourself, filter water
- Use filtered water for cooking, making tea, and coffee and soups
- Private well owners: If you have a private well, be sure to have your water tested so you know it's free of contaminants and toxins.
- Filter your water-- either at the sink or whole house, (whole home filtering may require replumbing the water pipes in your home if your pipes are older and corroded). Consider installing a filter in your shower as well.
- Don't use chlorine or bleach in your home
- Conserve your water use, install water saving faucets, appliances and toilets in your home, Fix leaking pipes, appliances.

SOLUTiONS WATER

Together we can keep water clean.

Get Involved

- Keep yourself hydrated with good quality water.
- Write to your Governor and Mayor as well as state and U.S. representatives asking that a comprehensive overhaul be implemented for our public drinking water filtration facilities. Compounding toxic water with more toxic chemicals to purify water is creating unnecessary exposure that is impairing health. Write letters.
- Protect yourself and your family by filtering your water, washing and peeling produce, and opting for organic food when possible.
- If you want to test your water for glyphosate, get this DIY kit available from National Testing Laboratories http://www.ntllabs.com/.
- Let's get the EPA to regulate all pesticides better.

Help Keep Stormwater Runoff Clean

"Stormwater runoff might seem harmless, but it can have significant environmental consequences. As it flows over streets, sidewalks, and other impervious surfaces, stormwater can pick up various pollutants, including sediment, chemicals, oils, phosphorous, fertilizers, salt, and bacteria. Stormwater runoff that goes down storm drains does not go through any treatment processes to remove contaminants before being discharged into local waterways."[505]

What we can do personally:
- Collect Rain: Use rainbarrels to capture runoff from your roof
- Responsible Lawn & Garden Care, use chemicals sparingly or not al all
- Proper disposal of household chemicals
- Manage pet waste, dispose of in trash cans to keep it out of water

Businesses and Industries:
- Create bioswales and creative landscaping to capture stormwater
- Use natural based landscaping to reduce toxins applied to grounds

SOLUTiONS
Holding Industry Accountable
- Keep chemicals out of the water and out of your personal care products. Learn more at www.waterkeeper.org.
- Shop responsibly and support companies that make things with the earth and *us* in mind.
- Let's reduce all toxic pollution emissions to zero. No more heavy metals, no more endocrine disruptors, no more neurotoxins, no more toxic pesticides, or PFAS, or BPA, or BADGE, or nanoparticles, excess fertilizer, or any toxic chemicals polluting our waterways.
- Let's get all fossil fuel corporations in compliance with good earth practices. This industry more than any other has the financial capability, the means and power to create technology that will prevent any future oil spills. They must take action and get going.
- The government must discontinue taxpayer subsidies for all industries that harm our drinking water or the air we breathe.
- Toxic Pollution must cease! Corporations must be held accountable for their discharges and pay for cleaning up any damage they have caused. Water treatment facilities are not capable of purifying many of the pollutants now entering our water.
- Help the whales and dolphins and other sea creatures harmed by ships and sonar noise. Go to **www.nrdc.org/water/oceans** and help bring sonar testing to an end!
- As much as possible, refrain from supporting corporations responsible for polluting the oceans, rivers, lakes, and streams. Water is sacred and vital to our existence! Healthy oceans and water ecosystems sustain us economically, spiritually, and physically. Buy products that do not contain toxic ingredients.
- In addition, we must consider fishing practices when we choose which fish to consume. We can contribute to healthy marine ecosystems through our purchases at grocery stores and dining out.
- Write to your Senators and Representatives, ask how they plan to bring water pollution to an end? Are they on board supporting human health?
- Do what you can at home to keep the water uncontaminated.
- Write your senators and congresspersons. Encourage them to introduce legislation that will end waivers for polluting industries and update our public water filtration methods.

WATER FILTERS

All of these filters purify your tap water. With a quality filter, you no longer need to buy bottled water except in emergencies. Remember, any filter is better than no filter.

Reverse Osmosis (RO)
RO systems typically push water through 3 stages of filters to effectively remove contaminants including heavy metals, pesticides, and DBPs. These filters can be installed under the sink or as a whole home filtration system.
Some brands that offer filters for home include:
- Aqua Tru: 3 filters include reverse osmosis, carbon and VOC filter. Removes over 80 contaminants including lead and 90% of fluoride.

Activated Carbon/ Carbon Block Filter/Gravity Filters
Activated carbon is a very dependable technology for removing contaminants from water. These can be installed in your shower also!
- Berkey is a carbon block gravity filter. Touted as removing most contaminants, 200+. Tip: filter speed is greatly improved if you get the air lock clip to mildly separate the two water reservoirs. Berkey has an excellent fluoride filter that can be added on as well.

Pitcher Filters
These have come a long way. Best results are seen with:
- Zero Filter
- Clearly Filter
- Larq Pure
- SOMA
- Pur and Brita Elite

Refrigerator Filters
These can be great. Replace them as needed.

Whole House Filters
These are excellent and filter water throughout the home. These are reverse osmosis systems.

SOLUTiONS WATER

FILTER MAINTENANCE
To keep filters working properly, they need to be cleaned and replaced from time to time. Filters have a life cycle, so any filter at the end of its useful life will need replacing. With gravity filters, it's good to clean out the drums holding the water. Make sure it's rinsed out well before refilling with water.

FILLING UP A GRAVITY FILTER
If you have a carbon block filter, it'll filter out impurities in your tap water. You fill up the reservoir with tap water. If you have a faucet with a hose, you can put the hose end in the top to fill it up. Otherwise, you have to place the device into the sink or fill it with a pitcher. Gravity filters can be slow if there's no air gap. Berkey sells a tiny airlock piece that fits in between the basins. This really helps speed up the filtering process and dispensing of water.

SHOWER FILTER
If you want to really reduce your exposure to water contaminants, consider installing a shower filter as well (unless you opt for the whole home filter in which case it will be filtered already). Inhaling steam from contaminated water can trigger health mishaps. There are many filters available that remove chloramines and fluoride. Vitamin C filters are very popular right now. Whatever filters you choose check their credentials and consumer reports for reviews. You may experiment with a few before you finally find the right shower filter for you.

REVERSE OSMOSIS
With RO, once it's connected properly, you can turn on the tap and what you receive will be filtered water.

Recycling Filters
Many filters are recyclable so can be put in the recycling bin.

SOLUTiONS Cleaning
NONTOXIC CLEANING

Natural Home Cleaner
You can clean just about anything in your home with a simple solution made of baking soda or Borax mixed with white vinegar and water. Add a drop or two of dish soap and some lavender essential oil.

Natural All-Purpose Cleaner
¼ cup lemon juice
2 cups water
¼ Cup hydrogen peroxide
add essential oils if desired

Natural Window Cleaner
½ cup white vinegar
1 cup water
½ tsp of dishwashing liquid
Mix together and pour into spray bottle.

DISINFECTANTS
Hydrogen Peroxide
Apple Cider Vinegar
- Heals wounds
- Disinfects cutting boards, countertops
- Mix with baking soda to remove stains on cookware
- Sterilizes toothbrushes
- Treats mold and fungus

Hydrogen Peroxide Whole Home Cleanser, Disinfectant
½ cup hydrogen peroxide
1 ½ cup water
Add ingredients together in spray bottle and away you go.

Natural Disinfectant and Stain Remover
Ditch the chlorine bleach, instead use the hydrogen peroxide cleanser above on fixtures and toilets.

Whitening Clothes
Add Borax along with your detergent to your load of clothes.

DIY Cleaner
Mix ½ cup White Vinegar, ½ cup water, a couple drops of dish soap and 20 drops of essential oil of your choice.

SOLUTiONS Plants

CLEAN WATER WITH FLOWERS AND PLANTS
Plants and wildflowers aren't just pretty, they're also helpful in absorbing pollutants, cleaning the water and the air! Plant more flowers America! And don't dump herbicides on them, let them exist and live naturally as God intended.

Plants that Filter Pollution out of Water[506]
Cat Tails: Zinc, Cadmium, Lead and Nitrate
Iris's: Absorbs Heavy Metals, reduce Algae growth
Moss: Absorbs Lead
    Moss Warnstofia fluitans: Absorbs Arsenic
Pine Trees: Xylem in Pine bark absorbs bacteria from water
Soft Rush (Juncus Effusus): Removes oil, bacteria, and heavy metals like cobalt, zinc, and copper
Water Lilies: Absorbs Heavy Metals, reduce Algae growth
Water Mint (Mentha Aquatica): Removes E. Coli and Salmonella
Cabomba and Hornwort: Submerged Plants that oxygenate water and help fish health.
(info thanks to Kellogg Garden Products

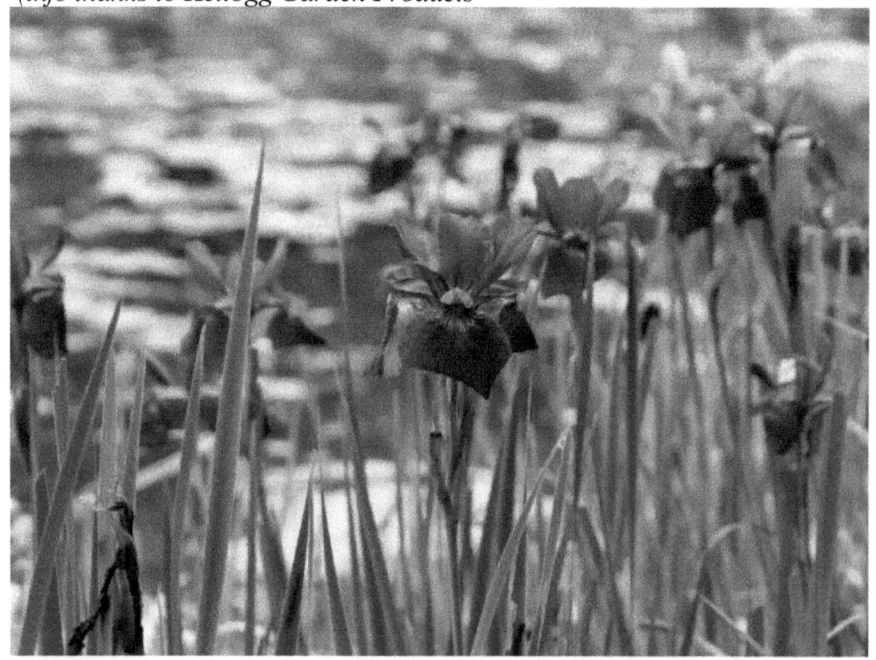

SOLUTiONS Gardening

Natural Lawn Fertilizer: Compost tea: Coffee grounds, egg shells, fruit and vegetable scraps make the perfect compost fertilizer and reduces food waste tossed into the trash.

Fungal Spray: If you notice plants developing fungus or mold, get some baking soda. Mix 2 Tbsp Baking Soda with 1 Gallon Water. Pour into spray container and spray plants where needed. Repeat for a few days until resolved.

Natural Pesticide Spray: Mix 1/2 cup white vinegar, 3 Tablespoons food grade diatomaceous earth, ½ cup water, 6 drops each essential oils of thyme, sage, citronella, lavender, lemongrass, and peppermint. Add to a spray bottle and spray where needed.

Neem Oil, Mild Insect Spray (Flea Eradicator too)
Mix 2 Tbsp Neem oil, dash of mild dish soap with 1 quart water. Put in spray bottle and use on plants as needed. Keep in fridge.

Natural insecticide, Diatomaceous Earth (Food Grade)
Please get Food Grade quality, very important!
Sprinkle this freely in your garden, it will not hurt your pets or plants. Sprinkle it around doorways to keep ant out. Clings to insects' exoskeleton and dehydrates them. Works most effectively when dry.

Rodale's Cayenne Pepper Recipe: Be careful, Avoid contact with eyes, wash hands thoroughly before touching face
Ingredients
1 garlic bulb and
1 small onion
1 teaspoon of powdered cayenne pepper
1 quart of water mixed with 1 tablespoon liquid dish soap
Chop garlic and onion. Add cayenne pepper and mix with soapy water mix. Steep 1 hour, then strain through cheesecloth. Mix well. Spray your plants thoroughly, including the undersides of the leaves. Store the mixture for up to a week in a labeled, covered container in the refrigerator.[507]

SOLUTiONS Toxins

TOXINS & POLLUTANTS
WHAT TO STOP BUYING:

- Toxic health harming pesticides
- Weed & feed fertilizer with atrazine, dicamba or 2,4-D
- Don't buy anything in Styrofoam
- Nanoparticles in sunscreen avoid avoid avoid!
- Hand Sanitizer with benzene or triclosan
- Anything with PFAS in it
- Anything containing disease-causing toxic chemicals
- Anything containing toxic pesticide residues
- Anything that brings harm to people, wildlife, and planet
- Anything that makes evil richer and stronger.
- Avoid food grown on fields with Sewage Sludge fertilizer
- Avoid PFAS, PFOA, Teflon, and all PFCs.
- Avoid BPA, BPS and BADGE
- Don't handle thermal paper receipts.
- Stop drinking fluoridated water
- Opt out of Food packaging, serving ware with PFAS.
- Avoid black plastic take out containers (e-waste)
- Government must cease funding all practices that add to declined forest health.
- Avoid endocrine disruptors, Avoid hormone disruptors
- Any product made by planet harming company
- Any product that causes harm to people
- Any product whose manufacturing harms our drinking water
- Any product that contains substances that harm babies and children
- _____
- _____

SOLUTiONS Replace

What to Buy Instead:
- Nontoxic cleaning products
- Support corporations that really do support clean air, clean water, healthy people and planet
- Furnishings and textiles without flame retardants
- Nontoxic personal care products, sundries, kitchenware
- Reef friendly sunscreen (see page 172)
- Recycled paper products
- Bamboo toilet paper and facial tissue
- Sustainable toilet paper saves Old Growth Forests!
- Nontoxic dish soap and detergent
- Nontoxic garden and lawn care products
- Organic cotton balls and cue tips
- Food grown without toxins, which in today's world is considered "organic", "biodynamic", or "regenerative"
- Shop at farmer's markets, look for farmers who use organic methods or IPM—integrated pest management
- Products without BPA or Badge or PFAS
- Products that are nontoxic
- Recycled paper saves trees☺
- Practice deep breathing daily.
- Take care of the planet
- Place plants in your home to absorb air pollution
- Trees and plants benefit us
- As we take care of the planet, the planet takes care of us.

Strengthen the Safe Drinking Water Act
- Can cities in the US switch to safer water purification methods—ones that don't use ammonia that causes nitrate pollution?
- No more loopholes for industrial toxic and agricultural polluters
- Help reduce toxic runoff pollution from lawns, farms and industry, Support farms that don't use toxic chemicals
- Let's get oil and gas operators to improve their processes from drilling and emissions to pipelines, transport, and shipping.
- Lets get all towns and industries on board this clean water train.

BOYCOTTING

- Certain companies and brands show disdain for our health. They deny the harm their products cause and resist improving their products to make them harmless. That leaves us with little choice, for we deserve good health, don't we? Those companies who refuse to care about our health, deserve to be boycotted. If they are not looking out for your health, why should you give them your money?
- Why boycott? Because what they create, how they create it, and what they are involved with is interfering with your and your family's health and happiness. In other words, they contribute to illness rather than health.
- In extreme times and under extreme circumstances Boycotting is an option we must enact. If every company and every product was good and harmless, this type of action would be unnecessary. Unfortunately, we live in a world where safety is often compromised and agencies that are designed to protect us fail to find the strength and courage to uphold their duty.
- Boycotting is a peaceful way to tell a company you expect them to do better. After all, money and profits should never be more important than the health and well-being of people. Answer this question: If the enemy is stealing your health and your happiness, do you let him continue and do nothing?
- Our government chooses not to enforce safety or caution when approving product and food additives (for example, nanoparticles, GRAS ingredients). Our government fails to display any interest enforcing rules (laws) that require labeling of dangerous ingredients, or banning dangerous chemicals from use. *Our* government is failing our health and our planet.
- Lobbyists (Corporate agents) have infiltrated our government. These lobbyists now hold posts in the government, yet they remain loyal to their corporation even though they are being paid with your tax dollars. Like crooks, they look out for their corporation's profits rather than your health.
- Our government is making very poor decisions and taking far too long to truly stop water pollution. When it comes to protecting our health, the government will only evolve if we require it.[508]

Are some companies profiting from cancer?
While ignoring efforts to prevent cancer by phasing out avoidable exposures to environmental and occupational carcinogens, The American Cancer Society remains silent about its intricate relationships with the wealthy cancer drug, chemical, and other industries. This reflects a virtually exclusive "blame-the-victim" philosophy. It emphasizes faulty lifestyles rather than unknowing and avoidable exposure to workplace or environmental carcinogens.

Giant corporations, which profit handsomely while they pollute the air, water, and food with a wide range of carcinogens, are greatly comforted by the silence of the ACS. This silence reflects a complex of mindsets fixated on diagnosis, treatment, and basic genetic research together with ignorance, indifference, and even hostility to prevention, coupled with conflicts of interest.

Indeed, despite promises to the public to do everything to "wipe out cancer in your lifetime," the ACS fails to make its voice heard in Congress and the regulatory arena. Instead, the ACS repeatedly rejects or ignores opportunities and requests from Congressional committees, regulatory agencies, unions, and environmental organizations to provide scientific testimony critical to efforts to legislate and regulate a wide range of occupational and environmental carcinogens.

The late Dr. Samuel Epstein
Prevent Cancer Coalition, *The Politics of Cancer*

SOLUTiONS 70%!
We are 70% Water, so is the Earth!
Being made mostly of water, doesn't it make sense to do all possible to keep our water clean?

Without question, water is our most precious and valuable resource. Without water, life cannot exist. While 72% of our planet is covered with water, only 2.6% is fresh water—and 2% of that is trapped in ice and glaciers. That means less than 1% of earth's water is accessible and available for drinking! With so little water to go around, we all need to do our share in taking care of it. That equates to adding as little pollutants to it as possible. People as well as industries must find better cleaner methods for doing just about everything. The EPA assesses and monitors most but not all water contaminants and sets thresholds. Yet safe thresholds for contaminants can change when evidence of health risks emerge.

QUALITY MATTERS
Quality matters. For your best health you don't need expensive or fancy water. You only need clean water. And clean water may be more difficult to find than ever. That's why this book is here to help clear up any misunderstandings about water, drinking water, tap water and clean water.

SAFE DRINKING WATER ACT (SDWA)
Protecting America's drinking water is a top priority. EPA has established protective drinking water standards for roughly 90 contaminants. We have a long way to go to regulate all the present contaminants not regulated and to stop the flow of toxic pollution into our waterways. In the meantime, do what you can to purify and filter your water!

SOLUTiONS, WATER

Heal the Ozone Layer and Reverse Climate Change

It's time to make some upgrades and help our world out.
What can companies, the Government, and regular folks do?

1. Reduce use of synthetic fertilizer
2. Reduce toxic chemical use in industry, hold industry accountable--require full transparency for toxic substances used.
3. **Fluorinated, Chlorinated Chemicals**: Ban or severely limit the industrial use and production of Fluorinated and Chlorinated Chemicals. At the very very least, any industry using or emitting these chemicals needs to install pollution capture technology.
4. **Ban PFAS, which means BIOSOLIDS will have to be banned as well. Ban Biosolid Fertilizer on American farmfields immediately.**
5. **Discontinue PFAS coatings on food packaging,**
6. **Ozone Depleting Substances** must be phased out from agriculture, as well as toxic farming chemicals
7. Change the Farm Bill so farmers are encouraged to nurture their soil, plant crops that suit their zone, and that endorses use earth-friendly, health-friendly substances on crops rather than toxic cancer-causing chemicals.
8. Reduce erosion and runoff by utilizing wetlands, bioswales and rain gardens on your property.
9. Nurture good water quality, human health, and the pollinators and wildlife by reducing use of toxic substances on your lawn.
10. **Reduce plastic waste and improve recycling technologies**
11. **Sustainable Farming Conversion**
12. Switching to Organic Farming Can Feed the World and Reduce the Effects of Climate Change as well as help end water pollution!
13. **Farmers can make money by making their soil a carbon capturing machine. In fact, doing farming healthier can reverse climate change.** [509]
14. **The EPA can start regulating all water pollution and emissions from all industries!**
15. **Save Trees, Save the Forests, use recycled paper and Choose bamboo toilet paper and paper towels.**
- Protect old growth woods from being harvested for toilet paper
- Be kind to animals

SOLUTiONS, WATER
PRIORITY LIST

What do you feel is the worst contaminant?

How does Water Pollution impact you and your family?

What concerns you most about water pollution?

Do you filter water at home?
How much water do you drink daily?

Is it filtered or bottled?

Do you cook with filtered water?

Toxic pollution of waterways must end. Thank you for Helping. You are part of the solution to end pollution.

Healing With Water

HEALING WATER

Hydration

Drink clean, filtered water.
Cook with clean, filtered water.
Drink 8 glasses of water or more daily. Drink water between meals. Drinking too much of any fluid with meals dilutes digestive juices and can hamper nutrient absorption.
Drinking water at room temperature may help with digestion.

> **Daily:
> Drink at least
> 8 glasses of
> clean water**

Shower with Clean Water

Let the Water pour over you and refresh you. Let the toxins and negative energy wash down the drain.

Cook with Clean Water

- Cook with clean, filtered water.
- Make baby formula with clean filtered water.
- Heat water on the stove or in the microwave.
- Do not hot tap water to make anything, unless you have reverse osmosis installed to your kitchen sink.

Clean Water:

- Filtered
- Spring water
- Uncontaminated
- Bottled water
- Distilled

Wash your hands with water and soap.

HEALING WATER

Water Therapy
FOOT BATH

Empower your body with minerals, instill calmness, connect with your well beingness.

Supplies Needed:
- foot bath basin (ceramic, stainless steel, glass bowl)
- transdermal magnesium (mg)
- hot water (or any temp will do)
- herbs and essential oils (optional)

When you have 25 minutes or more to soak your feet and relax and reset, set yourself a foot bath.

Directions
Step 1: Prepare the set: place a towel on the floor in front of you will be seated. Make sure your seat, chair is comfortable and makes you feel good. Bring blanket, pillow for support, cup of tea and water over to a table within reach. Turn on any music you wish, the lighting, whatever tools you need to work such as computer, notebook and pencil, what have you.
Intend to be comfortable. Wear comfy clothes that easily enough allow you to get your feet in the water without soaking your clothes. Some people wear a robe or a towel or a bathing suit. When the set is ready, you can prepare the foot bath.

Step 2: Fill foot-bath basin with hot water. Add 2 Tbsp transdermal magnesium or the cap filled just so. Add a few drops essential oils of lavender or frankincense or myrrh and rosemary if you like, or choose ones that resonate with you. Add a few fresh sprigs. Carry the bath over to the towel on the floor in front of your designated chair. Get yourself some tea or a notebook or laptop, whatever you want to do while soaking. Then sit back, dip your feet in the basin, relax and enjoy a little water therapy.

HEALING WATER

Water and Physical Health
There's a theory that most disease happens due to one thing--dehydration. Do we ever really get enough water? If we have ample water and are sufficiently hydrated would we avoid disease? With clean water, maybe so.

Sinus flush, Neti:
Be sure to use purified or distilled water

Humidifier and CPAP Devices:
Be sure to use purified or filtered water

Eyewash: Use cleanest, purest water available

Take a Bath and Relax

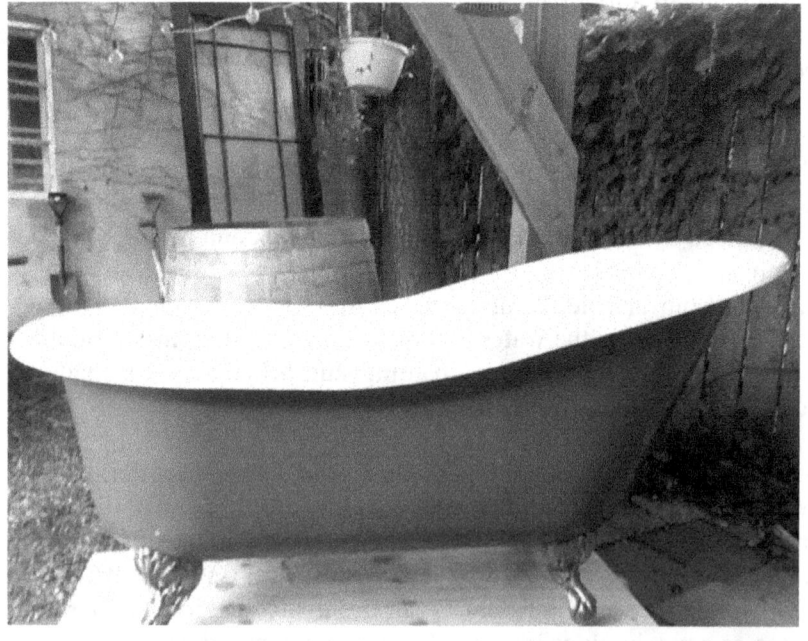

HEALING WATER

Water is Energy

By consciously treating water with care and thoughtfulness, we change the energy of everything, especially ourselves.

Water Reacts to Feelings and Thoughts

As Masaru Emoto showed us in *The Hidden Messages in Water*, water reacts to sounds, words, feelings, visions and images.

Pleasant words, beautiful sounds and thoughts create beautiful crystals. While angry, unhappy, harsh thoughts and words produced chaotic, angry looking, joyless, broken crystals.

> **Meditation for The Water: Ho'oponopono**
> I am sorry,
> please forgive me,
> I love you,
> Thank you.

As we are 70% water more or less, is it possible how we treat ourselves influences the water within us? This effect is seen in our health, our mood, how we see ourselves, how others perceive us.

Try an experiment with yourself to be kind, be nurturing, be gentle with yourself as well as with others. Visualize the water flowing beautifully and harmoniously within you and connecting you with others. Write words on a card and pin them to your shirt or pants if you like, or write love on your hand and see how it infuses your whole self with that vibration. Raise your frequency and tune in to all you are. Try it and let us know your stunning results!

Be like water, adaptable, forgiving, life giving, nonjudgemental.

HEALING WATER

Alkaline Water
Alkaline water may have some benefits but the evidence isn't entirely conclusive. Essentially, what makes it alkaline:
- pH at 8 or 9. (Regular water has neutral pH of 7).
- Water contains alkalizing minerals like calcium and magnesium carbonate[510]

Possible benefits: hydration, more endurance, keeps bones strong, reduces acid reflux, helps with athletic recovery

Ozonated Water	Ozone, O3, disinfects water, heals - must use purified water - helps with healing and infections, - can drink 1 8 oz glass daily on empty stomach, - useful on skin and for various infections	- limit to one glass daily - machine needs ventilation - requires training to use

Hydrogen Water
Hydrogen water appears to be a beneficial drink with numerous health benefits for the gut biome, acting as an antioxidant, antiapoptotic, good for metabolic syndrome, immune function, improving athletic performance. Advantages are seen in those with alcoholic fatty liver disease.[511]

What is pH: Potential Hydrogen

HEALING PEOPLE

BEST HEALTH SUGGESTIONS
From the President's Cancer Panel[512]:
"Filtering home tap or well water can decrease exposure to numerous known or suspected carcinogens and endocrine-disrupting chemicals. Unless the home water source is known to be contaminated, it is preferable to use filltered tap water instead of bottled water."

"Compounds found in dietary phytochemical preparations such as teas, garlic, herbs, grapes and cruciferous vegetables are now generally accepted to defend against the development of many different types of tumors as well as acting as epigenetic modulators that impact not only the initiation, but also the progression of oncogenesis."

"Family exposure to numerous occupational chemicals can be reduced by removing shoes before entering the home and washing work clothes separately from the other family laundry."

"From a National Level: 'A precautionary prevention-oriented approach… should be the cornerstone of a new national cancer prevention strategy… that eliminates toxic environmental exposures implicated in cancer causation'"

"A more integrated, coordinated, and transparent system for promulgating and enforcing environmental contaminant policy and regulations, driven by science and free of political or industry influence, must be developed to protect public health."

Corporations and Industry: Please stop polluting our water resources. Instead of using unsafe substances in making your products, please use health-friendly materials that help us all.
EPA and FDA: Please enforce the Clean Water Act and stop allowing industries to pollute our drinking water with disease-causing substances, or any untested unnatural toxic substance.

HEALING PEOPLE

REDUCE YOUR EXPOSURE TO TOXINS
Avoid these things:

Unfiltered tap water
Avoid drinking or cooking with, contains uber toxins including DBPs, PFAS, and neurotoxins

Nonstick Cookware
contains PFOA, PFAS, disease-causing water toxin

Plastic
harmful endocrine disruptors, most abundant persistant pollutant, harming animals, ecosystems, and people

Toxic Cleaning Products
These contain neurotoxins, carcinogens, endocrine disruptors, respiratory irritants, and VOCs. They poison water supplies, harm people and animals,. Avoid contact with chlorine bleach, harmful vapors, toxic substances, adhesives, ammonia, artificial scents, ethylene glygol, parabens, sodium laureth glycol, nitrosamines…

Pesticides
Neurotoxins, carcinogens, endocrine diruptors, repructive toxins

Receipts
Thermal receipts contain BPA

Ceramic Mugs with Lead
Avoid those with heavy metals in their glazing

Toxic Laundry Detergent
Go nontoxic, phosphate, endocrine disruptor free to bring wellness to nature and ourselves. Go a step further and use laundry sheets and skip the plastic jugs and waste. **Go to www.earthbreeze.com**

HEALING PEOPLE

In The Kitchen

Tea and Coffee:
Use purified or filtered water

Baby Formula:
Be sure to use purified or filtered water

Soup and Bone Broth:
Be sure to use purified or filtered water

Boiling Potatoes
Use filtered water!

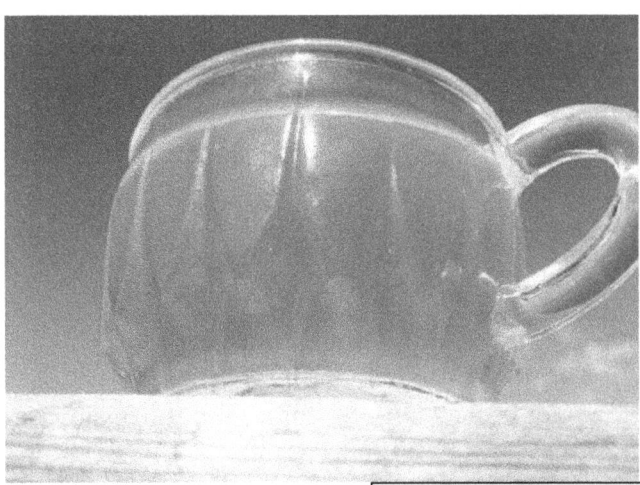

Herbal Organic Tea
Good for the body and good for the earth.
Good for Pollinators

LET THERE BE LIGHT!

Sunlight is so healing for all of us, people and animals. It's also a natural tool to help eliminate many diseases caused by microbes, fungus, mildew, mold, yeast, and pathogens. Don't slather on nanoparticle sunscreen though-- let sunlight absorb into your skin and reenergize you, boost your Vitamin D. Healthy Reef-friendly sunscreen is best for the day. Morning sun is ideal for healing; air is cleaner then too. Letting your tea brew in the sun is a nice way to infuse sunshine into your beverages. Red light therapy[513] is showing great promise for healing the body and brain[514].

VIBRATION and FREQUENCY

Everything is energy. Energy is healing or it's defeating. You decide what you want to be through your words, choices and actions. If you're shaken up with fear or confusion, or feel lost, or down, turn it around with different choices that will boost your vibration upward. Also, jumping up and down, clapping, stomping your feet to music all raise your vibration. Laughter is a wonderful high frequency tool. So is Sunshine.

MUSIC and SOUNDS

Music, uplifting music is energy. All music is energy, some may resonate with you more than others. That which makes you feel good inside is at a high vibration. Bird songs, high vibration. Beautiful sounds, beautiful words and thoughts are on a high vibration. If you feel blue, discouraged, hopeless, angry, practice raising your vibration. Get in the sunlight (high vibration), sing and dance (high vibration), smile, listen to the rain. Go on a nature walk and listen to the water, to the animals, to the leaves rustling on the trees, to the pebbles as you take your step, to your own breath. These are nature sounds, (high vibration).
Rain clears and charges your electrons. Walking barefoot on the earth recharges your electrons, so does copper.

COLOR: Colors are energy and vibrations too. Some make us feel happier than others. In nature, color abounds to bring us joy.

HEALING PEOPLE

HEALING FOODS

Food is health, if you choose the right foods for you. Everyone's health is different, we all have our own bio-individualist profile. What's good for you may not be good for another. One thing is true, a true nutritious diet can do wonders for your health. This is especially true if you want to boost your health or recover your health, or lower your risk of disease.

Holistic Healing Keys:

- Thoughts and energy
- Hydration—clean water, spring or filtered is essential.
- Reducing exposure to toxins — from water, air, food, home, any environments, indoor and out
- Nourish thyself with wholesome foods as nature created, grown and raised without toxins or artificial substances. Avoid factory farm raised meat, eggs, dairy and GMO foods of any kind if you want to heal.
- We want to make sure you're getting all the essential nutrients your body needs. Minerals, vitamins, omega oils, micronutrients, etc. We also make sure to heal stomach & clear any infection or overgrowth interfering with nutrient absorption.
- Consume healing nutrient-dense beverages in addition to clean water. These include: organic herbal tea, green tea, moringa…
- Indulge in the best foods available that are not only delicious and perfect for you, but also can be prepared in all sorts of ways to your fancy. Get imaginative☺
- Keep it simple, eat the rainbow in organic veges and fruits, enjoy homemade soup and supper when possible
- Have fun and also get lots of rest, relax more. Make this your best, most productive time. Use select supplements as needed.
- Laugh often.
- Every person is unique. We all have our own bioindividual, bioprivate profile. What's best for one won't necessarily be best for another. Seek personal guidance from a qualified naturopath, holistic healer, or natural nutrition guide.

WHEN YOU'RE HEALING, AVOID:

- Avoid artificial sweeteners, high fructose corn syrup (HFCS), junk food, sweets with no nutrients, GMOs and factory farm eggs, GMO milk and dairy products, avoid factory farm deli meats and hot dogs (top quality, organic can be okay), Avoid antibiotics, steroids or nitrites in meats, bacon, etc. Avoid 'egglands best'—as they abuse chickens and are really bad factory farm eggs[515] with marketing that makes them appear organic—they are not.
- Avoid consuming or cooking with unhealthy PUFA fats—they interfere with metabolism: canola oil, soybean oil, corn oil, sunflower, safflower oil, cottonseed oil, rice bran oil, grape seed oil.[516] The way these are processed contributes to weight gain and metabolic and immune system disorders.
- Lots of Healthy fats are preferred and essential for your best health. Healthy fats include: Extra virgin olive oil, unrefined coconut oil, butter (rBGH free), ghee, avocado oil, sesame oil, peanut oil, organic eggs, wild caught fish,
- Depending on your goals and conditions, you may opt to limit or restrict dairy, (if allergic, avoid it altogether). Some cancers[517], hormone-related diseases[518] and antibiotic-resistant infections[519] can be influenced by hormones in dairy.

FOODS ALLOWED INCLUDE:

Proteins: Organic eggs, wild caught salmon and halibut, tuna (sparingly), cod, canned tuna, salmon, grass fed meats and beef, organic chicken, organic turkey bacon, organic poultry, lamb. peanut oil, hummus, nuts, seeds, beans, grass fed meats, poultry, etc (No factory farm meat or eggs, absolutely no fake organic like *egglands best*[520]*!*)

Fats: Organic extra virgin olive oil, unrefined coconut oil, grass fed organic butter, ghee, lard, avocado, tallow, organic eggs, wild caught fish, tuna, sardines, sesame oil, peanut oil, flax seed oil, coconut milk

Vegetables: Organic Dark Leafy Greens, Broccoli, Cauliflower, Microgreens, Carrots, Kale, Celery, Beets, Chard, Squash, Hot Peppers, Beans, Peas, Asparagus, Potatoes, Tomatoes, Onion, Garlic, Green Onions, Sweet Potatoes, potatoes, olives, cucumber, parsley, cilantro, Spinach, Eggplant, Brussel Sprouts, Arugula, Lettuce...

Whole Grains (complex carbs): Brown Rice, Quinoa, Amaranth, Oats, Oatmeal, Buckwheat, Pasta, Organic corn (no wheat or wheat grains like spelt, try to avoid during healing protocol. Bread, roll, or bagel with plenty of olive oil or other healthy fat may be allowed).

Beans: Chickpeas, Pinto Beans, Kidney Beans, Lentils, Dal, Split pea, Hummus, bean spreads

Seaweed: Irish Moss, Bladderwack, Dulse, Kelp
Soup: Homemade soups, broth-based soups, bone broth, chili, vege
Dairy: unsweetened organic yogurt, cottage cheese, non-rBGH whole milk, organic cheese, goat milk cheese, pecorino
Fruit: Organic apples, goji berries, poached pears, green banana, blueberries, cherries, peaches, lemons, limes, oranges, grapefruit, etc
Nuts and Seeds: Organic almonds, walnuts, Brazil nuts, peanuts, pumpkin seeds, flax seeds, sunflower seeds, sesame seeds, pecans,
Beverages: Filtered and Spring Water, Mineral water, Organic Herbal Tea, Green tea and Matcha, Coconut water, herbal water, Moringa tea, Hot water with lemon and ginger, mineral water, unsweetened cranberry juice, unsweetened carbonated water, fresh fruit juice, vegetable broth

Fiber is important, brown rice, oats, vegetables, flax seeds, psyllium husks. PB shakes in morning ON an EMPTY Stomach are good to help detox and remove toxins. (Directions: 1Tbsp psyllium husks and 1Tbsp bentonite clay (food-grade) mixed well in 8 oz water. Follow with a few 8 oz glasses of water and other hydrating beverages afterward to keep things flowing)

Coffee is ok, but no refined sugar or artificial sweeteners. Raw honey is good, but suggest you lower intake of caffeine a bit, replace with green or herbal tea if and when you can. If you can go a few days or a week or two without coffee that is good and gives your endocrine system a break. Eliminating coffee depends on your situation. Going off sugar, caffeine, and alcohol at the same time does provide your entire system a break. If you also reduce intake of meat, you'll really give your digestive system a vacation too! Then the whole gang can reset in full.

If you're fasting, it's essential your water is purified and clean and you're consuming enough of it. Fresh organic vegetable juices and broths are encouraged for hydration benefits and electrolytes. Organic herbal teas are useful as well, especially herbs that improve lymph circulation, fresh squeezed lime or lemon, unsweetened cranberry juice, warm water with lemon.

This will get you started. If you'd like further guidance on meal planning, recipes, grocery shopping, morning routines, energy work, auto suggestion, nature therapy, personal growth and self care rituals, in other words the whole shabang, check out our *heal thyself* page at www.adoreyourplanet.com, or email hello@adoreyourplanet.com. This will all be included in our upcoming nutrients book as well!

HEALING ANIMALS

Give them love, treat them kindly. Play with them. Snuggle with them. Hold them and hug them. Say nice things to them. Dance and play music with them, for them. Give them toys and good treats. Give them fresh air and outdoor time if possible, sunlight and a nurturing environment, a soft bed to sleep on, an area to feel safe and secure. Like us, animals need a quiet environment for resting.

Give them fresh water and food
Daily, animals need fresh water and food

Filter their water
Give filtered clean water to your pets

Clean their bowls
Keep their water and food bowls clean, wash daily with soap.

Give them warm and dry shelter

Don't give them GMOs if you can help it.

Flea and Tick Prevention, Deworm
Give them appropriate flea and tick application or meds obtained from veterinarian. Give them de-wormer annually or more often if needed. Regular veterinarian check-ups.

To Help Prevent Disease:
- Make sure their food has all the essential nutrients they need Supplement with seaweed so they can be sure to get iodine.
- Don't give them sugar and unnatural things for animals
- Avoid toxic substances, avoid exposing them to toxic algae
- Help change pet food packaging: pet food bags contain PFAS.
- Vaccines: Not all vaccines are necessary for dogs and cats. Get a vet that's health conscious, only vaccinate when needed.

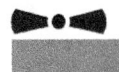

Drink Safe Water

After a natural disaster, water may not be safe to use.
Germs and chemicals may be in the water.
Listen to local officials to find out if your water is safe.

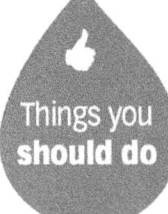

Things you should do

- Listen for announcements from local officials to find out what to do. They will tell you if there are germs and/or chemicals in the water.
- Boil water if instructed. Boil it for at least 1 minute (start counting when the water comes to a constant boil). Let the water cool sufficiently before drinking. Boiling kills germs in the water.
- Use bottled water if instructed. Sometimes after a disaster, there may be chemicals in the water that boiling cannot remove.

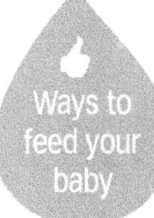

Ways to feed your baby

- Breast-feed or use ready-made formula.
- If you must use water to make formula, use only commercially-bottled water until officials say your tap water is safe to drink.

Things you should never do

- **Never** drink the water unless you know it is safe.
- **Never** wash or clean dishes, utensils, toys, or other objects in the water unless you know it is safe.
- **Never** bathe in the water unless you know it is safe.
- **Never** cook with the water unless you know it is safe.
- **Never** brush your teeth with the water unless you know it is safe.
- **Never** use the water to make ice unless you know it is safe.

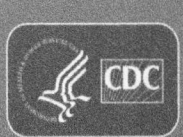

U.S. Department of Health and Human Services
Centers for Disease Control and Prevention

For more information on safe water after a natural disaster, please visit
http://www.cdc.gov/healthywater/emergency/drinking/emergency-water-supply-preparation.html

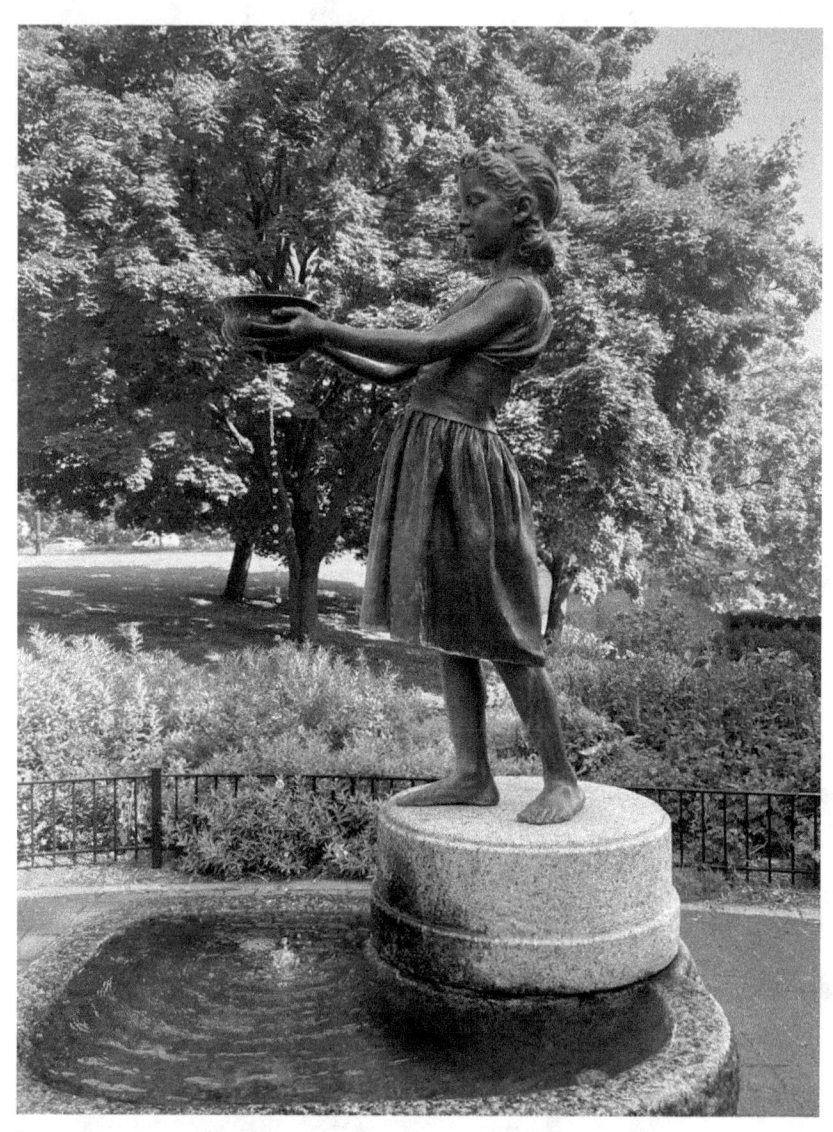

GOVERNMENT

> There is nothing wrong with America
> that the faith, love of freedom,
> intelligence and energy of
> her citizens cannot cure.
> **President Dwight David Eisenhower**

COMMUNICATION

In order to solve problems effectively, it will help to work together. To do that, we need good communication amongst ourselves, as well as with the government.

While we are a democracy run by the people for the people, many of the bills introduced and discussed in Congress, as well as open public opinion periods scheduled by government agencies are never broadcast to the general population. Oftentimes people don't find out anything until it's too late, a bill has already passed or the question and answer period has closed. If we had a better announcement system for all of us, we could all be engaged in the decision-making. You can bet the corporate interests are made aware of these opportunities, but strangely enough not the citizens whose lives are affected by such decisions? Let's fix this and make this truly a government for the people by the people

LET'S NEVER MISS A CHANCE TO BE INVOLVED

We propose a monthly and annual government calendar be made available and accessible by every citizen of this country.

- This Schedule will contain the agenda for both the House of Representatives and the Senate, issues to be discussed, bills introduced, bills pending signature, and understandable descriptions of the bills presented, as well as key people and government agency involved with the issue and contact information, etc. Additionally, each State shall provide to all of its residents the monthly agenda of its House and Senate issues, discussions, topics and bills being considered, pending resolutions, etc. If any last-minute riders to bills should be presented that are not mentioned on these annual or monthly schedules, the party proposing the bill will have the responsibility of informing the public, in all the US or respectively in only that State(s) addressed within 24 hours, but at least 48 hours before voting commences.
- Means of providing these aforementioned monthly and annual schedules will include a dedicated calendar website, internet postings on specified government websites and may also include media, emailing constituents, mailing reminders, flyers, posters,
- This calendar site will be updated often to provide true and complete information relating to the issues. in simple easy-to-read format, plainly and easily identified. This sharing of information will help us, the citizens and residents of this country to stay in the loop and be organized and to never miss an opportunity to be involved in our government's decision process again.

SOLUTiONS
YOUR GOVERNMENT PHONE LIST

NAME	PHONE
PRESIDENT's OFFICE	
President	(202) 456-6213
Vice President	(202) 456-1414
The Whitehouse	(202) 456-1111
Congress	1(800) FED-INFO
Senators	www.senate.gov
Representatives	www.house.gov
Governor, contact yours	www.nga.org
ATSDR	ATSDRIC@cdc.gov
Agency Toxic Substances	
CDC	(800) 311-3435
USDA	(202) 720-3631
FDA	1-888-463-6332
	www.fda.gov
HHS	(202) 619-0257
Health Human Services	
EPA	(800) 832-7828
Administrator	www.epa.gov
Hotline	(800) 426-4791
Lead Poisoning	(800) 424-5323
Pesticide Office	(703) 557-9307
Water Resource Center	(202) 566-1729
Water Admin	(202) 564-5700
	(202) 564-5700
FOREST SERVICE	
Stewardship Council	(202) 342-0413
OSHA	www.osha.gov
Dept of the Interior	(202) 208-3100
PROTECT AMERICA!	

ACCOUNTABILITY

When you look closely at the agencies created to protect us, you may be surprised to find policies based on risk and reaction rather than precaution and common sense. Most of us assume that the government shares our desire to keep us healthy and does what is necessary to keep us safe and sound. We assume that our country has done everything in its power to protect us, to keep our most cherished places untouched, that our tax dollars are used toward programs that help us, not hurt us. These beliefs once were true. Long ago, the United States was governed by people who genuinely cared about the wellbeing of its citizens, and it could be said that our country functioned in respectable and honorable ways. Today, however, our government's top priority does not always seem to be its people, nor is it our health.

Whether you know it or not, decisions have been made that are directly compromising your health, your family's health and the health of this planet. Lobbyists influence and oftentimes direct agency and congressional decisions. These decisions have been transforming America from a land founded on love and freedom to one corrupted with greed and arrogance.

Have you noticed in recent years just how many decisions are made behind closed doors? How public access to information has been dwindling? How many environmental regulations have been rolled back or altogether eliminated? You have two choices: You can close your eyes and let these violations continue, or you can prepare to rise and help change things peacefully.

Other countries endorse the policy known as the Precautionary Principle. When government and industries adopt this principle, the policies they create exercise caution and consideration for others. Additionally, any method or product they create is tested for safety *before* being exposed to the public. In America, we have not followed this principle. Instead, we have allowed risk to lead, and we follow with reaction. We have not required companies, notably chemical companies to prove that their products are safe before going to market. We've been their test subjects. It's time for action & reform of all our governmental houses of protection.
Nonpartisan U.S. Government Accountability Office, www.gao.gov, (202) 512-4800.

THE CDC, HHS

HHS, HEALTH AND HUMAN SERVICES

The U.S. Department of Health and Human Services (HHS) is the U.S. government's principal agency for protecting the health of all Americans and providing essential human services, especially for those who are least able to help themselves.

HHS: FDA, Food and Drug Administration
ATSDR, Agency Toxic Substances
CDC, Center for Disease Control
CFS, Children and Family Services
National Institutes of Health
Mental Health Services
Substance Abuse Administration

CDC: CENTER FOR DISEASE CONTROL manages:
Center for Global Health
National Institute for Occupational Safety and Health
Office for State, Tribal, Local, and Territorial Support
Office of Equal Employment Opportunity
Office of Infectious Diseases
- National Center for Emerging and Zoonotic Infectious Diseases
- National Center for HIV/AIDS, Viral Hepatitis, STD, and TB
- National Center for Immunization and Respiratory Diseases

Office of Minority Health and Health Equity
Office of Noncommunicable Diseases, Injury and Environmental Health
- National Center for Chronic Disease Prevention and Health Promotion
- National Center for Environmental Health/Agency for Toxic Substances and Disease Registry
- National Center for Injury Prevention and Control
- National Center on Birth Defects and Developmental Disabilities

Office of Public Health Preparedness and Response
Office of Public Health Scientific Services
- Center for Surveillance, Epidemiology and Laboratory Services

THE FDA & USDA

FDA: United States Food and Drug Administration
The FDA approves and oversees what goes in food, what's allowed to be used in food packaging, what's used in personal care products.

USDA: U.S. DEPARTMENT of AGRICULTURE
The USDA oversees factory farms, conditions for animals, as well as crop insurance and the forest service. They also have one of the cruelest agencies, Wildlife Services, that traps and kills millions of wild animals yearly. "We have a vision to promote agriculture production that better nourishes Americans while also helping feed others throughout the world; and to preserve our Nation's natural resources through conservation, restored forests, improved watersheds, and healthy private working lands.

FDA Manages:
- The Food Supply
- Bottled Water
- Infant Formulas
- Food Safety
- GMOS
- Nanoparticles in foods, drugs, pesticides
- Pharmaceuticals, Drugs, Vaccines, medical supplies and equipment
- Supplements, Vitamins and Minerals
- Cosmetics
- Veterinary Products
- Tobacco

USDA Manages:
Agriculture, Animal & Plant Health
Animal Welfare
Factory Farms
Farm Inspections
Crop Insurance
Center for Nutrition Policy
Food Safety and Inspection Service
Foreign Agricultural Service
U.S. Forest Service
Wildlife Services
Grain inspection, Stockyards
Risk Management Agency
Rural Development
National Inst for Food & Agriculture

Department of the Interior

The Department of the Interior oversees our Public Lands, Fish and Wildlife Service, The Endangered Species Act, US Geological Service, and more. Through the Bureau of Land Management (BLM), they decide who gets to lease our public lands and generally is favorable to oil and gas leases over wild animal welfare. Currently they have the BLM harshly removing thousands of wild horses and free roaming burros from our Public Lands yearly. They prefer to lease the land to oil and gas and cattle ranchers than to allow horses to remain free. Horses don't pay rent. This policy is costly and un-American. There are better ways to holistically manage horse populations instead of rounding them up by helicopter by people who abuse animals. Their current policy divides the colts from the herds, causing massive horse injuries and casualties. We must help these animals who are defenseless against the despicable helicopter hunting methods the BLM employs. Incidentally, **the BLM is breaking the Law: 1971 Wild Horse and Burro Protection Act !**

Endangered Species Act
The U.S. Fish and Wildlife Service oversees the ESA.
- conservation incentives
- Increase public participation through grants & partnerships

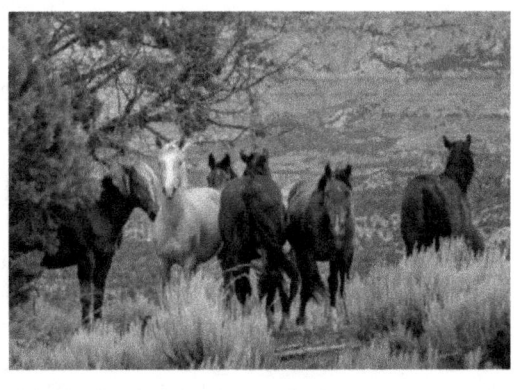

The Department of the Interior includes:
- Bureau of Land Management (BLM) (Public Lands, Wild Horses)
- US Fish & Wildlife Service (Manages Endangered Species Act)
- USGS US Geological Survey
- Bureau Ocean Energy Management approves offshore drilling
- Bureau of Reclamation
- Bureau of Safety and Environmental Enforcement
- FOIA Program
- Indian Water Rights Office
- Land Buy-Back Program for Tribal Nations
- National Invasive Species Council
- National Park Service

The EPA
Environmental Protection Agency

President Nixon established the EPA on December 2, 1970. Its mission included gathering information related to pollution, and then using that information to strengthen environmental protection programs and to make pollution cease.

> EPA History of the Clean Water Act: Into and page 11

It is claimed the EPA's mission is to protect human health and the environment

1. all Americans are protected from significant risks to human health and the environment where they live, learn and work;
2. national efforts to reduce environmental risk are based on the best available scientific information;
3. federal laws protecting human health and the environment are enforced fairly and effectively;
4. environmental protection is an integral consideration in U.S. policies concerning natural resources, human health, economic growth, energy, transportation, agriculture, industry, and international trade, and these factors are similarly considered in establishing environmental policy;
5. all parts of society -- communities, individuals, businesses, and state, local and tribal governments -- have access to accurate information sufficient to effectively participate in managing human health and environmental risks;
6. environmental protection contributes to making our communities and ecosystems diverse, sustainable and economically productive;
7. the United States plays a leadership role in working with other nations to protect the global environment. www.epa.gov

Once serving as the guardian of the public's health, the EPA has bounced back some from being an under-funded agency, yet still falling short from wholeheartedly protecting people or natural resources. The loopholes and exemptions for horrible polluters makes no sense, the failure to restrict and ban pesticides is truly an insult to everyone's health, the agency's hypocritical position as an agency designed to protect the environment, yet still allowing pesticide manufacturers to supply their own studies as evidence of no harm. Sub-par enforcement and favors for industry just doesn't work for us.

EPA Office of Water

The laws and regulations were designed to protect people and animals. How can the EPA so easily let Neonicotinoid, Atrazine, and Glyphosate use continue? Where do your loyalties lie?

The EPA was significantly weakened under the Bush/Cheney Administration from 2000 -2008. Many EPA heroes were forced to resign, for they were unwilling to carry out orders that contradicted their beliefs. Former EPA scientist Michele Merkel stated, "Once the Bush team came in, I was not allowed to pursue any further air lawsuits against CAFOs [concentrated animal feeding operations]. It wasn't just coming from my EPA superiors, it was coming from the White House."[521]

How many contaminants does the EPA Regulate?

Currently the EPA monitors and regulates about 90 contaminants in our drinking water. Yet, there are hundreds, in some places thousands of contaminants, and older and emerging contaminants that pose a health danger. The process to include a new contaminant on the EPA list is long and often bungled by red tape and lobbyists. The result is that there's much more in our water threatening our health than the EPA tells us about.

Industry, Agriculture, and Corporations have a lot of room for improvement. Ultimately, we need to prevent pollution as much as possible. Using nontoxic earth-friendly materials and methods is ideal for everything. If you went to a Waldorf School you have a good awareness of nature's magical gifts.

We must persist. It may be tough at times, but if we all keep strong and keep going after the bad guys, we will end toxic pollution. By so doing we will have helped countless children, animals, and people of all ages have better health for years to come.
[522]The Office of Water (OW) ensures drinking water is safe, and restores and maintains oceans, watersheds, and their aquatic ecosystems to protect human health, support economic and recreational activities, and provide healthy habitat for fish, plants and wildlife. OW is responsible for implementing the Clean Water Act and Safe Drinking Water Act, and portions of the Coastal Zone Act Reauthorization Amendments of 1990.[523] We must protect America and one another.

EPA: Contaminants Chart

The following charts contain the lists of Contaminants Regulated by the EPA, their potential health effects as well as the source.
www.epa.gov/safewater/hfacts.html#Volatile

Disinfection Byproducts

Contaminant	MCLG[1] (mg/L)[2]	MCL or TT[1] (mg/L)[2]	Potential Health Effects from Ingestion of Water	Sources of Contaminant in Drinking Water
Bromate	Zero	0.010	Increased risk of cancer	Byproduct of drinking water disinfection
Chlorite	0.8	1.0	Anemia; infants & young children: nervous system effects	Byproduct of drinking water disinfection
Haloacetic acids (HAA5)	n/a[6]	0.060	Increased risk of cancer	Byproduct of drinking water disinfection
Total **Trihalomethanes (TTHMs)**	None[7] ---------- n/a[6]	0.10 --------- -0.080	Liver, kidney or central nervous system problems; increased risk of cancer	Byproduct of drinking water disinfection

Disinfectants

Contaminant	MRDLG[1] (mg/L)[2]	MRDL[1] (mg/L)[2]	Potential Health Effects from Ingestion of Water	Sources of Contaminant in Drinking Water
Chloramines (as Cl_2)	MRDLG=4[1]	MRDL=4.0[1]	Eye/nose irritation; stomach discomfort, EPanemia, DNA damage	Water additive used to control microbes
Chlorine (as Cl_2)	MRDLG=4[1]	MRDL=4.0[1]	Eye/nose irritation; stomach discomfort	Water additive used to control microbes
Chlorine dioxide (as ClO_2)	MRDLG=0.8[1]	MRDL=0.8[1]	Anemia; infants & young children: nervous system effects	Water additive used to control microbes

Inorganic Chemicals

Contaminant	MCLG[1] (mg/L)[2]	MCL or TT[1] (mg/L)[2]	Potential Health Effects from Ingestion of Water	Sources of Contaminant in Drinking Water
Antimony	0.006	0.006	Increase in blood cholesterol; decrease in blood sugar	Discharge from petroleum refineries; fire retardants; ceramics; electronics; solder
Arsenic	0[7]	0.010 as of 01/23/06	Skin damage or problems with circulatory systems, and may have	Erosion of natural deposits; runoff from orchards, runoff from glass & electronics

287

			increased risk of getting cancer	production wastes
Asbestos (fiber >10 micrometers)	7 million fibers	7 MFL	Increased risk of developing benign intestinal polyps	Decay of asbestos cement in water mains; erosion of natural deposits
Barium	2	2	Increase in blood pressure	Discharge of drilling wastes; discharge from metal refineries; erosion of natural deposits
Beryllium	0.004	0.004	Intestinal lesions	Discharge from metal refineries and coal-burning factories; discharge from electrical, aerospace, and defense industries
Cadmium	0.005	0.005	Kidney damage	Corrosion of galvanized pipes; erosion of natural deposits; discharge from metal refineries; runoff from waste batteries and paints
Chromium (total)	0.1	0.1	Allergic dermatitis	Discharge from steel and pulp mills; erosion of natural deposits
Copper	1.3	TT[8]; Action	Short term exposure:	Corrosion of household

		Level =1.3	Gastrointestinal distress Long term exposure: Liver or kidney damage. People with Wilson's Disease should consult their doctor if the amount of copper in their water exceeds the action level	plumbing systems; erosion of natural deposits
Cyanide (as free cyanide)	0.2	0.2	Nerve damage or thyroid problems	Discharge from steel/metal factories; discharge from plastic and fertilizer factories
Fluoride	4.0	4.0	Bone disease (pain and tenderness of the bones); Children may get mottled teeth	Water additive which promotes strong teeth; erosion of natural deposits; discharge from fertilizer and aluminum factories
Lead	Zero	TT[8]; Action Level =0.015	Infants and children: Delays in physical or mental development; deficits in attention span and learning abilities. Adults: Kidney problems; high blood pressure	Corrosion of household plumbing systems; erosion of natural deposits

Mercury (inorganic)	0.002	0.002	Kidney damage	Erosion of natural deposits; discharge from refineries and factories; runoff from landfills and croplands
Nitrate (measured as Nitrogen)	10	10	Infants below the age of six months who drink water containing nitrate in excess of the MCL could become seriously ill and, if untreated, may die. Symptoms include shortness of breath and blue-baby syndrome.	Runoff from fertilizer use; leaching from septic tanks, sewage; erosion of natural deposits
Nitrite (measured as Nitrogen)	1	1	Infants below the age of six months who drink water containing nitrite in excess of the MCL could become seriously ill and, if untreated, may die. Symptoms include shortness of breath and blue-baby syndrome.	Runoff from fertilizer use; leaching from septic tanks, sewage; erosion of natural deposits
Selenium	0.05	0.05	Hair or fingernail loss; numbness in	Discharge from petroleum refineries;

			fingers or toes; circulatory problems	erosion of natural deposits; discharge from mines
Thallium	0.0005	0.002	Hair loss; changes in blood; kidney, intestine, or liver problems	Leaching from ore-processing sites; discharge from electronics, glass, and drug factories

Volatile Organic Chemicals (including Pesticides)

Contaminant	MCLG[1] (mg/L)[2]	MCL or TT[1] (mg/L)[2]	Potential Health Effects from Ingestion of Water	Sources of Contaminant in Drinking Water
Acrylamide	Zero	TT[2]	Nervous system or blood problems; increased risk of cancer	Added to water during sewage/waste water treatment
Alachlor	Zero	0.002	Eye, liver, kidney or spleen problems; anemia; increased risk of cancer	Runoff from herbicide used on row crops
Atrazine	0.003	0.003	Cardiovascular system or reproductive problems	Runoff from herbicide used on row crops
Benzene	Zero	0.005	Anemia; decrease in blood platelets; increased risk of cancer	Discharge from factories; leaching from gas storage tanks and landfills

Benzo(a)pyrene (PAHs)	Zero	0.0002	Reproductive difficulties; increased risk of cancer	Leaching from linings of water storage tanks and distribution lines
Carbofuran	0.04	0.04	Problems with blood, nervous system, or reproductive system	Leaching of soil fumigant used on rice and alfalfa
Carbon tetrachloride	Zero	0.005	Liver problems; increased risk of cancer	Discharge from chemical plants and other industrial activities
Chlordane	Zero	0.002	Liver or nervous system problems; increased cancer risk	Residue of banned termiticide
Chlorobenzene	0.1	0.1	Liver or kidney problems	Discharge from chemical and agricultural chemical factories
2,4-D	0.07	0.07	Kidney, liver, or adrenal gland problems	Runoff from herbicide used on row crops
Dalapon	0.2	0.2	Minor kidney changes	Runoff from herbicide used on rights of way
1,2-Dibromo-3-chloropropane (DBCP)	Zero	0.0002	Reproductive difficulties; increased risk of cancer	Runoff/leaching from soil fumigant used on soybeans, cotton,

				pineapples, and orchards
o-Dichlorobenzene	0.6	0.6	Liver, kidney, or circulatory system problems	Discharge from industrial chemical factories
p-Dichlorobenzene	0.075	0.075	Anemia; liver, kidney or spleen damage; changes in blood	Discharge from industrial chemical factories
1,2-Dichloroethane	Zero	0.005	Increased risk of cancer	Discharge from industrial chemical factories
1,1-Dichloroethylene	0.007	0.007	Liver problems	Discharge from industrial chemical factories
cis-1,2-Dichloroethylene	0.07	0.07	Liver problems	Discharge from industrial chem factories
trans-1,2-Dichloroethylene	0.1	0.1	Liver problems	Discharge from industrial chemical factories
Dichloromethane	Zero	0.005	Liver problems; increased risk of cancer	Discharge from drug and chemical factories
1,2-Dichloropropane	Zero	0.005	Increased risk of cancer	Discharge from industrial chemical factories

Di(2-ethylhexyl) adipate	0.4	0.4	Weight loss, liver problems, or possible reproductive difficulties.	Discharge from chemical factories
Di(2-ethylhexyl) phthalate	Zero	0.006	Reproductive difficulties; liver problems; increased risk of cancer	Discharge from rubber and chemical factories
Dinoseb	0.007	0.007	Reproductive difficulties	Runoff from herbicide used on soybeans and vegetables
Dioxin (2,3,7,8-TCDD)	Zero	0.00000003	Reproductive difficulties; increased risk of cancer	Emissions from waste incineration and combustion; discharge from chemical factories
Diquat	0.02	0.02	Cataracts	Runoff from herbicide use
Endothall	0.1	0.1	Stomach and intestinal problems	Runoff from herbicide use
Endrin	0.002	0.002	Liver problems	Residue of banned insecticide
Epichlorohydrin	Zero	TT[2]	Increased cancer risk, and over a long period of time, stomach problems	Discharge from chemical factories; impure water treatment chemicals
Ethylbenzene	0.7	0.7	Liver or kidneys problems	Discharge from

				petroleum refineries
Ethylene dibromide	Zero	0.00005	Problems with liver, stomach, reproductive system, or kidneys; increased risk of cancer	Discharge from petroleum refineries
Glyphosate	0.7	0.7	Kidney problems; reproductive difficulties	Runoff from herbicide use
Heptachlor	Zero	0.0004	Liver damage; increased risk of cancer	Residue of banned termiticide
Heptachlor epoxide	Zero	0.0002	Liver damage; increased risk of cancer	Breakdown of heptachlor
Hexachlorobenzene	Zero	0.001	Liver or kidney problems; reproductive difficulties; increased risk of cancer	Discharge from metal refineries, agricultural chem factories
Hexachlorocyclopentadiene	0.05	0.05	Kidney or stomach problems	Discharge from chemical factories
Lindane	0.0002	0.0002	Liver or kidney problems	Runoff/leaching from insecticide used on cattle, lumber, gardens
Methoxychlor	0.04	0.04	Reproductive difficulties	Runoff/leachin insecticide fruits, veges alfalfa, livestock

Oxamyl (Vydate)	0.2	0.2	Slight nervous system effects	Runoff/leaching from insecticide used on apples, potatoes, and tomatoes
Polychlorinated biphenyls (PCBs)	Zero	0.0005	Skin changes; thymus gland problems; immune deficiencies; reproductive or nervous system difficulties; cancer risk	Runoff from landfills; discharge of waste chemicals
Pentachlorophenol	Zero	0.001	Liver or kidney problems; increased cancer risk	Discharge from wood preserving factories
Picloram	0.5	0.5	Liver problems	Herbicide runoff
Simazine	0.004	0.004	Problems with blood	Herbicide runoff
Styrene	0.1	0.1	Liver, kidney, or circulatory system problems	Discharge from rubber, plastic factories; leaching from landfills
Tetrachloroethylene	Zero	0.005	Liver problems; increased risk of cancer	Discharge from factories and dry cleaners
Toluene	1	1	Nervous system, kidney, or liver problems	Discharge from petroleum factories

Toxaphene	Zero	0.003	Kidney, liver, or thyroid problems; increased risk of cancer	Runoff/leaching from insecticide used on cotton and cattle
2,4,5-TP (Silvex)	0.05	0.05	Liver problems	Residue of banned herbicide
1,2,4-Trichlorobenzene	0.07	0.07	Changes in adrenal glands	Discharge from textile finishing factories
1,1,1-Trichloroethane	0.20	0.2	Liver, nervous system, or circulatory problems	Discharge from metal degreasing sites other factories
1,1,2-Trichloroethane	0.003	0.005	Liver, kidney, or immune system problems	Discharge from industrial chemical factories
Trichloroethylene	Zero	0.005	Liver problems; increased risk of cancer	Discharge from metal degreasing sites other factories
Vinyl chloride	Zero	0.002	Increased risk of cancer	Leaching from PVC pipes; discharge from plastic factories
Xylenes (total)	10	10	Nervous system damage	Discharge from petroleum, chemical factories

What do you feel the EPA can do to help our water?
1. Hold industries accountable to manage their wastewater properly, with care for the planet and care for people
2. Ban the use of sewage sludge and biosolids as fertilizer!
3. Ban the use of flame retardants on furniture & clothing!
4. Work with the FDA to ban Nanoparticles
5. Do everything possible to keep waterways clean
6. Restrict use of pesticides and herbicides that cause disease
7. Penalize corporations and industries that pollute
8. Work with the USDA and FDA to change how factory farms operate so animals are not confined in unsuitable, unsanitary conditions and locked inside indefinitely
9. Fill in your own ideas:
10. _____
11. _____
12. _____
13. _____
14. _____
15. _____
16. _____
17. _____
18.

BELIEVE and WE WILL ACHIEVE.

Periodic Table

1 H 1.008 Hydrogen																	2 He 4.003 Helium
3 Li 6.94 Lithium	4 Be 9.012 Beryllium											5 B 10.81 Boron	6 C 12.011 Carbon	7 N 14.007 Nitrogen	8 O 15.999 Oxygen	9 F 18.998 Fluorine	10 Ne 20.180 Neon
11 Na 22.990 Sodium	12 Mg 24.305 Magnesium											13 Al 26.982 Aluminum	14 Si 28.085 Silicon	15 P 30.974 Phosphorus	16 S 32.06 Sulfur	17 Cl 35.45 Chlorine	18 Ar 39.948 Argon
19 K 39.098 Potassium	20 Ca 40.078 Calcium	21 Sc 44.956 Scandium	22 Ti 47.867 Titanium	23 V 50.942 Vanadium	24 Cr 51.996 Chromium	25 Mn 54.938 Manganese	26 Fe 55.845 Iron	27 Co 58.933 Cobalt	28 Ni 58.693 Nickel	29 Cu 63.546 Copper	30 Zn 65.38 Zinc	31 Ga 69.723 Gallium	32 Ge 72.630 Germanium	33 As 74.922 Arsenic	34 Se 78.971 Selenium	35 Br 79.904 Bromine	36 Kr 83.798 Krypton
37 Rb 85.468 Rubidium	38 Sr 87.62 Strontium	39 Y 88.906 Yttrium	40 Zr 91.224 Zirconium	41 Nb 92.906 Niobium	42 Mo 95.95 Molybdenum	43 Tc (98) Technetium	44 Ru 101.07 Ruthenium	45 Rh 102.906 Rhodium	46 Pd 106.42 Palladium	47 Ag 107.868 Silver	48 Cd 112.414 Cadmium	49 In 114.818 Indium	50 Sn 118.710 Tin	51 Sb 121.760 Antimony	52 Te 127.60 Tellurium	53 I 126.904 Iodine	54 Xe 131.293 Xenon
55 Cs 132.905 Cesium	56 Ba 137.327 Barium	57/71	72 Hf 178.49 Hafnium	73 Ta 180.948 Tantalum	74 W 183.84 Tungsten	75 Re 186.207 Rhenium	76 Os 190.23 Osmium	77 Ir 192.217 Iridium	78 Pt 195.084 Platinum	79 Au 196.967 Gold	80 Hg 200.592 Mercury	81 Tl 204.38 Thallium	82 Pb 207.2 Lead	83 Bi 208.980 Bismuth	84 Po (209) Polonium	85 At (210) Astatine	86 Rn (222) Radon
87 Fr (223) Francium	88 Ra (226) Radium	89/103	104 Rf (267) Rutherfordium	105 Db (268) Dubnium	106 Sg (271) Seaborgium	107 Bh (270) Bohrium	108 Hs (269) Hassium	109 Mt (278) Meitnerium	110 Ds (281) Darmstadtium	111 Rg (282) Roentgenium	112 Cn (285) Copernicium	113 Nh (286) Nihonium	114 Fl (289) Flerovium	115 Mc (289) Moscovium	116 Lv (293) Livermorium	117 Ts (294) Tennessine	118 Og (294) Oganesson

Lanthanide Series: 57 La 138.905 Lanthanum | 58 Ce 140.116 Cerium | 59 Pr 140.908 Praseodymium | 60 Nd 144.242 Neodymium | 61 Pm (145) Promethium | 62 Sm 150.36 Samarium | 63 Eu 151.964 Europium | 64 Gd 157.25 Gadolinium | 65 Tb 158.925 Terbium | 66 Dy 162.500 Dysprosium | 67 Ho 164.930 Holmium | 68 Er 167.259 Erbium | 69 Tm 168.934 Thulium | 70 Yb 173.045 Ytterbium | 71 Lu 174.967 Lutetium

Actinide Series: 89 Ac (227) Actinium | 90 Th 232.038 Thorium | 91 Pa 231.036 Protactinium | 92 U 238.029 Uranium | 93 Np (237) Neptunium | 94 Pu (244) Plutonium | 95 Am (243) Americium | 96 Cm (247) Curium | 97 Bk (247) Berkelium | 98 Cf (251) Californium | 99 Es (252) Einsteinium | 100 Fm (257) Fermium | 101 Md (258) Mendelevium | 102 No (259) Nobelium | 103 Lr (266) Lawrencium

Legend:
- Alkali metals
- Alkali earth metals
- Transition metals
- Post-transition metals
- Metalloid
- Lanthanides
- Actinides
- Nonmetals
- Halogens
- Noble gases

SYMBOL box: Atomic Number / SYMBOL / Atomic Weight * / Name

*() indicates the mass number of the longest-lived isotope.

Based on NIST 2017 Periodic Table

The Precautionary Principle

When an activity (or product) raises threats of harm to human health or the environment, precautionary measures should be taken even if some cause-and-effect relationships are not fully established scientifically. In this context, the proponents of an activity (the product manufacturer), rather than the public, should bear the burden of proof (to prove that the product is safe). The process of applying the Precautionary Principle must be open, informed and democratic and must include potentially affected parties (the public and consumers)."

www.ecologycenter.org

Why does our government not follow the advice of the President's Cancer Panel to consider the Precautionary Principle with a precautionary approach?

President's Cancer Panel Report excerpt:
"An alternative approach to regulation that supports primary cancer and other disease prevention is precautionary. In 1998, a conference of international environmental scientists, scholars, activists, treaty negotiators, and others convened to discuss implementation of the Precautionary Principle asserted in a consensus statement that 'when an activity raises threats of harm to human health or the environment, precautionary measures should be taken even if some cause and effect relationships are not fully established scientifically.' The core tenets of the Precautionary Principle are:
- Taking preventive action in the face of uncertainty.
- Shifting the burden of proof to proponents of an activity.
- Exploring a wide range of alternatives to possibly harmful actions.
- Including public participation in decision making."[421]

LAWS

"Government of the
People, by the People,
for the People,
Shall not perish from the earth.
President Abraham Lincoln
Gettysburg Address

HOW LAWS ARE MADE

Most laws in the United States begin as bills. A bill begins with an idea. That idea can come from anyone—including you! The idea is sent to Congress, where a Member of the U.S. House of Representatives researches the idea and writes a bill.
Once the bill is written, it is placed in the hopper, and introduced to the rest of the Members of the U.S. House of Representatives. The Members debate the bill, then vote on whether it should become a law or not using the electronic voting system.

After the bill has passed in the House, it is sent to the U.S. Senate. The Members of the Senate debate and vote on the bill. If the bill passes, it is sent to the President of the United States for approval. Once the President signs the bill, it is a law. Now that the bill has become a law, it is a rule that all Americans must follow.

WHAT IS CONGRESS?

The U.S. government is made up of the executive branch, the judicial branch, and the legislative branch. The executive branch, led by the President and the Vice President, enforces our laws. The judicial branch, led by the Supreme Court, interprets our laws. The legislative branch, which makes our laws, is the Congress.

Congress has two parts: the U.S. Senate and the U.S. House of Representatives. Each state has two U.S. Senators and at least one U.S. Representative; the more residents a state has, the more U.S. Representatives it is allowed. There are 100 U.S. Senators and 435 U.S. Representatives.

The laws Congress makes help Americans. There are laws that say kids have to go to school, laws that set standards for vehicle and highway safety, and laws that protect animals and nature. Congress meets in the Capitol in Washington, D.C.

http://kids.clerk.house.gov

LAWS & REGULATIONS

Laws are created in this country through a process as described below. Regulations are implemented after a law is created. Here is the process as described by the EPA[524]:

The Basics of the Regulatory Process

Have you ever wondered how EPA protects the environment? They use a variety of tools and approaches, like partnerships, educational programs, and grants. One of their most significant tools is writing regulations. Regulations are mandatory requirements that can apply to individuals, businesses, state or local governments, non-profit institutions, or others. Congress passes the laws that govern the United States, but Congress also authorizes agencies like the EPA to regulate them. Below, you'll find a basic description of how laws and regulations are developed.

Creating a law
Step 1: Congress Writes a Bill
A member of Congress proposes a bill. A bill is a document that, if approved, will become law. To see the text of bills Congress is considering or has considered, go to Congress.gov

Step 2: The President Approves or Vetoes the Bill
If both houses of Congress approve a bill, it goes to the President who has the option to either approve it or veto it. If approved, the new law is called an act or statute.

Step 3: The Act is Codified in the *United States Code*
Once an act is passed, the House of Representatives standardizes the text of the law and publishes it in the *United States Code* (U.S.C.). The U.S.C. is the codification by subject matter of the general and permanent laws of the United States. Since 1926, the U.S.C. has been published every six years. In between editions, annual cumulative supplements are published in order to present the most current information. **United States Code:** This database is available from the Government Printing Office (GPO).

Once a law is official, here's how it is put into practice: Laws often do not include all the details needed to explain how an individual, business, state or local government, or others might follow the law. In order to make the laws work on a day-to-day level, Congress authorizes certain government agencies - including EPA - to create regulations.

LAWS

HEALTH AND ENVIRONMENT

AIR

THE CLEAN AIR ACT

"The Clean Air Act (CAA) is the comprehensive federal law that regulates air emissions from stationary and mobile sources. Among other things, this law authorizes EPA to establish National Ambient Air Quality Standards (NAAQS) to protect public health and public welfare and to regulate emissions of hazardous air pollutants.

One of the goals of the Act was to set and achieve NAAQS in every state by 1975 in order to address the public health and welfare risks posed by certain widespread air pollutants. The setting of these pollutant standards was coupled with directing the states to develop state implementation plans (SIPs), applicable to appropriate industrial sources in the state, in order to achieve these standards. The Act was amended in 1977 and 1990 primarily to set new goals (dates) for achieving attainment of NAAQS since many areas of the country had failed to meet the deadlines."[525]

ANIMALS

ENDANGERED SPECIES ACT

"The purpose of the ESA is to protect and recover imperiled species and the ecosystems upon which they depend. It is administered by the U.S. Fish and Wildlife Service and the Commerce Department's National Marine Fisheries Service (NMFS). The FWS has primary responsibility for terrestrial and freshwater organisms, while the responsibilities of NMFS are mainly marine wildlife such as whales and anadromons fish such as salmon," states the U.S. Fish and Wildlife Service, http://www.fws.gov/endangered/laws-policies/index.html.

ANIMAL WELFARE ACT

The Animal Welfare Act (AWA) requires that minimum standards of care and treatment be provided for certain animals bred for commercial sale, used in research, transported commercially or exhibited to the public. Let's get all animals including farm animals and all animals trapped or held in captivity included in this.

MARINE MAMMALS PROTECTION ACT
The Marine Mammal Protection Act (MMPA) was enacted on October 21, 1972. All marine mammals are protected under the MMPA. The MMPA prohibits, with certain exceptions, the "take" of marine mammals in U.S. waters and by U.S. citizens on the high seas, and the importation of marine mammals and marine mammal products into the U.S.
Congress passed the Marine Mammal Protection Act of 1972 based on the following findings and policies:
- Some marine mammal species or stocks may be in danger of extinction or depletion as a result of human activities;
- These species or stocks must not be permitted to fall below their optimum sustainable population level ("depleted");
- Measures should be taken to replenish these species or stocks;
- Marine mammals have proven to be resources of great international significance.[526]

ENVIRONMENT
NEPA, National Environmental Policy Act
"The National Environmental Policy Act (NEPA) was one of the first laws ever written that establishes the broad national framework for protecting our environment. NEPA's basic policy is to assure that all branches of government give proper consideration to the environment prior to undertaking any major federal action that significantly affects the environment.
NEPA requirements are invoked when airports, buildings, military complexes, highways, parkland purchases, and other federal activities are proposed. Environmental Assessments (EAs) and Environmental Impact Statements (EISs), which are assessments of the likelihood of impacts from alternative courses of action, are required from all Federal agencies and are the most visible NEPA requirements." [527]

American Antiquities Act of 1906
Be it enacted by the Senate and House of Representatives of the United States of America in Congress assembled, That any person

who shall appropriate, excavate, injure, or destroy any historic or prehistoric ruin or monument, or any object of antiquity, situated on lands owned or controlled by the Government of the United States, without the permission of the Secretary of the Department of the Government having jurisdiction over the lands on which said antiquities are situated, shall, upon conviction, be fined in a sum of not more than five hundred dollars or be imprisoned for a period of not more than ninety days, or shall suffer both fine and imprisonment, in the discretion of the court.

Sec. 2. That the President of the United States is hereby authorized, in his discretion, to declare by public proclamation historic landmarks, historic and prehistoric structures, and other objects of historic or scientific interest that are situated upon the lands owned or controlled by the Government of the United States to be national monuments, and may reserve as a part thereof parcels of land, the limits of which in all cases shall be confined to the smallest area compatible with proper care and management of the objects to be protected: Provided, That when such objects are situated upon a tract covered by a bona fide unperfected claim or held in private ownership, the tract, or so much thereof as may be necessary for the proper care and management of the object, may be relinquished to the Government, and the Secretary of the Interior is hereby authorized to accept the relinquishment of such tracts in behalf of the Government of the United States.

Sec. 3. That permits for the examination of ruins, the excavation of archaeological sites, and the gathering of objects of antiquity upon the lands under their respective jurisdictions may be granted by the Secretaries of the Interior, Agriculture, and War to institutions which the may deem properly qualified to conduct such examination, excavation, or gathering, subject to such rules and regulation as they may prescribe: Provided, That the examinations, excavations, and gatherings are undertaken for the benefit of reputable museums, universities, colleges, or other recognized scientific or educational institutions, with a view to increasing the knowledge of such objects, and that the gatherings shall be made for permanent preservation in public museums.

Sec. 4. That the Secretaries of the Departments aforesaid shall make and publish from time to time uniform rules and regulations for the purpose of carrying out the provisions of this Act. Approved, June 8, 1906[528]

PESTICIDES
Laws Regulating Pesticide Use
Federal Insecticide, Fungicide, and Rodenticide Act (FIFRA): Gives the EPA authority to regulate the sale, use and distribution of pesticides.
Federal Food, Drug, and Cosmetic Act (FFDCA): Gives the EPA authority to set limits on the amount of pesticide residues allowed on food or animal feed. These limits are called tolerances (link to tolerance page).
Food Quality Protection Act of 1996 (FQPA): This act amended FIFRA and FFDCA by increasing the safety standards for new pesticides used on foods. FQPA also required older pesticides and previously established tolerances (link) to be periodically re-assessed using the new, tougher standards.
Pesticide Registration Improvement Act (PRIA): Establishes the fees and time-lines associated with pesticide registration (link to registration page) actions.
Endangered Species Act (ESA): Requires the EPA to assess the risk of pesticides to threatened or endangered species and their habitats.[529]

Information Source: http://www.epa.gov/pesticide-registration/about-pesticide-registration
<u>Federal Insecticide, Fungicide, and Rodenticide Act (FIFRA)</u> – Requires all pesticides sold or distributed in the United States (including imported pesticides) to be registered by EPA.
    Registration is based on evaluation of scientific data and assessment of risks and benefits of a product's use.
    Label directions control how products are used.
- We can authorize limited use of unregistered pesticides or pesticides registered for other uses to address emergencies and special local needs.

- We can suspend or cancel a product's registration.
- Training is required for workers in pesticide-treated areas and certification and training for applicators of restricted use pesticides.

<u>Federal Food, Drug and Cosmetic Act (FFDCA)</u> – Requires us to set pesticide tolerances for all pesticides used in or on food or in a manner that will result in a residue in or on food or animal feed. A tolerance is the maximum permissible level for pesticide residues allowed in or on human food and animal feed.
- Includes strong provisions for protecting infants and children, as well as other sensitive subpopulations.
- Provides for exemption from the requirement for a tolerance.

Under the <u>Food Quality Protection Act, of 1996</u>, which amended both FIFRA and FFDCA, we must find that a pesticide poses a "reasonable certainty of no harm" before it can be registered for use on food or feed. We must review each pesticide registration at least once every 15 years.
- Several factors must be addressed before a tolerance can be established, including:
- the aggregate, non-occupational exposure from the pesticide (exposure through diet and drinking water and from using pesticides in and around the home);
- the cumulative effects from exposure to pesticides that have a common mechanism of toxicity, that is, two or more pesticide chemicals or other substances that cause a common toxic effect(s) by the same, or essentially the same, sequence of major biochemical events (i.e., interpreted as mode of action);
- whether there is increased susceptibility to infants and children, or other sensitive subpopulations, from exposure to the pesticide; and
- whether the pesticide produces an effect in humans similar to an effect produced by a naturally-occurring estrogen or produces other endocrine-disruption effects.

The Pesticide Registration Improvement Act of 2003 (PRIA) also amended FIFRA and FFDCA. PRIA was reauthorized by the Pesticide Registration Improvement Renewal Act of 2007 and the Pesticide Registration Improvement Extension Act of 2012. Under PRIA:
- Companies must pay service fees according to the category of the registration
- EPA must meet decision review time periods, which result in a more predictable evaluation process for companies.
- Shorter decision review periods are provided for reduced-risk registration applications.

The Endangered Species Act (ESA) requires federal agencies to ensure that any action they authorize, fund, or carry out, will not likely jeopardize the continued existence of any listed species, or destroy or adversely modify any critical habitat for those species. EPA is responsible for reviewing information and data to determine whether a pesticide product may be registered for a particular use. As part of that determination, we assess whether listed endangered or threatened species or their designated critical habitat may be affected by use of the product. All pesticide products that EPA determines "may affect" a listed species or its designated critical habitat may be subject to EPA's Endangered Species Protection Program.

GRAS: Generally Recognized as Safe

How are toxic chemicals allowed in the food supply? Well over 10,000 untested toxins are allowed through the GRAS loophole. Help the FDA get better, press them to be transparent, to be leaders, and to prevent disease and cancer. The Generally Recognized as Safe Clause to the 1958 Food Additives Amendment was signed into law by President Eisenhower. Over the years, the implementation of the law has allowed industry to take advantage of this seemingly innocent loophole. Similar to the EPA's role with the Toxic Substance Control Act, The FDA does not require safety testing or honesty from the food manufacturer. The TSCA as well as these food laws were designed with the assumption that honest information would be provided by manufacturers. And that just ain't happening. "The agency's (FDA's) attempts to limit these undisclosed GRAS determinations by asking industry to voluntarily inform the FDA about their chemicals are insufficient to ensure the safety of our food in today's global marketplace with a complex food supply. Furthermore, no other developed country in the world has a system like GRAS to provide oversight of food ingredients."[530]

TOXIC SUBSTANCES
TSCA, TOXIC SUBSTANCES CONTROL ACT
Established in 1976, the TSCA was designed to give the EPA the framework to monitor the thousands of chemicals in use, produced, and imported into the country.
While the EPA theoretically has the power to screen and monitor these chemicals, many slip through the cracks and end up in various consumer products. For this and other reasons that favor industry over our own health, safety and wellbeing, many organizations have been seeking to reform the TSCA. In the 114th Congress that opportunity became realized through the Lautenberg Chemical Safety Act.

FRANK R. LAUTENBERG CHEMICAL SAFETY ACT FOR THE 21ST CENTURY ACT became law June 22, 2016
- Mandates safety reviews for all chemicals in commerce.
- Requires a safety finding for new chemicals before they can enter the market.
- Replaces TSCA's burdensome cost-benefit safety standard
- Explicitly requires protection of vulnerable populations like children and pregnant women.
- Gives EPA enhanced authority to require testing of both new and existing chemicals.
- Sets aggressive, judicially enforceable deadlines for EPA decisions.
- Makes more information about chemicals available, by limiting companies' ability to claim information as confidential, and by giving states and health and environmental professionals access to confidential information they need to do their jobs."[531]

CERCLA, SUPERFUND
"The Comprehensive Environmental Response, Compensation, and Liability Act -- otherwise known as CERCLA or Superfund -- provides a Federal "Superfund" to clean up uncontrolled or abandoned hazardous-waste sites as well as accidents, spills, and other emergency releases of pollutants and contaminants into the environment. Through CERCLA, EPA was given power to seek out those parties responsible for any release and assure their cooperation in the cleanup."[532]

RCRA, Resource Conservation and Recovery Act [533]
The Resource Conservation and Recovery Act (RCRA) gives EPA the authority to control hazardous waste from the "cradle-to-grave." This includes the generation, transportation, treatment, storage, and disposal of hazardous waste. RCRA also set forth a framework for the management of non-hazardous solid wastes. The 1986 amendments to RCRA enabled EPA to address environmental problems that could result from underground tanks storing petroleum and other hazardous substances.

WATER

HISTORY OF THE CLEAN WATER ACT[534]
The Federal Water Pollution Control Act of 1948 was the first major U.S. law to address water pollution. Growing public awareness and concern for controlling water pollution led to sweeping amendments in 1972. As amended in 1972, the law became commonly known as the Clean Water Act (CWA). The 1972 amendments:
1. Established the basic structure for regulating pollutant discharges into the waters of the United States. 2. Gave EPA the authority to implement pollution control programs such as setting wastewater standards for industry. 3. Maintained existing requirements to set water quality standards for all contaminants in surface waters. 4. Made it unlawful for any person to discharge any pollutant from a point source into navigable waters, unless a permit was obtained under its provisions.
5. Funded the construction of sewage treatment plants under the construction grants program. 6. Recognized the need for planning to address the critical problems posed by nonpoint source pollution.

THE SAFE DRINKING WATER ACT

"The Safe Drinking Water Act (SDWA) was established to protect the quality of drinking water in the U.S. This law focuses on all waters actually or potentially designed for drinking use, whether from above ground or underground sources. The Act authorizes EPA to establish minimum standards to protect tap water and requires all owners or operators of public water systems to comply with these primary (health-related) standards. The 1996 amendments to SDWA require that EPA consider a detailed risk and cost assessment, and best available peer-reviewed science, when developing these standards. State governments, which can be approved to implement these rules for EPA, also encourage attainment of secondary standards (nuisance-related). Under the Act, EPA also establishes minimum standards for state programs to protect underground sources of drinking water from endangerment by underground injection of fluids."[535]

EPA AND FRACKING:
Natural gas and shale gas extraction, including hydraulic fracturing, operations can result in a number of potential impacts to the environment, our drinking water and our health including:
- Stress on surface water and ground water supplies from the withdrawal of large volumes of water used in drilling and hydraulic fracturing;
- Contamination of underground sources of drinking water and surface waters resulting from spills, faulty well construction, or by other means;
- Adverse impacts from discharges into surface waters or from disposal into underground injection wells;

Recycling of Wastewater
Some drilling operators elect to re-use a portion of the wastewater to replace and/or supplement fresh water in formulating fracturing fluid for a future well or re-fracturing the same well. Re-use of shale gas wastewater is, in part, dependent on the levels of pollutants in the wastewater and the proximity of other fracturing sites that might re-use the wastewater. This practice has the potential to reduce discharges to treatment facilities or surface waters, minimize underground injection of wastewater and conserve water resources.[536]

Water Reclamation Act History
"Inadequate precipitation in the American West required settlers to use irrigation for agriculture. At first, settlers simply diverted water from

streams, but in many areas demand outstripped supply. As demand for water increased, settlers wanted to store "wasted" runoff from rains and snow for later use, thus maximizing use by making more water available in drier seasons. At that time, private and state-sponsored storage and irrigation ventures were pursued, but often failed because of lack of money and/or lack of engineering skill.

"Pressure mounted for the Federal Government to undertake storage and irrigation projects. Congress had already invested in America's infrastructure through subsidies to roads, river navigation, harbors, canals, and railroads. Westerners wanted the Federal Government also to invest in irrigation projects in the West. The irrigation movement demonstrated its strength when pro-irrigation planks found their way into both Democratic and Republican platforms in 1900. Eastern and Midwestern opposition in the Congress quieted when Westerners filibustered and killed a bill containing rivers and harbors projects favored by opponents of Western irrigation. Congress passed the Reclamation Act of June17, 1902. The Act required that water users repay construction costs from which they received benefits. In July of 1902, in accordance with the Reclamation Act, Secretary of the Interior Ethan Allen Hitchcock established the United States Reclamation Service within the U. S.Geological Survey (USGS)."[537]

GLOBAL AGREEMENTS ******
PERTAINING TO TOXIC POLLUTANTS
Montreal Protocol
Substances that Deplete the Ozone Layer[538]
September 1987, went into force January 1, 1989, Signed by 197 Nations including United States. Seeks to eliminate substances that cause depletion of the Earth's Ozone Layer allowing the hole in the ozone layer above Antarctica to fully heal by 2050. The Ozone layer is earth's protective shield that keeps harmful UV rays out.

Stockholm Convention
Persistent Organic Pollutants
May 22, 2001 went into force May 17, 2004. The U.S. signed in 2001, but has not ratified. According to the Secretary of State's website, "The United States signed the Stockholm Convention in 2001, but has yet to ratify because we currently lack the authority to implement all of its provisions. The United States participates as an observer."[539]
- The Stockholm Convention on Persistent Organic Pollutants is a global treaty to protect human health and the environment from chemicals that

remain intact in the environment for long periods, become widely distributed geographically, accumulate in the fatty tissue of humans and wildlife, and have harmful impacts on human health or on the environment.[540]

Kyoto Protocol

United States joined 1997, withdrew in 2001
- Became official February 16, 2005
- Goal: to limit Green House Gas Emissions
- Developed countries to reduce emissions between 2008 – 2012 by average of 5.2% below 1990 levels
- Countries encouraged to develop emission credit trading program[541]

Paris Climate Accord

US signed April 22, 2016. Governments agreed
- a long-term goal of keeping the increase in global average temperature to well below 2°C above pre-industrial levels;
  - to aim to limit the increase to 1.5°C, since this would significantly reduce risks and the impacts of climate change
  - on the need for global emissions to peak as soon as possible, recognizing that this will take longer for developing countries to undertake rapid reductions hereafter in accordance with the best available science.[542]

Kunming-Montreal Global Biodiversity Framework

Through this agreement reached on December 19, 2022, 196 countries across the world committed to saving animals and preventing loss of nature and biodiversity. The natural systems are in grave danger, "in the last 50 years, wildlife populations have declined by 69%!"[543] This Framework agreement aims to halt and reverse nature loss by 2030!

HEALTH &
Planet Friendly
SHOPPING GUIDE

HEALTH-FRIENDLY
Products free of health harming toxins
From Companies who Care about the Planet and You

Personal Care	
Toothpaste	Avoid antimicrobials, fluoride
Dental Floss	Smart Floss, avoid any containing Triclosan
Sunscreen	Reef Friendly, No Nanos, Badger,
Moisturizer	Avoid any containing nanoparticles
Soap	Goat Milk, Dr. Bronner's, Seventh Generation
Shampoo	Shampoo bars are good, Kitsch, no plastic
Hair Care	Avoid those containing phosphates, parabens…
Make Up	Avoid nanoparticles, heavy metals, PEG
Cleaning Products	Wash cloths, sponges Zero Waste Outlet.com,
All Purpose	Seventh Generation, Thrive Market, Myers
Dishwasher	Seventh Generation, Myers
Dishwashing Soap	Seventh Generation, Biokleen, Honest Co.
Scrubbing	Bon Ami
Bathroom Cleaner	Seventh Gen, Myers, Thrive Market, Vinegar
Shower Cleaner	DIY Vinegar spray,
Mildew Cleaner	Meyers Probiotic Shower Spray, UV light, EC3
Drain Cleaner	Baking soda, white vinegar follow with hot H2O, get it rodded periodically, Myers Probiotic
Oven Cleaner	Best nontoxic: Use apple cider vinegar, orange peels and baking soda, see how here.
Laundry Detergent	Molly's Suds, Laundry Sheets, Earth Breeze
Window Cleaner	Seventh Generation, White vinegar + H2O
Air Purifier	Molekule, Air Oasis, Coway Airmega, Blueair
Paper Products	
Paper towels	Seventh Generation, Bim Bam Boo
Toilet tissue	Bim Bam Boo Bamboo Paper

Facial tissue	Bim Bam Boo, Seventh Generation, 365
Writing Paper	Choose recycled content
Printer Paper	Source Recycled content
Office Supplies	Shop on EarthHero.com
Beverages	
Bottled water	Mountain Springs, Evian, Smart Water
Coffee	Café Mam, Grounds for Change, Forecast
Mineral water	San Pelligrino, Perrier, Gerolsteiner
Water filters	RO, Berkey, zero water, cloud, see chart pg 20
Drink mixes	Look for organic, no gmos, no artificial swtnrs
Juices	Choose Organic or fresh squeezed
Coconut water	Harmless Harvest, VitaCoco
Coconut milk	Look for packaging without BPA
Non dairy milks	Hemp, Almond, Rice
Organic Herbal Tea	Hippocrateas, Traditional Medicinals, Eden
Green Tea organic	Yogi, Traditional Medicinals, Eden organic
Traditional Tea	Equal Exchange, The Republic of Tea, Numi
Kombucha	Aqua Vitae, GT's, Brew Dr, Remedy

Food Essentials	
Fruit	Organic, local farmers market, source that with fewest pesticides
Vegetables	Organic, farmers market, source that with fewest pesticides
Eggs	Local, organic, pasture raised, organic valley
Dairy	Local or organic, avoid rBGH, rBST
Butter	Organic nonrBGH
Milk	Organic nonrBGH
Yogurt	Organic nonrBGH
Grains Bread	Organic, avoid GMO desiccated/glyphosate residues
Rice	Organic, Lundberg, avoid roundup residues
Quinoa	Organic avoids roundup residues
Amaranth	Organic avoids roundup residues
Oats	Organic avoids roundup residues
Millet	Organic avoids roundup residues
Tortilla	Organic avoids roundup residues

Pantry	
Dried Fruit	Organic avoids pesticide residues
Honey	Local and Raw is best
Salad Dressing	Primal, Simple Truth, Mother Raw
Seeds and Nuts	Organic avoids pesticide residues
Organic Chips	Garden of Eatin, Late July, Siete (grain free!)
Organic Beans	Eden, Westbrae, Amy's
Organic Soups	Amy's
Tuna dolphin safe	Find dolphin safe Safe Catch, Wild Planet
Condiments	Choose organic nonGMO, without high fructose corn syrup, nanoparticles of titanium dioxide
Mayo	Choose organic and avoid PUFA oils (hateful8)- they interfere with metabolism
Ketchup	Organic, nonGmo, avoid single serv packets
Kimchi/sauerkraut	Eden, Ocean's Halo, Wise Goat
Dark Chocolate	There are heavy metal concerns, so eat sparingly perhaps, choose organic, fair trade
Candy	Avoid nanoparticles of Titanium Dioxide, HFCS
Frozen Food	
Frozen Pizza	Amy's, Monteli, Simple Mills (almond flour)
Fruit	Cascadian Farms
Frozen Fish	Studies show freezing fish first is ideal to kill off any pathogens, microbes
Frozen Dinners	Organic: Aunt Ethel's, Amy's Blake's,
Ice Cream	Organic: Alden's, Dee Bee's Gelato
Pet Food	Pets food are very low in iodine, add seaweed
Cat Food	Source nonGMO, full nutrient, raw is good
Dog Food	Source nonGMO, full nutrient, raw is good
Housewares	
Cleaning	Choose nontoxic
Cookware	Avoid nonstick coatings, nanoparticles
Candles	Avoid synthetic scents, phthalates, EDCs
Paint	Avoid VOCs, heavy metals,
Flooring	Avoid VOCs, formaldehyde
Window Treatments	Avoid vinyl fabric, or wrinklefree, stain free, any coatings containing PFAS

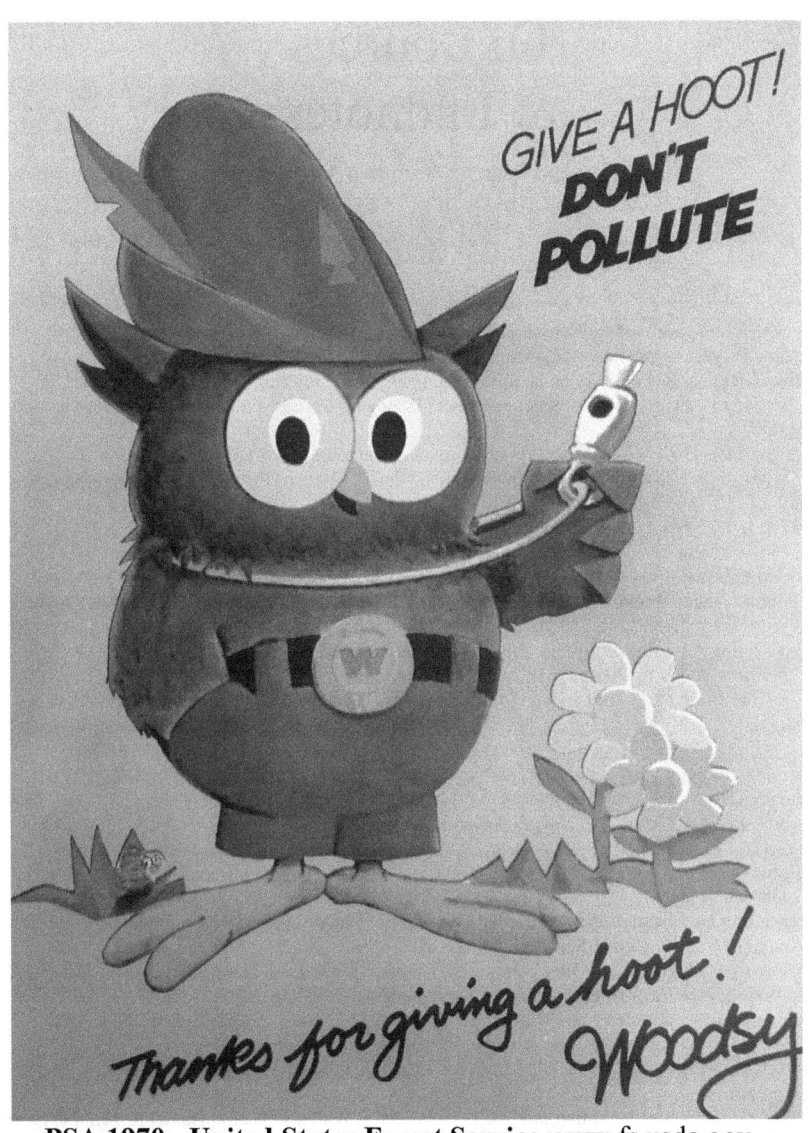

PSA 1970: United States Forest Service www.fs.usda.gov

List Of Sources & Endnotes

[1] President John F. Kennedy's Natural Resource speech to Congress, February, 1961, The Presidency Project, University of California Santa Barbara, www.presidency.ucsb.edu.
[2] "Special Message to Congress on Natural Resources," The American Presidency Project, UC Santa Barbara, https://www.presidency.ucsb.edu/documents/special-message-the-congress-natural-resources
[3] "History of the 1972 Clean Water Act and How it Became Law- Part 3," Online Safety Trainer, https://www.onlinesafetytrainer.com/the-history-of-the-1972-clean-water-act-and-how-it-became-law-part-3/#:~:text=In%20his%20first%20address%20to,Control%20Act%20Amendments%20of%201961.
[4] https://www.health.ny.gov/environmental/water/drinking/boilwater/response_information_public_health_professional.htm
[5] "25 Popular Water Brands, Ranked Worst to Best," Noelle Caliguri, Tasting Table, Feb 2, 2023, https://www.tastingtable.com/756881/popular-bottled-water-brands-ranked-worst-to-best/
[6] "Pepsi Admits Aquafina is Bottled Tap Water," Plumbing Today, September 19, 2019, https://plumbingtoday.biz/blog/aquafina-bottled-tap-water
[7] "Toxic Chromium Found in Chicago Drinking Water," Michael Hawthorne, Chicago Tribune, August 6, 2011, https://www.chicagotribune.com/lifestyles/ct-xpm-2011-08-06-ct-met-drinking-water-chromium-20110806-story.html
[8] https://deainfo.nci.nih.gov/advisory/pcp/annualreports/pcp08-09rpt/pcp_report_08-09_508.pdf
[9] "Pesticide Use and Exposure Extensive Worldwide," Michael C.R. Alavanja, Sept 27, 2010, Rev Environ Health. 2009 Oct-Dec;24(4):303-9. doi: 10.1515/reveh.2009.24.4.303. PMID: 20384038; PMCID: PMC2946267. https://www.ncbi.nlm.nih.gov/entrez/eutils/elink.fcgi?dbfrom=pubmed&retmode=ref&cmd=prlinks&id=20384038
[10] "Controlling Nitrification in Chloraminated Drinking Water Supplies," New Hampshire Department of Environmental Services, January 2021, https://www.des.nh.gov/sites/g/files/ehbemt341/files/documents/wd-21-02.pdf
[11] Zero Water, https://zerowater.co.uk/pages/how-it-works
[12] "How to Remove Nitrates from Water," Brock Robinson, Clean Water Systems, Jan 6, 2020, https://www.freshwatersystems.com/blogs/blog/how-to-remove-nitrates-from-water#:~:text=Nitrates%20can%20be%20removed%20from,membrane%20of%20an%20ultrafiltration%20system.
[13] Shallow Groundwater Sampling in Kane County, 2015, Walter R. Kelly, Daniel R. Hadley, Devin H. Mannix, Illinois State Water Survey, Prairie Research Institute, University of Illinois at Urbana-Champaign, https://www.isws.illinois.edu/pubdoc/CR/ISWSCR2016-04.pdf
[14] http://www.epa.gov/agriculture/lcwa.html
[15] EPA, History of the Clean Water Act, https://www.epa.gov/laws-regulations/history-clean-water-act
[16] www.epa.gov/region5/water/cwa.htm
[17] "How Much Water is There on Earth," Water Science School, USGS, Nov 13, 2019, https://www.usgs.gov/special-topics/water-science-school/science/how-much-water-there-earth
[18] Ozone Disinfection," Wastewater Technology Fact Sheet, EPA, https://www3.epa.gov/npdes/pubs/ozon.pdf

[19] (18)
[20] "Environmental Rules Stoke Anger as California Lets Precious Stormwater Wash Out to Sea," Hayley Smith, Los Angeles Times, Jan 20, 2023, https://www.latimes.com/california/story/2023-01-20/anger-flares-as-california-stormwater-washes-out-to-sea
[21] "Chart: Globally 70% of Freshwater is Used for Agriculture,"Tariq Khokhar, World Bank Blog, March 22, 2017, https://blogs.worldbank.org/en/opendata/chart-globally-70-freshwater-used-for-agriculture
[22] "Conservation Agriculture," Arizona Department of Water Resources,https://www.azwater.gov/conservation/agriculture#:~:text=Irrigated%20agriculture%20is%20the%20largest,of%20the%20available%20water%20supply
[23] https://www.propublica.org/article/california-drought-colorado-river-water-crisis-explained
[24] United Nations World Water Development Report 2023, UN, https://unesdoc.unesco.org/ark:/48223/pf0000384567
[25] https://projects.propublica.org/killing-the-colorado/story/arizona-cotton-drought-crisis
[26] (24)
[27] "What to Know About Rising Rates of Early Onset Cancer," Kathy Katella, Yale Medicine, August 1, 2024, https://www.yalemedicine.org/news/early-onset-cancer-in-younger-people-on-the-rise
[28] Cancer and the Environment, What You Need to Know, National Institutes of Health, August 2003, https://www.niehs.nih.gov/health/materials/cancer_and_the_environment_508.pdf
[29] Reducing Environmental Cancer Risk, President's Cancer Panel Annual Report 2008-2009, https://deainfo.nci.nih.gov/advisory/pcp/annualreports/pcp08-09rpt/pcp_report_08-09_508.pdf
[30] 'Cancer Rates Set to Rise 77 Percent by 2050,"United Nations, Feb 1, 2024, https://news.un.org/en/story/2024/02/1146127
[31] "Water- At the Center of the Climate Crisis,United Nations Climate Action, https://www.un.org/en/climatechange/science/climate-issues/water
[32] United Nations World Water Development Report 2023, UN, https://unesdoc.unesco.org/ark:/48223/pf0000384567
[33] "Nitrogen Emissions from Rising Fertilizer Use Threaten Climate Goals," Thin Lei Win, Reuters, Oct 7, 2020, https://www.reuters.com/article/us-global-climatechange-agriculture/nitrogen-emissions-from-rising-fertiliser-use-threaten-climate-goals-idUSKBN26S2HV
[34] "White House Releases Report on Reflecting Sunlight to Cool the Earth, No Formal Study Planned Now," Catherine Gifford, CNBC, June 30, 2023, https://www.cnbc.com/2023/06/30/white-house-releases-report-on-solar-geoengineering.html
[35] USGS, Groundwater Contaminants, https://www.usgs.gov/special-topics/water-science-school/science/contamination-groundwater
Agricultural Runoff
[36] "Large-scale factory farms have become the biggest source of water pollution in the U.S.." Gina Goldberg, https://pirg.org/articles/large-scale-factory-farms-have-become-the-biggest-source-of-water-pollution-in-the-u-s/
[37] "How Drug-Resistant Bacteria Travel from the Farm to Your Table," Melinda Wenner Moyer, Scientific American, Dec 1, 2016, https://www.scientificamerican.com/article/how-drug-resistant-bacteria-travel-from-the-farm-to-your-table/
[38] "About Antimicrobial Resistance,"Centers for Disease Control and Prevention, https://www.cdc.gov/drugresistance/about.html

Sewage
[39] NPDES CAFO Permitting Status Report: National Summary, Endyear 2013, May 14, 2024, https://www.epa.gov/system/files/documents/2024-06/cafo-status-report-2023.pdf
[40] "Who Will Keep the Poop Out of the Water? The Latest in the Saga of CAFO Regulation Under the Clean Water Act," Bill Shultz, Georgetown Environmental Law Review, Dec 4, 2023, https://www.law.georgetown.edu/environmental-law-review/blog/who-will-keep-the-poop-out-of-the-water-the-latest-in-the-saga-of-cafo-regulation-under-the-clean-water-act/

Aluminum
[41] "The Age of Aluminum, ALCOA," Claire Xu, Pennsylvania Center for the Book, Spring 2010, https://pabook.libraries.psu.edu/literary-cultural-heritage-map-pa/feature-articles/age-aluminum-alcoa

[42] "Growth of ALumnium Industry, Key to Clean Energy, Puts Climate, Air, Water and Heatlh at Risk,Environmental Intergrity Project, September 27, 2023,
https://environmentalintegrity.org/news/growth-of-aluminum-industry-key-to-clean-energy-puts-climate-air-water-and-health-at
risk/#:~:text=Mining%20the%20ore%20that%20contains,creates%20toxic%20dust%20and%20waste.

[43] "Public Health Statement for Aluminum," US Agency for Toxic Substances and Disease Registry,"
https://wwwn.cdc.gov/TSP/PHS/PHS.aspx?phsid=1076&toxid=34#:~:text=The%20EPA%20has%20recommended%20a,for%20aluminum%20in%20drinking%20water.

[44] "Evaluating Nanoparticle Breakthrough During Water Treatment," Talia E Abbott Chalew, Gaurav S Ajmani, Jaiou Huang, Kellogg J Schwab, Environmental Health Perspectives, Vol. 121, Issue 10, Aug 9, 2013,
https://ehp.niehs.nih.gov/doi/10.1289/ehp.1306574#:~:text=into%20the%20future.-,Conclusions,and%20advanced%20drinking%20water%20treatment.

[45] "Neurotoxicity of aluminum oxide nanoparticles and their mechanistic role in dopaminergic neuron injury involving p53-related pathways," Huanliang Lui, Wei shang, Yanjun Fang, Honglian Yang, Lei Tian, Kang Li, Wenqing Lai, Liping Bian, Bencheng Lin, Xiaohua Liu, Zhuge Xi, Journal of Hazardous Materials, June 15, 2020,
https://www.sciencedirect.com/science/article/abs/pii/S0304389420303009#:~:text=Nano%2DAl2O3%20is%20deposited%20in%20olfactory%20bulb,cell%20cycle%20arrest%20and%20apoptosis.

[46] "Aluminum Oxide Nanoparticle," Robert Y. Pelgrift, Adam J Friedman, Advanced Drug Delivery Reviews, 2013, https://www.sciencedirect.com/topics/pharmacology-toxicology-and-pharmaceutical-science/aluminium-oxide-nanoparticle#:~:text=2.7%20Aluminum%20oxide%20nanoparticles&text=Al2O3%20nanoparticles%20are%20well%20known%20for%20their,foundations%20%5B123%2C3%5D.

[47] "Nanoparticles and Their Interactions with the Dermal Barrier," March Schneider, Frank Stracke, Steffi Hansen, Ulrich F Schaefer, Dermato Endocrinology, July-August, 2009,
https://www.ncbi.nlm.nih.gov/pmc/articles/PMC2835875/

[48] "Hippocampus in Health and Disease: An Overview," Kuljeet Singh Anand, Vikas Dhikav, Ann Indian Acad Neurol, Oct-Dec, 2015,
https://www.ncbi.nlm.nih.gov/pmc/articles/PMC3548359/#:~:text=Hippocampus%20is%20a%20complex%20brain,of%20neurological%20and%20psychiatric%20disorders.

[49] Toxicity of Nanoparticles and an Overview of Current Experimental Models, Haji Bahadar, Faheem Maqbool, Kamal Niaz, Mohammed Abdollahi, Iran Biomed J, Jan, 2016,
https://www.ncbi.nlm.nih.gov/pmc/articles/PMC4689276/#:~:text=Titanium%20dioxide%20NPs%20(%3C100%20nm,animals%5B55%2C56%5D.

[50] "Aluminum in Drinking Water, Everything You Need to Know," Sasha Sosnowski,Tap Score, March 15, 2023, https://mytapscore.com/blogs/tips-for-taps/aluminium-in-drinking-water-everything-you-need-to-know?utm_term=&utm_campaign=&utm_source=adwords&utm_medium=ppc&hsa_acc=4622273785&hsa_cam=18532191078&hsa_grp=&hsa_ad=&hsa_src=x&hsa_tgt=&hsa_kw=&hsa_mt=&hsa_net=adwords&hsa_ver=3&gad_source=1&gbraid=0AAAAADhlnKm1t6L7uH8AI2zfpmZA2rzu5&gclid=Cj0KCQjw0Oq2BhCCARIsAA5hubUigwPCNkLOqkJj6-QaxOxp4Evk8l0mzyQ-FTH5mgBlrkQm8Avu1MQaAjfGEALw_wcB

[51] "Environmental Aluminum Oxide Inducing Neurodegeneration in Human Neurovascular Unit with Immunity," Yingqu Xue, Minh Tran, Yen N Diep, Seonghun Shin, Jinkee Lee, Hansang Cho, You Jung Kang, Scientific Reports, Jan 7, 2024, https://www.nature.com/articles/s41598-024-51206-4

[52] "Aluminum in Drinking Water," Guidelines for Drinking Water Quality, World Health Organization, 1998,
https://iris.who.int/bitstream/handle/10665/75362/WHO_SDE_WSH_03.04_53_eng.pdf

AMR
[53] "Antibiotic resistance levels in soils from urban and rural land uses in Great Britain," Osbiston K, Oxbrough A, Fernández-Martínez LT. Access Microbiol. 2020 Nov 23;3(1):acmi000181. doi: 10.1099/acmi.0.000181. PMID: 33997612; PMCID:

PMC8115975, https://www.ncbi.nlm.nih.gov/pmc/articles/PMC8115975/#:~:text=In%20addition%2C%20other%20anthropogenic%20activities,(ARGs)%20in%20these%20soils.
[54] "Antimicrobial Resistance Genes (ARGs), the Gut Microbiome, and Infant Nutrition. Nutrients," Theophilus RJ, Taft DH. 2023 Jul 18;15(14):3177. doi: https://www.ncbi.nlm.nih.gov/pmc/articles/PMC10383493/
[55] "Antimicrobial Resistance," World Health Organization, Nov 21, 2023, https://www.who.int/news-room/fact-sheets/detail/antimicrobial-resistance
[56] "Antibiotic Resistance Levels in soils from urban and rural land uses in Great Britain," Osbiston K, Oxbrough A, Fernández-Martínez LT. Access Microbiol, Nov, 2020,https://www.ncbi.nlm.nih.gov/pmc/articles/PMC8115975/#:~:text=In%20addition%2C%20other%20anthropogenic%20activities,(ARGs)%20in%20these%20soils.

Ammonia
[57] National Library of Medicine, Medline Plus, https://medlineplus.gov/ency/article/002759.htm
[58] http://www.nlm.nih.gov/medlineplus/ency/article/002759.htm

Arsenic
[59] "LED Products Billed as Eco-Friendly Contain Toxic Metals, study finds, University of California- Irvine, Feb 11, 2011, https://www.sciencedaily.com/releases/2011/02/110210124136.htm
[60] "How to Reduce Arsenic in Rice, and Why it Matters,"Devon Wagner, Ohio State Wexner Medical Center, https://health.osu.edu/wellness/exercise-and-nutrition/how-to-reduce-arsenic-in-rice

Atrazine
[61] https://www.nrdc.org/sites/default/files/atrazine.pdf https://www.organicconsumers.org/news/us-drinking-water-and-watersheds-widely-contaminated-hormone-disrupting-pesticide-atrazine
[62] http://www.pnas.org/content/107/10/4612.full, Atrazine induces complete feminization and chemical castration in male African clawed frogs (*Xenopus laevis*)
[63] "Atrazine and Human Health," R.K. Pathak, A.K.Dikshit, International Journal of Ecosystem, 2011; 1(1): 14-23 DOI: 10. 5923/j.ije.20110101.03 , https://outside.vermont.gov/agency/agriculture/vpac/Shared%20Documents/January_2014/pathak_humaneffects_10%205923%20j%20ije%2020110101%2003%20(2).pdf

Bacteria and Parasites
[64] "Protozoan Parasites in Drinking Water: A System Approach for Improved Water, Sanitation and Hygiene in Developing Countries," Alua Omarova, Kamshat Tussupova, Ronny Berndtsson, Marat Kalishev, Kulyash Sharapatova, International J Environ Res Public Health, March, 2018, https://www.ncbi.nlm.nih.gov/pmc/articles/PMC5877040/
[65] "Efficiency of Chlorine and UV in the Inactivation of Cryptosporidium and Giardia in Wastewater," Folasade E Adeyemo, Gulshan Singh, Poovendhree Reddy, Faizal Bux, Thor Axel Stenstrom, PloS One 2019, May 13, 2019, https://www.ncbi.nlm.nih.gov/pmc/articles/PMC6513095/
[66] "Infectious Disease, A Surprising Cause of Cancer," Julie Parsonnet, MD, professor of infectious diseases and geographic medicine, Stanford University June 20, 2008, https://med.stanford.edu/news/all-news/2008/06/infectious-disease-a-surprising-cause-of-cancer.html
[67] "Lung Flukes, Paragonimiasis: An Emerging Foodborne Parasitic Disease of Public Health Concern, Anita Tewari, Mahendra Pal, Reference Model in Food Science, 2023, https://www.sciencedirect.com/topics/agricultural-and-biological-sciences/lung-flukes#:~:text=Paragonimiasis%20affects%2022%20million%20people,harbour%20metacercariae%20of%20the%20parasite.
[68] "Parasites," CDC.gov, https://www.cdc.gov/parasites/fasciola/index.html
[69] "Intestinal Parasites," Mount Sinai Health Center, https://www.mountsinai.org/health-library/condition/intestinal-parasites#:~:text=Parasites%20can%20live%20in%20the,Diarrhea

[70] "Parasitic Infections Also Occur in the United States, Millions of People Infected," CDC Press Release, May 8, 2014, https://archive.cdc.gov/www_cdc_gov/media/releases/2014/p0508-npi.html
[71] "How Undiagnosed Parasite Infections Cause Chronic Health Conditions," Dr. Shawn Greenan, Rupa Health Magazine, July 12, 2024, https://www.rupahealth.com/post/parasites-a-possible-underlying-reason-behind-chronic-health-conditions
[72] "Parasitic Infection, Carcinogenesis and Human Malignancy, Hoang van Tong, Paul J. Brindley, Christian G Meyer, Thirumalaisamy P Velavan, The Lancet, Feb, 2017 Volume 15, https://www.thelancet.com/article/S2352-3964(16)30551-5/fulltext
[73] "Environmental Reservoirs of the Drug-Resistant Pathogenic Yeast Candida Auris," Ayorinde B Akinbobola, Ryan Kean, Syed Manzoor Ahmed Hanifi, Richard S. Quilliam, N. Luisa Hiller, PloS Pathog. April 19, 2023, https://www.ncbi.nlm.nih.gov/pmc/articles/PMC10101498/
[74] http://www.cancer.org/cancer/cancercauses/othercarcinogens/infectiousagents/infectiousagentsandcancer/infectious-agents-and-cancer-parasites
[75] http://www.cdc.gov/dpdx/
[76] "Ozone Disinfection," Wastewater Technology Fact Sheet, https://www3.epa.gov/npdes/pubs/ozon.pdf
[77] "Bisphenols exert detrimental effects on neuronal signaling in mature vertebrate brains, Elizabeth Schirmer, Stefan Schuster, Peter Machnik, Communications Biology, 4 Article 465, April 12, 2021, https://www.nature.com/articles/s42003-021-01966-w
[78] Bisphenol S in Food Causes Hormonal and Obesogenic Effects Comparable to or Worse than Bisphenol A: A Literature Review," Michael Thone, Ewa Dzika, Slawomir Gonkowski, Joanna Wojtkiewicz, Nutrients, February 2020, https://www.ncbi.nlm.nih.gov/pmc/articles/PMC7071457/
[79] Estrogen Receptor "Estrogen receptors and endocrine diseases: Lessons from Estrogen Receptor Knockout Mice," Stefan O Mueller, Kenneth S Korach, Pharmacology, 2001, https://www.sciencedirect.com/topics/pharmacology-toxicology-and-pharmaceutical-science/estrogen-receptor#:~:text=ERs%20are%20classified%20as%20estrogen,bone%2C%20and%20central%20nervous%20system.
[80] "EU Gets Ready to Ban Most BPA Uses. Once Again: Where's FDA?,"EDF Blogs, Environmental Defense Fund, March 1, 2024, https://blogs.edf.org/health/2024/03/01/eu-gets-ready-to-ban-most-bpa-uses-once-again-wheres-fda/
[81] **BPA: Cancer "Letter to Dr. Dennis Keefe, Director, Office of Food Additive Safety,"** Center for Food Safety, January 27, 2021, https://blogs.edf.org/health/wp-content/blogs.dir/11/files/2022/01/EDF-et-al-BPA-Food-Additive-Petition-FINAL-1-27-22.docx.pdf
[82] **BPA: Cancer "Letter to Dr. Dennis Keefe, Director, Office of Food Additive Safety,"** Center for Food Safety, January 27, 2021, https://blogs.edf.org/health/wp-content/blogs.dir/11/files/2022/01/EDF-et-al-BPA-Food-Additive-Petition-FINAL-1-27-22.docx.pdf
[83] "BPA's Evil Cousin, An ongoing series examining BADGE — an unregulated danger in epoxy resins," EHN Editors, Environmental Health News, April 4, 2023, https://www.ehn.org/epoxy-chemicals-2660287969.html#:~:text=BADGE%2C%20short%20for%20bisphenol%2DA,liver%20and%20kidney%20effects%20and
[84] "Triclosan Technical Fact Sheet," Connecticut Deparment of Public Health, January 2014, https://portal.ct.gov/-/media/departments-and-agencies/dph/dph/environmental_health/eoha/pdf/triclosantechfspdf.pdf

Benzene
[85] http://stateimpact.npr.org/pennsylvania/2014/08/28/new-study-shows-gas-workers-could-be-exposed-to-dangerous-levels-of-benzene/

Biosolids

[86] "Our Sewage Often Becomes Fertilizer. Problem is, It's Tainted with PFAS, Barbara Moran, WBUR, March 30, 2023, https://www.wbur.org/news/2023/03/30/boston-massachusetts-pfas-forever-chemicals-sludge-deer-island#

[87] "Our Sewage Often Becomes Fertilizer. Problem is, It's Tainted with PFAS, Barbara Moran, WBUR, March 30, 2023, https://www.wbur.org/news/2023/03/30/boston-massachusetts-pfas-forever-chemicals-sludge-deer-island#

[88] "Maine Passes First PFAS Biosolids Ban, Taking Stand Against Forever Chemicals," Brook Hays, UPI, May 4, 2022, https://www.upi.com/Science_News/2022/05/04/maine-forever-chemicals-farms-food-health/3291651077538/

[89] "What are the Health Effects of PFAS?," Agency for Toxic Substances and Disease Registry, https://www.atsdr.cdc.gov/pfas/health-effects/index.html

[90] "*EPA Unable to Assess the Impact of Hundreds of Unregulated Pollutants in Land-Applied Biosolids on Human Health and the Environment,"Office of the Inspector General*, 19-P-0002 November 15, 2018, https://www.epa.gov/sites/default/files/2018-11/documents/_epaoig_20181115-19-p-0002.pdf

[91] "Farmers File Suit Over PFAS Contamination," Brigit Rollins, The National Agricultural Law Center, April 2, 2024, https://nationalaglawcenter.org/farmers-file-suit-over-pfas-contamination/

[92] From the Archives: Adrienne Anderson, University Libraries, University of Colorado Boulder, https://www.colorado.edu/libraries/2018/04/06/archives-adrienne-anderson

[93] "Keep unregulated chemical pollutants off our farmland and waterways," Phillip Thompson, Mari Winkler, Seattle Times, April 15, 2022, https://www.seattletimes.com/opinion/keep-unregulated-chemical-pollutants-off-our-farmland-and-waterways/

[94] "Maine Legislature Passes Bill Prohibiting Land Application of Biosolids, Governor Expected to Sign," NACWA, April 20, 2022, https://www.nacwa.org/news-publications/news-detail/2022/04/20/maine-legislature-passes-bill-prohibiting-land-application-of-biosolids-governor-expected-to-sign

[95] The National Academy of Sciences, "Direct Detection of Atmospheric Atomic Bromine Leading to Mercury and Ozone Depletion, Siyuan Wang, Stephen McNamara, Christopher Moore, Kerri A. Pratt, Mark Thiemens, University of California San Diego, PNAS Earth, Atmospheric, and Planetary Sciences, May 29, 2019

Bromine

[96] "Flame Retardant Transfers from U.S. Households (Dust and Laundry Wastewater) to the Aquatic Environment, Erika D. Schreder, Mark J. LaGuardia, Environmental Science Technology, 2014, 48, 19, 11575-11583, ACS Publications, https://pubs.acs.org/doi/abs/10.1021/es502227h, September 17, 2014.

[97] https://www.cspinet.org/new/bromate.html, https://www.huffingtonpost.com/dr-mercola/thyroid-health_b_472953.html

Chlorine

[98] http://www.thenutritionalhealingcenter.com/iodine-the-fountain-of-youth-part-two/

[99] Water Technology, Joe Cotruvo, Joe Cotruvo and Associates, Water, Environment, and Public Health Consultants, Former Director of the EPA Drinking Water Standards Division,https://www.watertechonline.com/process-water/article/15549694/contaminant-of-the-month-bromine-and-bromine-disinfection

[100] "Chlorination: A Link Between Heart Disease and Cancer," Martin Fox PhD, The Pure Water Gazette, Feb 29, 2012, http://www.purewatergazette.net/blog/chlorination-a-link-between-heart-disease-and-cancer/

[101] "Tap Water and Trihalomethanes: Flow of Concerns Continues," Ernie Hood, Environ Health Perspectives, July 2005, https://www.ncbi.nlm.nih.gov/pmc/articles/PMC1257669/

[102] "Chlorinated Water Exposure May Boost Cancer Risk," Reuters, Aug 9, 2007, https://www.reuters.com/article/business/healthcare-pharmaceuticals/chlorinated-water-exposure-may-boost-cancer-risk-idUSTON885665/#:~:text=Study%20participants%20who%20drank%20chlorinated,also%20at%20an%20increased%20cancer%20risk.

[103] "Wastewater Technology Fact Sheet, Ozone Disinfection," EPA, https://www3.epa.gov/npdes/pubs/ozon.pdf
[104] "Wastewater Technology Fact Sheet, Ozone Disinfection," EPA, https://www3.epa.gov/npdes/pubs/ozon.pdf
[105] "Long-Term Exposure to Nitrate and Trihalomethanes in Drinking Water and Prostate Cancer: A Multicase-Control Study in Spain," Donat-Vargas C, Kogevinas M, Castaño-Vinyals G, Pérez-Gómez B, Llorca J, Vanaclocha-Espí M, Fernandez-Tardon G, Costas L, Aragonés N, Gómez-Acebo I, Moreno V, Pollan M, Villanueva CM, Environ Health Perspect. March 13, 2023, https://www.ncbi.nlm.nih.gov/pmc/articles/PMC9994181/
[106] "Nitrate," Cancer Trends Progress Report, National Cancer Institute, March, 2024, https://progressreport.cancer.gov/prevention/chemical_exposures/nitrate#:~:text=Studies%20have%20shown%20increased%20risks,results%20in%20increased%20NOC%20formation.
[107] "Common Water Disinfecting Method May Result in Toxic Byproducts, Study Finds,"Chanapa Tantibanchachai, John Hopkins University Hub, Jan 29, 2020, https://hub.jhu.edu/2020/01/29/toxic-chlorinated-water-649-em1-art1-rel-science/
[108] "Colorectal Cancers and Chlorinated Water,"Ahmed Mahmoud El-Tawil, World J Gastrointest Oncology, April 15, 2016, https://www.ncbi.nlm.nih.gov/pmc/articles/PMC4824718/
[109] Total Trihalomethanes (TTHMs), EWG Tap Water Database, https://www.ewg.org/tapwater/contaminant.php?contamcode=2950
[110] "Chlorination: A Link Between Heart Disease and Cancer," Martin Fox PhD, The Pure Water Gazette, Feb 29, 2012, http://www.purewatergazette.net/blog/chlorination-a-link-between-heart-disease-and-cancer/
[111] "Tap Water Linked to Miscarriages,"Jim Newton, Julie Marquis, Los Angeles Times, Feb 10, 1998, https://www.latimes.com/archives/la-xpm-1998-feb-10-mn-17476-story.html#:~:text=Drinking%20five%20or%20more%20glasses,water%20by%20California%20state%20researchers.

Chloramines

[112] "Chloramines and Drinking Water Safety,"Nate Seltenrich, Berkeley Engineering, June 10, 2016, https://engineering.berkeley.edu/news/2016/06/qa-lead-chloramines-and-drinking-water-safety/#:~:text=Chloramines%20are%20used%20in%20many,and%20solder%20in%20household%20plumbing.
[113] "Byproduct of water-disinfection process found to be Highly Toxic," Jim Barlow, University of Illinois Urbana, Sept 14, https://news.illinois.edu/view/6367/2075032004,
[114] "Controlling Nitrification in Public Water Systems with Chloramines," Texas Commission on Environmental Quality, https://www.tceq.texas.gov/drinkingwater/disinfection/nitrification.html#
[115] "Nitrate in Drinking Water, 2003-2017: Illinois," Environmental Working Group, https://www.ewg.org/interactive-maps/2020-nitrate-pollution-of-drinking-water-for-more-than-20-million-americans-is-getting-worse/il/#:~:text=Source%3A%20EWG%2C%20from%20Illinois%20Environmental,4.61%20mg%2FL%20in%202017.

Chlorpyrifos

[116] "What You Need to Know About Chlorpyrifos," Earthjustice, April 9, 2024, https://earthjustice.org/feature/chlorpyrifos-what-you-need-to-know
[117] 88
[118] "88
[119] Chlorpyrifos, Pesticide Action Network North America, https://www.panna.org/resources/chlorpyrifos-facts/#:~:text=EPA%20indicates%20that%20a%20single,vulnerable%20to%20the%20potent%20insecticide.
[120] "Pesticides and Water Quality," Water Resources Mission Area, USGS, March 1, 2019, https://www.usgs.gov/mission-areas/water-resources/science/pesticides-and-water-quality
[121] (60) (61)
[122] Food Quality Protection Act, USDA, https://www.ams.usda.gov/rules-regulations/fqpa#:~:text=The%20Food%20Quality%20Protection%20Act,monitoring%20to%20support%20this%20requirement.

123 "Celebrated 2021 Ag Ban of Deadly Pesticide, Chlorpyrifos, Reversed!", Beyond Pesticides, https://beyondpesticides.org/dailynewsblog/2023/11/2021-ag-ban-of-deadly-pesticide-chlorpyrifos-reversed-by-court-despite-decades-of-review-and-litigation/
124 Results to Petition filed with the Court,vs the EPA, https://cdn.ca9.uscourts.gov/datastore/opinions/2021/04/29/19-71979.pdf
125 "Celebrated 2021 Ag Ban of Deadly Pesticide, Chlorpyrifos, Reversed!", Beyond Pesticides, https://beyondpesticides.org/dailynewsblog/2023/11/2021-ag-ban-of-deadly-pesticide-chlorpyrifos-reversed-by-court-despite-decades-of-review-and-litigation/
126 "Europe Shipping Banned Pesticide Linked to Child Brain Damage To Global South," Unearthed, Green Peace, https://unearthed.greenpeace.org/2023/03/28/eu-banned-pesticide-global-south/
127 "The USA Lags Behind Other Agricultural Nations in Banning Harmful Pesticides, Nathan Donley, Environmental Health, June 07, 2019, https://ehjournal.biomedcentral.com/articles/10.1186/s12940-019-0488-0
128 http://www.swrcb.ca.gov/lahontan/water_issues/projects/pge/
129 http://www.ewg.org/research/chromium6-in-tap-water

Chromium-6

130 "High Levels of Chromium Found in Chicago-Area Tap Water," Michael Hawthorne, Chicago Tribune, December 22, 2010, https://www.chicagotribune.com/news/ct-xpm-2010-12-22-ct-met-chromium-water-contamination-20101220-story.html
131 http://www.ewg.org/research/chromium6-in-tap-water
132 "California on Path (Again) toward Regulating Hexavalent Chromium (Chromium-6) in Drinking Water; Follows EPA Scientific Workshop in September 2021," National Law Review, March 30, 2022, https://www.natlawreview.com/article/california-path-again-toward-regulating-hexavalent-chromium-chromium-6-drinking
133 http://www.chicagotribune.com/lifestyles/health/ct-met-drinking-water-chromium-20110806-story.html

Coal Ash

134 Southeast Coal Ash, http://www.southeastcoalash.org/about-coal-ash/coal-ash-storage/
135 https://earthobservatory.nasa.gov/NaturalHazards/view.php?id=36352
136 https://water.usgs.gov/nawqa/mercury/MercuryFAQ.html
137 Testimony of Stephen A. Smith, DVM, Executive Director, Southern Alliance for Clean Energy, Submitted to U.S. Senate Committee on Environment and Public Works, January 8, 2009, http://www.southeastcoalash.org

Cosmetics

138 "How Do I Know if Microbeads Are in My Products," Kylie Matthews, Choice, November 22, 2021, https://www.choice.com.au/health-and-body/beauty-and-personal-care/skin-care-and-cosmetics/articles/microplastics-and-microbeads-in-toothpaste-facial-body-scrubs#:~:text=Microbeads%20are%20present%20in%20some,and%20other%20personal%20care%20products.
139 "Cancer Prevention Coalition: Multiple Carcinogens in Johnson and Johnson's Baby Shampoo," Dr. Samuel Epstein, Dec 15, 2011, Fierce Pharma, https://www.fiercepharma.com/pharma/cancer-prevention-coalition-multiple-carcinogens-johnson-johnson-s-baby-shampoo
140 "Fluorinated Compounds in North American Cosmetics," *Environ. Sci. Technol. Lett.* 2021, 8, 7, 538–544, Publication Date: June 15, 2021
https://doi.org/10.1021/acs.estlett.1c00240, Copyright © 2022 The Authors. Published by American Chemical Society. This publication is licensed under
CC-BY-NC-ND 4.0.
141 "Quaternary Ammonium Compounds: A Chemical Class of Emerging Concern," Environ Sci Technol. 2023 May 23; 57(20): 7645–7665.
Published online 2023 May 9. doi: 10.1021/acs.est.2c08244, William A. Arnold,[†] Arlene Blum,[‡,§] Jennifer Branyan,[∥] Thomas A. Bruton,[∥] Courtney C. Carignan,[⊥] Gino Cortopassi,[#] Sandipan Datta,[#,⊞] Jamie DeWitt,[∇] Anne-Cooper Doherty,[∥] Rolf U. Halden,[○] Homero Harari,[♦] Erica M. Hartmann,[¶] Terry C. Hrubec,[⋈] Shoba Iyer,[⊙◨] Carol F. Kwiatkowski,[*,‡,●] Jonas LaPier,[‡] Dingsheng

Li,° Li Li,° Jorge G. Muñiz Ortiz,⊡Amina Salamova,◘ Ted Schettler,ᵛ Ryan P. Seguin,▫ Anna Soehl,‡ Rebecca Sutton,⊖ Libin Xu,▫ and Guomao Zheng, https://www.ncbi.nlm.nih.gov/pmc/articles/PMC10210541/

[142] https://www.fda.gov/Cosmetics/Labeling/Regulations/ucm126444.htm#clgl2

[143] "Draft Guidance for Industry: Lead in Cosmetic Lip Products and Externally Applied Cosmetics: Recommended Maximum Level," December 2016, Docket Number FDA-2014-D-2275, Center for Food Safety and Applied Nutrition, Office of Cosmetics and Colors, https://www.fda.gov/regulatory-information/search-fda-guidance-documents/draft-guidance-industry-lead-cosmetic-lip-products-and-externally-applied-cosmetics-recommended

[144] "Prohibited & Restricted Ingredients in Cosmetics, FDA, https://www.fda.gov/cosmetics/cosmetics-laws-regulations/prohibited-restricted-ingredients-cosmetics

DBPs

[145] http://www.who.int/water_sanitation_health/dwq/chemicals/mx.pdf
MX is the common name for 3-chloro-4-dichloromethyl-5-hydroxy-2(5H)-furanone)

[146] The Water Research Foundation, "The Role and Behavior of Chloramines in Drinking Water, Djanette Khiari, May 2019. https://www.waterrf.org/sites/default/files/file/2019-12/Chloramines_StateOfTheScience.pdf

[147] What's in Your Water, Researchers Identify New Toxic Byproducts of Disinfecting Drinking Water, John Hopkins University, January 28, 2020, ,https://phys.org/news/2020-01-toxic-byproducts-disinfecting.html

[148] https://phys.org/news/2020-01-toxic-byproducts-disinfecting.html

[149] Trihalomethanes, Delaware Health and Social Services, https://dhss.delaware.gov/dph/files/trihalomfaq.pdf

[150] "Get Informed, What are Chloroform and Trichloromethane?, Know Your H2O, Water Research Center, https://www.knowyourh2o.com/indoor-6/chloroform-and-trichloromethane

[151] https://www.knowyourh2o.com/indoor-6/chloroform-and-trichloromethane

Dicamba

[152] "Dicamba Use and Cancer Incidence in the Agricultural Health Study, An Updated Analysis," Lerro CC, Hofmann JN, Andreotti G, Koutros S, Parks CG, Blair A, Albert PS, Lubin JH, Sandler DP, Beane Freeman LE, Int J Epidemiol. 2020 Aug 1;49(4):1326-1337. doi: 10.1093/ije/dyaa066. PMID: 32357211; PMCID: PMC7660157, https://www.ncbi.nlm.nih.gov/pmc/articles/PMC7660157/

[153] Dicamba, EPA, https://www.epa.gov/pesticides/dicamba#:~:text=Dicamba%20has%20been%20used%20as,soybeans%2C%20sugarcane%20and%20wheat%20crops.

[154] "What is Roundup for Lawns?" Jennie Silver, University of Wisconsin-Madison, April 24, 2017, https://richland.extension.wisc.edu/2017/04/24/what-is-roundup-for-lawns/#:~:text=Roundup%20for%20Lawns%20contains%20the,small%20or%20prior%20to%20emergence.

[155] "Bayer Trying Again with Dicamba," Pesticide Action Network, June 7, 2024, https://www.panna.org/news/bayer-dicamba-again/

[156] "GMO Crops, Animal Food, and Beyond," US Food and Drug Administration, https://www.fda.gov/food/agricultural-biotechnology/gmo-crops-animal-food-and-beyond#:~:text=Most%20soy%20grown%20in%20the,and%20proteins)%20in%20processed%20foods.

[157] "2024 Dicamba Update," Minnesota Dept of Agriculture, https://www.mda.state.mn.us/pesticide-fertilizer/dicamba-general-information#:~:text=It%20was%20first%20registered%20by,dicamba%20tolerant%20(DT)%20soybeans.

[158] "Study Finds An Association Between Dicamba Use and Increased Risk of Developing Various Cancers," Beyond Pesticides, May 21, 2020, beyondpesticides.org

Dichlorobenzene

[159] "Deadly Pesticide Poses an Increased Risk of Hormone-Associated Reproductive Cancers in Women, Beyond Pesticides, https://beyondpesticides.org/dailynewsblog/2023/07/deadly-pesticide-poses-an-increased-risk-of-hormone-associated-reproductive-cancers-in-women/#:~:text=(Beyond%20Pesticides%2C%20July%2013%2C,of%20common%20endocrine%20(hormone)%2D

[160] Deadly Pesticide Poses an Increased Risk of Hormone-Associated Reproductive Cancers in Women, Beyond Pesticides, https://beyondpesticides.org/dailynewsblog/2023/07/deadly-pesticide-poses-an-increased-risk-of-hormone-associated-reproductive-cancers-in-women/#:~:text=(Beyond%20Pesticides%2C%20July%2013%2C,of%20common%20endocrine%20(hormone)%2D

Dioxin

[161] "Learn About Dioxin," EPA, https://www.epa.gov/dioxin/learn-about-dioxin

[162] (146)

[163] "Delaware's Rivers and Streams Are the Most Polluted in the U.S., a New Report Says, Zoe Read, PBS, WHYY, March 17 2022, https://whyy.org/articles/delawares-rivers-and-streams-pollution-enviornmental-integrity-project-water-safety/

[164] "Dioxins and Human Toxicity,"Natalija Marinkovic, Daria Pasalic, Goran Ferencak, Branka Grskovic, Ana Stavlijenic Rukavina, Arh Hig Rada Toksikol, Dec, 2010, https://pubmed.ncbi.nlm.nih.gov/21183436/

[165] "The American's People Dioxin Report," The Center for Health, Environment, & Justice, https://chej.org/wp-content/uploads/American%20Peoples%20Dioxin%20Report.pdf

[166] "Dioxins," World Health Organization, Nov 29, 2023, https://www.who.int/news-room/fact-sheets/detail/dioxins-and-their-effects-on-human-health#:~:text=Their%20half%2Dlife%20in%20the,tetrachlorodibenzo%20para%20dioxin%20(TCDD).

[167] "Dioxins," World Health Organization, https://www.who.int/news-room/fact-sheets/detail/dioxins-and-their-effects-on-human-health

[168] "Water Use by Ethanol Plants,"Institute for Agriculture and Trade Policy, October, 2006, https://www.iatp.org/sites/default/files/258_2_89449.pdf

[169] "More Ethanol Means More Toxic Water Pollution," Emily Cassidy, EWG, Jan 19, 2016, https://www.ewg.org/news-insights/news/more-ethanol-means-more-toxic-water-pollution

[170] "Iowa Town's Drinking Water Contamination Returns After Testing Ends," Jared Strong, Iowa Capital Dispatch, Jan 22, 2023, https://www.desmoinesregister.com/story/news/2023/01/22/iowa-towns-drinking-water-contamination-returns-after-testing-ends/69825931007/

Ethanol

[171] https://news.agu.org/press-release/ethanol-refining-may-release-more-of-some-pollutants-than-previously-thought/

[172] "Growing health concerns surrounding pesticides, including two commonly used in Iowa," Lauren Mills, Iowa Watch, Investigate Midwest, July 22, 2016, https://investigatemidwest.org/2016/07/22/growing-health-concerns-surrounding-pesticides-including-two-commonly-used-in-iowa/

[173] "EPA Renewable Fuels "Set Rule" to Destroy Habitat, Kill Endangered Species, Degrade Water Quality," Brett Hartl, Center for Biological Diversity, Dec 1, 2022, https://biologicaldiversity.org/w/news/press-releases/epa-renewable-fuels-set-rule-to-destroy-habitat-kill-endangered-species-degrade-water-quality-2022-12-01/

[174] "Toxic Blue-Green Algae: A Threat to Iowa Beaches and Beachgoers," Iowa Environmental Council, January, 2017, https://www.iaenvironment.org/webres/File/IEC_Cyanobacteria_Facts_2017_Final.pdf

[175] "US EPA Allows Temporary Expansion of Higher-Ethanol Gasoline Blend This Summer," Stephanie Kelly, Reuters, April 22, 2024, https://www.reuters.com/business/energy/us-epa-allows-

temporary-expansion-higher-ethanol-gasoline-blend-this-summer-2024-04-19/#:~:text=Adding%20ethanol%20to%20gasoline%20is,more%2Dwidely%20available%20E10%20blends.

[176] "More Ethanol Means More Toxic Water Pollution," Emily Cassidy, January 19, 2016, EWG, https://www.ewg.org/news-insights/news/more-ethanol-means-more-toxic-water-pollution#:~:text=Planting%20massive%20amounts%20of%20corn,and%20too%20toxic%20to%20drink.

[177] Hazardous Substance Fact Sheet, New Jersey Department of Health, Right to Know Factsheet, 2-Butoxy Ethanol, http://nj.gov/health/eoh/rtkweb/documents/fs/0275.pdf
Ethylene Glycol

[178] "A Dense PEG Coating Improves Penetration of Large Polymeric Nanoparticles within Brain Tissue," Elizabeth A Nance, Graweme F. Woodworth, and team, Sci Transl Med, Aug 29, 2013, https://www.ncbi.nlm.nih.gov/pmc/articles/PMC3718558/

[179] Agency for Toxic Substances, Environmental Health and Medicine Education, Ethylene Glycol, Propylene Glycol Toxicity, https://www.atsdr.cdc.gov/csem/ethylene-propylene-glycol/regulations_guidelines.html

Factory Farms

[180] https://deainfo.nci.nih.gov/advisory/pcp/annualreports/pcp08-09rpt/pcp_report_08-09_508.pdf

[181] NPDES CAFO Permitting Status Report: National Summary, Endyear 2013, May 14, 2024, https://www.epa.gov/system/files/documents/2024-06/cafo-status-report-2023.pdf

[182] "Factory Farm Gas:What is it and Why is it Harmful?" Hannah Trembley, Farm Aid, June 6, 2024, https://www.farmaid.org/blog/fact-sheet/factory-farm-gas-what-it-is-and-why-its-harmful/

[183] "Report: Indiana Has the Most Polluted Rivers, Streams of Any State, Rebecca Thiele, PBS WFYI Indianapolis, March 17, 2022, https://www.wfyi.org/news/articles/report-indiana-has-the-most-polluted-rivers-streams-of-any-state#:~:text=deemed%20%22impaired.%22-,Indiana%20has%20the%20most%20miles%20of%20rivers%20and%20streams%20deemed,coli%20and%20toxic%20algae.

[184] "Report: Indiana Has the Most Polluted Rivers, Streams of Any State, Rebecca Thiele, PBS WFYI Indianapolis, March 17, 2022, https://www.wfyi.org/news/articles/report-indiana-has-the-most-polluted-rivers-streams-of-any-state#:~:text=deemed%20%22impaired.%22-,Indiana%20has%20the%20most%20miles%20of%20rivers%20and%20streams%20deemed,coli%20and%20toxic%20algae.

[185] Dr. Epstein: https://www.huffingtonpost.com/entry/american-publlic-health-a_b_399147.html

Fertilizer Runoff

[186] "How to Spot the Toxic Algae that's Killing Dogs in the Southeast," Susan Scutti, CNN, Aug 12, 2019, https://www.cnn.com/2019/08/12/health/toxic-algae-dog-deaths-trnd/index.html

[187] "Pesticides as a Cause of Soil Degradation,"John Kempf, March 27, 2020, https://johnkempf.com/pesticides-as-a-cause-of-soil-degradation/

[188] "Here's the Scoop on Chemical and Organic Fertilizers, Oregon State University, https://extension.oregonstate.edu/news/heres-scoop-chemical-organic-fertilizers

[189] "Largest Ever Study Reveals Environmental Impact of Genetically Modified Crops," Caroline Newman, , *UVA Today*, University of Virginia, Sept 14, 2016, https://news.virginia.edu/content/largest-ever-study-reveals-environmental-impact-genetically-modified-crops

[190] Nitrogen Fertilizer and Natural Gas Bombshell
https://www.fertilizerseurope.com/fertilizers-in-europe/how-fertilizers-are-made/#:~:text=For%20nitrogen%2Dbased%20fertilizers%2C%20the,to%20power%20the%20synthesis%20process.

[191] Monsanto's Evil Twin, Disturbing Facts About the Fertlizer Industry, Martha Rosenberg, Ronnie Cummins, April 5, 2016, Organic Consumers Association,
https://www.organicconsumers.org/essays/monsanto%E2%80%99s-evil-twin-disturbing-facts-about-fertilizer-industry

[192] "Contaminated Water from Florida Mining Facility Dumped a Year's Worth of Hazardous Nutrients into Tamp Bay in just 10 Days, study shows," Li Cohen, CBS News, April 25, 2022,

https://www.cbsnews.com/news/piney-point-mining-facility-dumped-years-worth-hazardous-nutrients-tampa-bay-10-days-study/
[193] Radioactive Material From Fertilizer Production, EPA, https://www.epa.gov/radtown/radioactive-material-fertilizer-production
[194] The Clock is Ticking on Florida's Mountains of Hazardous Phosphate Waste,Craig Pittman, Sarasota Magazine, April 26, 2017, https://www.sarasotamagazine.com/articles/2017/4/26/florida-phosphate

Flame Retardants

[195] "Flame Retardant Chemicals Found in More People," Julia Calderone, Consumer Reports, February 13, 2017, https://www.consumerreports.org/toxic-chemicals-substances/flame-retardant-chemicals-found-in-more-people/
[196] "First-Of-Its-Kind Study Finds Toxic Flame Retardants From Consumer Products Are Significant Source Of Pollution To Waterways," Toxic-Free Future, September 16, 2014, https://toxicfreefuture.org/press-room/first-of-its-kind-study-finds-toxic-flame-retardants-from-consumer-products-are-significant-source-of-pollution-to-waterways/
[197] "Breast Cancer: The risks of brominated flame retardants," Institut national de la recherche scientifique -INRS, Science News, March 12, 2021, https://www.sciencedaily.com/releases/2021/03/210312084702.htm
[198] "Fear Fans Flames for Chemical Makers," Patricia Callahan, Sam Roe, Chicago Tribune, May 6, 2021, https://www.chicagotribune.com/investigations/ct-met-flame-retardants-20120506-story.html
[199] Excerpted from the book *Wildfire* by The Foundation for Deep Ecology.

Fluoride

[200] US Government Report Says Fluoride at Twice the Recommended Limit is Linked to Lower IQ,"Mike Stobbe, AP News, Aug 22, 2024, https://apnews.com/article/fluoride-water-brain-neurology-iq-0a671d2de3b386947e2bd5a661f437a5
[201] "Is Fluoridated Drinking Water Safe?,"Harvard Public Health Magazine, Spring 2016, https://www.hsph.harvard.edu/magazine/magazine_article/fluoridated-drinking-water/
[202] "Water Fluoridation, What Does the Rest of the World Think?," Oliver Milman, The Guardian, Sept 16, 2013, https://www.theguardian.com/world/2013/sep/17/water-fluoridation
[203] "Benefits of Oral Probiotics & Best Strains,"Mark Burhenne, DDS, October 26, 2021, Ask the Dentist, https://askthedentist.com/oral-probiotics/#:~:text=One%20of%20the%20most%20problematic,version%20and%20prevent%20plaque%20buildup.
[204] http://www.who.int/ipcs/features/fluoride.pdf?ua=1
[205] Is Fluoridated Drinking Water Safe?,"Harvard Public Health Magazine, Spring 2016, https://www.hsph.harvard.edu/magazine/magazine_article/fluoridated-drinking-water
[206] Fluoridated Milk Scheme, Blackpool Council, March 14, 2024, https://www.blackpool.gov.uk/Residents/Education-and-schools/School-meals/Fluoridated-milk-scheme.aspx#:~:text=Fluoridated%20milk%20has%20been%20offered,no%20additional%20cost%20to%20parents.
[207] "Exploring the Role of Excess Fluoride in Chronic Kidney Disease: A Review," R.W. Dharmaratne, Hum Exp Toxicol. 2019 Mar;38(3):269-279. doi: 10.1177/0960327118814161. Epub 2018 Nov 25. PMID: 30472891,
National Institute of Health
[208] "Fluoride Occurrences, Health Problems, Detection, and Remediation Methods for Drinking Wtaer: A Comprehensive Review," Yogendra Singh Solanki, Madhu Agarwal, AB Gupta, Sanjeeva Gupta, Pushkar Shukla, National Library of Medicine, Science Total Environment, February 10, 2022,
https://pubmed.ncbi.nlm.nih.gov/34597567/
[209] "US Government Report Says Fluoride at Twice the Recommended Limit is Linked to Lower IQ in Kids," Mike Stobbe, AP News, August 22, 2024, https://apnews.com/article/fluoride-water-brain-neurology-iq-0a671d2de3b386947e2bd5a661f437a5#
[210] Mandatory State Laws on Fluoridation, Tom Reeves, CDC Fluoridation Engineer, December 1, 2000, Fluoride Alert and Juneau Fluoride Study Commission, Exhibit C, pages 97-101, July 11, 2006, https://fluoridealert.org/content/mandatory-fluoridation-in-the-u-s/
[211] http://fluoridealert.org/content/oecd_nations/

Hazardous Waste
[212] http://www.epa.gov/brownfields/brownfield-overview-and-definition

Fracking
[213] "In Fracking's Wake: New Rules are Needed to Protect Our Health and Environment from Contaminated Water," Rebecca Hammer, Jeanne VanBriesen, Larry Levine, Natural Resources Defense Council, May, 2012, https://www.nrdc.org/sites/default/files/Fracking-Wastewater-FullReport.pdf
[214] https://www.epa.gov/sites/production/files/2016-12/documents/hfdwa_executive_summary.pdf
[215] "Feds Link Water Contamination to Fracking for the First Time," ProPublica, Abrahm Lustgarten, Nicholas Kusentz, Dec.8,2011, , http://www.propublica.org/article/feds-link-water-contamination-to-fracking-for-first-time
[216] https://energy.gov/sites/prod/files/2013/04/f0/shale_gas_challenges_water.pdf
[217] https://www.epa.gov/hw/special-wastes
[218] https://www.huffingtonpost.com/entry/epa-fracking-waste-lawsuit_us_572a29f1e4b096e9f08fe5ae
[219] "How to Tackle Fracking in Your Community," Alexandra Zissu, NRDC, January 27, 2016, https://www.nrdc.org/stories/how-tackle-fracking-your-community
[220] "How Fracking Has Contaminated Drinking Water," Elena Bruess, Consumer Reports, December 3, 2020, https://www.consumerreports.org/water-contamination/how-fracking-has-contaminated-drinking-water-a1256135490/
[221] "Why Frack Wastewater Injected Underground Doesn't Always Stay There," Julie Grant, The Alleghany Front, March 19 2021, https://www.alleghenyfront.org/why-frack-wastewater-injected-underground-doesnt-always-stay-there/
[222] "How to Tackle Fracking in Your Community," NRDC, Alexandra Zissu, January 27, 2016, https://www.nrdc.org/stories/how-tackle-fracking-your-community

Gen X
[223] Fact Sheet: Human Health Toxicity Assessment for GenX Chemicals, EPA United States Environmental Protection Agency, https://www.epa.gov/system/files/documents/2021-10/genx-final-tox-assessment-general_factsheet-2021.pdf

Glyphosate
[224] "Toxic Effects of Glyphosate on the Nervous System: A Systematic Review," Carmen Costas-Ferreira, Rafael Duran, Lilian R.F. Faro,Joao Pedro Silva, International Journal Molecular Science, May 23, 2022, https://www.ncbi.nlm.nih.gov/pmc/articles/PMC9101768/
[225] AMPA, What is Aminomethylphospohonic Acid?, Wisconsin Department of Health Services, https://www.dhs.wisconsin.gov/publications/p02434k-2.pdf
[226] "Toxic Effects of Glyphosate on the Nervous System: A Systematic Review," Carmen Costas-Ferreira, Rafael Duran, Lilian R.F. Faro,Joao Pedro Silva, International Journal Molecular Science, May 23, 2022, https://www.ncbi.nlm.nih.gov/pmc/articles/PMC9101768/
[227] "What the Monsanto Papers Tell Us About Corporate Science," Corporate Europe Observatory, Jan 3, 2018, https://corporateeurope.org/en/food-and-agriculture/2018/03/what-monsanto-papers-tell-us-about-corporate-science#:~:text=This%20means%20that%2C%20for%20glyphosate,herbicide%20because%20it%20is%20inefficient).
[228] "Glyphosate infiltrates the Brain and Increases Pro-inflammatory Cytokine TNFa: implications for Neurodegenerative disorders, Winstone JK, Pathak KV, Winslow W,

Piras IS, White J, Sharma R, Huentelman MJ, Pirrotte P, Velazquez R. 2022 Jul 28;19(1):193. doi: 10.1186/s12974-022-02544-5. Erratum in: J Neuroinflammation. 2024 Ja, https://pubmed.ncbi.nlm.nih.gov/35897073/

Special Report: Herbicides

[229] Dicamba Use and Cancer Incidence in the Agricultural Health Study, An Updated Analysis," Lerro CC, Hofmann JN, Andreotti G, Koutros S, Parks CG, Blair A, Albert PS, Lubin JH, Sandler DP, Beane Freeman LE, Int J Epidemiol. 2020 Aug 1;49(4):1326-1337. doi: 10.1093/ije/dyaa066. PMID: 32357211; PMCID: PMC7660157, https://www.ncbi.nlm.nih.gov/pmc/articles/PMC7660157/

[230] "A Method for the Analysis of Glyphosate, Aminomethylphosphonic Acid, and Glufosinate in Human Urine Using Liquid Chromatography-Tandem Mass Spectrometry," Zhong-Min Li, Kurunthachalam Kannan, Int J Environ Res Public Health. 2022 May; 19(9): 4966,doi: 10.3390/ijerph19094966, https://www.ncbi.nlm.nih.gov/pmc/articles/PMC9104544/#:~:text=Glufosinate%20is%20mainly%20used%20to,annually%20since%202016%20%5B3%5D.

[231] "Dicamba Use and Cancer Incidence in the Agricultural Health Study, An Updated Analysis," Lerro CC, Hofmann JN, Andreotti G, Koutros S, Parks CG, Blair A, Albert PS, Lubin JH, Sandler DP, Beane Freeman LE, Int J Epidemiol. 2020 Aug 1;49(4):1326-1337. doi: 10.1093/ije/dyaa066. PMID: 32357211; PMCID: PMC7660157, https://www.ncbi.nlm.nih.gov/pmc/articles/PMC7660157/

[232] "33 Countries Ban the Use of Glyphosate – the key ingredient in Roundup," Biodx, May 22, 2019, https://biodx.co/28-countries-ban-the-use-of-glyphosate-key-ingredient-in-roundup/#:~:text=The%20following%20countries%20have%20banned,%3B%20Oman%3B%20Qatar%3B%20St.

Hand Sanitizers

[233] "Valisure Detects Benzene in Hand Sanitizers," March 24, 2021, https://www.valisure.com/valisure-newsroom/valisure-detects-benzene-in-hand-sanitizers

[234] "Triclosan Facts," EPA, March 2010, https://archive.epa.gov/pesticides/reregistration/web/html/triclosan_fs.html#:~:text=Triclosan%20was%20first%20registered%20as,available%20on%20EPA's%20Web%20site.

[235] EU to Ban Triclosan, While U.S EPA and FDA Reject Calls for U.S. Ban, AgNews, June 26, 2015, https://news.agropages.com/News/NewsDetail---15177.htm#:~:text=Focus%20on%20Ecuador-,EU%20to%20ban%20triclosan%2C%20while%20U.S.%20EPA%20and,reject%20calls%20for%20U.S.%20ban&text=The%20agency%20responsible%20for%20chemical,replaced%20by%20more%20suitable%20alternatives.

[236] "Triclosan Exposure, Transformation, and Human Health Effects," Lisa M. Weatherly, Julie A. Gosse, Journal Toxicology Environmental Health, Sept 6, 2018, https://www.ncbi.nlm.nih.gov/pmc/articles/PMC6126357/

[237] "Long-term exposure to triclosan increases migration and invasion of human breast epithelial cells in vitro," Abdullah Farasani, Philippa D. Darbre, Applied Toxicology, Nov 10, 2020, https://analyticalsciencejournals.onlinelibrary.wiley.com/doi/full/10.1002/jat.4097

Heavy Metals

[238] "Human Health Effects of Heavy Metals," Center for Hazardous Substance Research, March 2009, https://engg.k-state.edu/chsr/files/chsr/outreach-resources/15HumanHealthEffectsofHeavyMetals.pdf

Landscaping

[239] "Lawsuit Challenges TruGreen Chemical Lawn Care Company for Deceptive Safety Claims; Pesticide Applications Stopped by Some States During Covid-19 Crisis as Nonessential," Beyone Pesticides, March 30 2020, https://beyondpesticides.org/dailynewsblog/2020/03/lawsuit-challenges-trugreen-

chemical-lawn-care-company-for-deceptive-safety-claims-pesticide-applications-stopped-by-some-states-during-covid-19-crisis-as-nonessential/
[240] "Phytotoxicity: Chemical Damage to Garden Plants,"University of Maryland Extension, June 7, 2024, https://extension.umd.edu/resource/phytotoxicity-chemical-damage-garden-plants/

Lead
[241] "Profiting from Poison: How the US Lead Industry Knowingly Created a Water Crisis," Erin McCormick, Aliya Uteuova, The Guardian, September 22, 2022, https://www.theguardian.com/us-news/2022/sep/22/us-lead-industry-history-water-crisis
[242] "The Lead Industry and Lead Water Pipes, A Modest Campaign," Richard Rabin, Amerian Journal of Public Health, 2008, September; 98((): 1584-1592, https://www.ncbi.nlm.nih.gov/pmc/articles/PMC2509614/
[243] "Revealed, the Shocking Levels of Toxic Lead in Chicago Tap Water, Erin McCormick, Aliya Uteuova, Taylor Moore, Jamie Kelter Davis, the Guardian, September 21, 2022, https://www.theguardian.com/us-news/2022/sep/21/lead-contamination-chicago-tap-water-revealed
[244] https://www.nrdc.org/onearth/go-easy-salt
[245] "Time Bomb Lead Pipes Will Be Removed. But First Water Utilities Have to Find Them," Allison Kite, NPR, July 20, 2022, https://www.npr.org/sections/health-shots/2022/07/20/1112049811/lead-pipe-removal
[246] Heavy Metal Poisoning, Cleveland Clinic, https://my.clevelandclinic.org/health/diseases/23424-heavy-metal-poisoning-toxicity

Light Bulbs
[247] "Do LED Lights Contain Hazardous Materials," LED Lights Unlimited, February 15, 2021, https://www.ledlightsunlimited.net/2021/02/15/do-led-lights-have-hazard-materials/#:~:text=LED%20lights%20do%20contain%20hazardous,categorized%20as%20toxic%20by%20law.
[248] The Hour of Lead, "A Brief History of Lead Poisoning in the United States over the Past Century and of Efforts by the Lead Industry to Delay Regulation," Peter Reich, Environmental Defense Fund, June 1992, https://www.edf.org/sites/default/files/the-hour-of-lead.pdf
[249] "Decades After The Dangers of Lead Became Clear, Cities Are Leaving Lead Pipe In The Ground," Michael Phillis, AP News, July 8, 2023, https://apnews.com/article/toxic-lead-pipes-epa-providence-health-bc793dea64ab59d26e27620d3c2338c9
[250] "Ramped-Up US Construction Exposes Workers to An Unregulated Toxic," Meg Wilcox, Environmental Health News, August 3, 2023, https://www.ehn.org/epoxy-chemical-exposure-2660276391.html
[251] "A Popular Underground Pipe Fix is Making People Sick: Here's What We Learned From Our Investigation," Emily Le Coz, Monique O. Madan, USA Today, April 1, 2023, https://www.usatoday.com/story/news/investigations/2023/04/01/cured-place-pipe-lining-making-people-sick-heres-what-we-found/11571878002/
Manganese
[252] "Lead and Manganese Pollution May Lead to Life of Crime," Lead Action News, Alsion Motluk, May 31, 1997, https://www.lead.org.au/lanv5n3/lan5n3-3.html
[253] Drinking Water Contaminant Candidate List (CCL) and Regulatory Determination, https://www.epa.gov/ccl
[254] "Tap Water's Toxic Secret," Christine Mehta, Harvard Public Health, August 31, 2023, https://harvardpublichealth.org/environmental-health/manganese-in-water-a-threat-to-americans-health/#:~:text=Manganese%20is%20naturally%20occurring%2C%20but,water%20and%20cause%20manganese%20pollution.
[255] "Metals and Neurodegeneration," Pan Chen, Mahfuzur Rahman Miah, Michael Aschner, Version 1. F1000Res. 2016; 5: F1000 Faculty Rev-366, March 17, 2016, https://www.ncbi.nlm.nih.gov/pmc/articles/PMC4798150/
[256] Manganese in Water, Risks & Treatment, https://tataandhoward.com/manganese-in-water-risks-treatment-2/
[257] "Black Water: How Industry Fights Controls of Little-Known Drinking Water Contaminant," Natasha Gilbert, Public Health Watch, Aug 29, 2023,

https://publichealthwatch.org/2023/08/29/drinking-water-contaminant-manganese-epa-pennsylvania/

Mercury

[258] "Mercury in Home Products," Thurston Country Public Health and Social Services, Olympia, Washington, https://www.co.thurston.wa.us/health/ehhm/mercury.html
[259] http://oceana.org/sites/default/files/reports/PoisonPlants1.pdf
[260] "How Industries Can Reduce Water Pollution More Effectively," Keiken Engineering, https://www.keiken-engineering.com/news/how-industries-can-reduce-water-pollution-more-effectively#:~:text=Reducing%20the%20waste%20produced%20so,the%20waste%20produced%20from%20them.&text=Reduce%20or%20completely%20eliminate%20the%20dangerous%20materials%20used%20in%20the%20production%20process.
[261] What Are Microplastics? National Oceanic and Atmospheric Administration, National Ocean Service, https://oceanservice.noaa.gov/facts/microplastics.html

Microplastics

[262] MicroPlastics Are Turning Up Everywhere, Even in Human Excrement, Jill Neimark, NPR, WBEZ, https://www.npr.org/sections/thesalt/2018/10/22/659568662/microplastics-are-turning-up-everywhere-even-in-human-excrement
[263] In A First, Microplastics Found in Human Poop, Laura Parker, National Geographic, Oct 22, 2018, https://www.nationalgeographic.com/environment/2018/10/news-plastics-microplastics-human-feces/
[264] Styrene, ToxNet, National Institutes of Health, https://toxnet.nlm.nih.gov/cgi-bin/sis/search/a?dbs+hsdb:@term+@DOCNO+171
[265] "A Common Plastic Comes Under Scrutiny," Health Encyclopedia, University of Rochester Medical Center, https://www.urmc.rochester.edu/encyclopedia/content.aspx?contenttypeid=1&contentid=4248
[266] Cooking Safely in Microwave Oven, USDA, https://www.fsis.usda.gov/wps/portal/fsis/topics/food-safety-education/get-answers/food-safety-fact-sheets/appliances-and-thermometers/cooking-safely-in-the-microwave/cooking-safely-in-the-microwave-oven

Nanoparticles

[267] "FDA Releases Final Guidance on Nanotechnology in Food," Center for Food Safety, June 25, 2014, https://www.centerforfoodsafety.org/press-releases/3262/fda-releases-final-guidance-on-nanotechnology-in-food
[268] "Assessing the direct occupational and public health impacts of solar radiation management with stratospheric aerosols," Effiong, U., Neitzel, R.L. *Environ Health* **15**, 7 (2016). https://doi.org/10.1186/s12940-016-0089-0, https://link.springer.com/article/10.1186/s12940-016-0089-0#citeas
[269] "Nanoparticles Can Damage DNA, Increase Cancer Risk," American Association for Cancer Research, Science Daily, April 18, 2007, https://www.sciencedaily.com/releases/2007/04/070417154357.htm
[270] "Face Masks and Nanotechnology: Keep the Blue Side Up," Valentina Palmieri, Flavio De Maio, Marco De Spirito, Massimilano Papi, Nano Today, Jan 13, 2021, https://www.ncbi.nlm.nih.gov/pmc/articles/PMC7833187/
[271] "Toxicity Spectrum and Detrimental Effects of Titanium Dioxide Nanoparticles As An Emerging Pollutant: A Review," Qaisar Manzoor, Arfaa Sajid, Zulfiqar Ali, Arif Nazir, Anam Sajid, Faiza Imtiaz, Shahid Iqbal, Umer Younas, Hamza Arif, Munawar Iqbal, Desalination and Water Treatment, Jan 2024,

https://www.sciencedirect.com/science/article/pii/S1944398624000250#:~:text=Research%20sugge sted%20that%20exposure%20of,and%20ovarian%20function%20%5B70%5D.

[272] "A Dose Response Effect of Oral Aluminum Nanoparticle on Novel Object Recognition Memory, Hippocampal Caspase-3 and MAPKs Signaling in Mice," Nahid Mehrbeheshti, Zahra Esmaili, Mojdeh Ahmadi, Mayam Moosavi, Behavioral Brain Research, Jan 24, 2022, https://www.sciencedirect.com/science/article/abs/pii/S0166432821005039#:~:text=The%20increas ing%20use%20of%20aluminum,cognitive%20function%20and%20brain%20health.

[273] "Reef Friendly Sunscreens," Surfrider Organization, https://www.surfrider.org/news/your-guide-to-reef-friendly-sunscreens-0,

[274] "Nanomaterial Cleans Toxic Water Within 3 Minutes," Prashant Rupera, The Times of India, April 8, 2024, https://timesofindia.indiatimes.com/city/ahmedabad/nanomaterial-cleans-toxic-water-within-3-minutes/articleshow/109117332.cms

[275] "Forget Microplastics, We Have A Much Smaller Problem," Anna Turns, The Guardian, April 25, 2022, https://www.theguardian.com/environment/2022/apr/25/nano-state-tiny-and-now-everywhere-how-big-a-problem-are-nanoparticles

[276] "Forget Microplastics, We Have A Much Smaller Problem," Anna Turns, The Guardian, April 25, 2022, https://www.theguardian.com/environment/2022/apr/25/nano-state-tiny-and-now-everywhere-how-big-a-problem-are-nanoparticles

[277] EPA Finalizes Biological Evaluations Assessing Potential Effects of Three Neonicotinoid Pesticides on Endangered Species, EPA, June 16, 2022, https://www.epa.gov/pesticides/epa-finalizes-biological-evaluations-assessing-potential-effects-three-neonicotinoid

Neonicotinoids

[278] Insect "Apocalypse' In US Driven by 50x Increase in Toxic Pesticides," Stephen Leahy, National Geographic, August 6, 2019, https://www.nationalgeographic.com/environment/article/insect-apocalypse-under-way-toxic-pesticides-agriculture

[279] EPA Finalizes Biological Evaluations Assessing Potential Effects of Three Neonicotinoid Pesticides on Endangered Species, EPA, June 16, 2022, https://www.epa.gov/pesticides/epa-finalizes-biological-evaluations-assessing-potential-effects-three-neonicotinoid

[280] EPA: Neonic Likely Harms Nearly 80% of Listed Species, Lucas Rhoads, NRDC, Sept 1, 202, https://www.nrdc.org/bio/lucas-rhoads/epa-neonic-likely-harms-nearly-80-listed-species

Nitrate

[281] http://www.health.state.mn.us/divs/eh/wells/waterquality/nitrate.html

[282] "Four Reasons Why the World Needs to Limit Nitrogen Pollution," Jan 16, 2023, United Nations Environment Program (UNEP), https://www.unep.org/news-and-stories/story/four-reasons-why-world-needs-limit-nitrogen-pollution#:~:text=Nitrogen%20is%20a%20key%20contributor%20to%20climate%20change&text=This%20gas%20is%20300%20times,off%2C%20also%20emit%20greenhouse%20gases.

Nitrogen Fertilizer

[283] "Drinking Water Nitrate and Human Health, An Updated Review, Mary H. Ward, Rena R Jones, Jean D Brender, Theo M deKok, Peter J. Weyer, Bernard T. Nolan, Cristina M. Villaneueva, Simone G. van Breda, National Library of Medicine, Int J Environ Res Public Health. 2018 Jul; 15(7): 1557, https://www.ncbi.nlm.nih.gov/pmc/articles/PMC6068531/
Published online 2018 Jul 23. doi: 10.3390/ijerph15071557
" https://www.ncbi.nlm.nih.gov/pmc/articles/PMC6068531/

[284] "Fertilizer Management Could Reduce Ammonia Pollution From 3 Staple Crops: Study," Claire Asher, Mongabay, March 18, 2024,
https://news.mongabay.com/2024/03/fertilizer-management-could-reduce-ammonia-pollution-from-3-staple-crops
study/#:~:text=Nitrogen%20fertilizers%20are%20applied%20to,lung%20cancer%20and%20cardiovascul ar%20disease.

[285] Nature Conservancy, https://www.nature.org/en-us/what-we-do/our-priorities/provide-food-and-water-sustainably/

Nitrous Oxide

[286] Overview of Greenhouse Gases, https://www.epa.gov/ghgemissions/overview-greenhouse-gases
[287] "The Causes of Climate Change," NASA, https://climate.nasa.gov/causes/
Nutrient Pollution
[288] Nutrient Pollution, "Water Pollution: Everything You Need to Know," Melissa Dunchak, Natural Resources Defense Council, January 11, 2023, https://www.nrdc.org/stories/water-pollution-everything-you-need-know#whatis
[289] Elaine Shannon, http://www.ewg.org/enviroblog/2015/01/toxic-chemicals-oil-and-gas-drilling-waste-list-grows-longer
[290] "Report Exposes Vast Amounts of Unregulated Pollution from Oil Refineries," Environmental Integrity Project, January 26, 2023, https://environmentalintegrity.org/news/report-exposes-vast-amount-of-unregulated-water-pollution-from-oil-refineries/
[291] "Oil's Unchecked Outfalls," Environmental Integrity Project, Jan 26, 2023, https://environmentalintegrity.org/reports/oils-unchecked-outfalls/
[292] "Petroleum Refining Effluent Guidelines," United States EPA, https://www.epa.gov/eg/petroleum-refining-effluent-guidelines
[293] "Report Exposes Vast Amounts of Unregulated Pollution from Oil Refineries," Environmental Integrity Project, January 26, 2023, https://environmentalintegrity.org/news/report-exposes-vast-amount-of-unregulated-water-pollution-from-oil-refineries/

Cancer Alley

[294] "Real-Time Data Show the Air in Louisiana's 'Cancer Alley' Is Even Worse Than Expected," Navenna Sadasivam, Grist, June 12, 2024, https://lailluminator.com/2024/06/12/cancer-alley-4/#:~:text=Since%20the%201980s%2C%20the%2085,cancer%20than%20the%20average%20American.
[295] "US: Louisiana's 'Cancer Alley,' Dire Health Crisis From Government Failure to Rein in Fossil Fuels," Human Rights Watch, Jan 25, 2024, https://www.hrw.org/news/2024/01/25/us-louisianas-cancer-alley
[296] "Six Houston-Based Refineries Dump Millions of Gallons of Contaminated Wastewater With Little Penalty, Report Finds, Rebecca Noel, Houston Public Media, Jan 30, 2023, https://www.houstonpublicmedia.org/articles/news/energy-environment/2023/01/30/442559/six-houston-based-refineries-dump-millions-of-gallons-of-contaminated-wastewater-with-little-penalty-report-finds/#:~:text=Six%20specific%20refineries%20in%20the,and%20Kinder%20Morgan%20Galena%20Park.
[297] "Report Exposes Vast Amounts of Unregulated Water Pollution from Oil Refineries," Environmental Integrity Project, January 26, 2023, https://environmentalintegrity.org/news/report-exposes-vast-amount-of-unregulated-water-pollution-from-oil-refineries/
[298] "Holding Fossil Fuel Companies Liable for Climate Harms in California: Law, Science, and Justice," Fowler Museum at UCLA, January 25, 2018, https://law.ucla.edu/academics/centers/emmett-institute-climate-change-environment/holding-fossil-fuel-companies-liable-climate-change-harms-california

Pipeline Spills

[299] "Enbridge Line 5 Pipeline in the Great Lakes," For Love of Water, https://forloveofwater.org/line5/
[300] "Biden Administration Says Federal Court Should Reconsider Line 5 Shutdown Order," Danielle Kaeding, Superior Telegram, Wisconsin Public Radio, April 11, 2024, https://www.superiortelegram.com/news/wisconsin/biden-administration-says-federal-court-should-reconsider-line-5-shutdown-order
[301] "Keystone Pipeline Raises Concerns After Third Major Spill in Five Years," Michael Sainato, the Guardian, Dec 21, 2022, https://www.theguardian.com/environment/2022/dec/21/oil-spills-keystone-pipeline-seem-worse-kansas#:~:text=Keystone%20pipeline%20raises%20concerns%20after%20third%20major%20spill

%20in%20five%20years,-This%20article%20is&text=The%20Keystone%20pipeline%2C%20which%20traverses,%2C%20Kansas%2C%20on%207%20December.

302 Kalamazoo River Watershed Council, https://kalamazooriver.org/learn/what-are-the-problems/oil-spill-2/

303 "A Battle for the Future of the Great Lakes," Donovan Hohn, Geoff McGee, Adam Joseph Wells, Sierra Club, March 16, 2023, https://www.sierraclub.org/sierra/battle-future-great-lakes-enbridge-line-5-resisters

304 "Future of Controversial Dakota Access Pipeline's River Crossing Remains Unclear, Associated Press, NPR, Sept 8, 2023, https://www.npr.org/2023/09/08/1198492185/dakota-access-pipeline-river-crossing-environmental-review

305 "Stopping Line 5: What's Going on Now, and What Happens Next?" Sierra Club, Wisconsin, April 14, 2024, https://www.sierraclub.org/wisconsin/blog/2024/04/stopping-line-5-what-s-going-now-and-what-happens-next

306 "The Dakota Access Pipeline: What You Need to Know," Shelia Hu, June 12, 2024, https://www.nrdc.org/stories/dakota-access-pipeline-what-you-need-know

Oil Spills

307 "Petroleum," Soil Science Society of America, https://www.soils.org/about-soils/contaminants/petroleum/#:~:text=Petroleum%20products%20have%20the%20greatest,and%20xylene%20can%20cause%20cancer.

308 http://ocean.si.edu/gulf-oil-spill ,Smithsonian Museum of Natural History

309 Dr. Rikki Ott Seeks to Change How We Respond to Oil Spills, Cherri Foytlin, June 5, 2014, http://bridgethegulfproject.org/blog/2014/dr-riki-ott-seeks-change-how-we-respond-oil-spills

Packaging Waste

310 "Toxic Chemicals Used in Food Preparation Leach into Human Bodies, Study Finds," Sandee LaMotte, CNN, Sept 16, 2024, https://www.cnn.com/2024/09/16/health/food-packaging-chemical-toxins-study-wellness/index.html

311 "You Could Be Eating a Side of E-Waste with Your Takeout," Kat Eschner, Popular Science, May 31, 2018, https://www.popsci.com/e-waste-black-plastic/

312 "Farming Without Pesticides is Possible, The Contribution of Biodynamic Farming to the Earth's Health,"Sebastian Jungel, Goetheanum Section for Agriculture, June 11, 2011, https://www.sektion-landwirtschaft.org/en/news/sv/farming-without-pesticides-is-possible

Paraquat and 2,4-D

313 "Pesticides," USGS, March 23, 2017, https://www.usgs.gov/centers/ohio-kentucky-indiana-water-science-center/science/pesticides

314 "Breathing Pesticides Can Trigger MS and Parkinson's Disease," Sean Poulter, Daily Mail, Aug 9, 2006, https://www.dailymail.co.uk/health/article-399684/Breathing-pesticides-trigger-MS-Parkinsons-disease.html

315 "What is 2-4-D," Wisconsin Department of Health Services, Weed B Gone, Acme, AquaKleen, https://www.dhs.wisconsin.gov/chemical/24d.htm#:~:text=However%2C%20studies%20have%20found%20that,been%20observed%20in%20laboratory%20animals.

316 "Paraquat as a Cause of Parkinson's Disease," Priyanshu Sharma, Payal Mittal, Parkinsonism & Related Disorders, Feb, 2024, https://www.sciencedirect.com/science/article/abs/pii/S1353802023010118#:~:text=Due%20to%20the%20unique%20neurotoxicity,time%2C%20according%20to%20epidemiological%20studies.

317 "EPA-Registered Herbicide Found to Trigger Inflammation Linked to Onset of Multiple Sclerosis,"Beyond Pesticides, Feb 5, 2019, https://beyondpesticides.org/dailynewsblog/2019/02/epa-registered-herbicide-found-to-trigger-inflammation-linked-to-onset-of-multiple-sclerosis/

318 "Screening Enviromental Chemicals That May Influence MS," MS International Federation, Feb 26, 2019, https://www.msif.org/news/2019/02/26/screening-environmental-chemicals-that-may-influence-ms/#:~:text=Finally%2C%20to%20ensure%20this%20was,may%20also%20contribute%20to%20MS.

[319] "The Manufacturers of Paraquat, What Did They Know?" MadeKSho Law May 3, 2021, https://www.madeksholaw.com/post/the-manufacturers-of-paraquat

[320] "What is 2-4-D," Wisconsin Department of Health Services, Weed B Gone, Acme, AquaKleen, https://www.dhs.wisconsin.gov/chemical/24d.htm#:~:text=However%2C%20studies%20have%20found%20that,been%20observed%20in%20laboratory%20animals.

[321] "2,4-D: The Most Dangerous Pesticide You've Never Heard Of,"NRDC, March 15, 2016, https://www.nrdc.org/stories/24-d-most-dangerous-pesticide-youve-never-heard#:~:text=It's%20used%20widely%20in%20agriculture,be%20safe%20by%20today's%20standards.

[322] "Which Crops is Parquat Sprayed On?"ELG Law, https://www.elglaw.com/faq/which-crops-is-paraquat-sprayed-on/

[323] "Linuron," G Chen, Encyclopedia of Toxicology, 2014, https://www.sciencedirect.com/topics/nursing-and-health-professions/linuron#:~:text=It%20is%20used%20in%20soybean,%2C%20carrot%2C%20and%20fruit%20crops.

[324] https://www.ewg.org/research/suspect-salads/rocket-fuel-winter-lettuce#.Wm-JbpM-f64

Perchlorate

[325] "Perchlorate in the Pacific Southwest," Region 9, EPA, https://archive.epa.gov/region9/toxic/web/html/per_nv.html

PERC, TCE

[326] "Study Finds Elevated Rates of Cancer in Crestwood," Michael Hawthorne, Chicago Tribune, March 5, 2010, https://www.chicagotribune.com/lifestyles/health/ct-met-crestwood-cancer-20100305-story.html

[327] "Trichloroethylene (TCE), National Cancer Institute, https://www.cancer.gov/about-cancer/causes-prevention/risk/substances/trichloroethylene#:~:text=Trichloroethylene%20(TCE)%20is%20a%20volatile,degreasing%20solvent%20for%20metal%20equipment.

[328] "Tetrachloroethylene (PERC), State of North Carolina, Department of Health and Human Services, https://epi.dph.ncdhhs.gov/oee/docs/perc_facts.pdf

[329] "Camp Lejeune Water Contamination Claims," https://www.camplejeuneclaimscenter.com

[330] Tetrachloroethylene (Perchloroethylene) Hazard Summary 127-18-4, Cdc.gov, January 2000, https://www.epa.gov/sites/default/files/2016-09/documents/tetrachloroethylene.pdf

[331] Dry Cleaning Chemicals and a Cluster of Parkinson's Disease and Cancer: A Retrospective Study, E. Ray Dorsey MD, Dan Kinel JD, Meghan E. Pawlik BA, Maryam Zafar BS, Samantha E. Lettenberger BS, Madeleine Coffey BA, Peggy Auinger MS, Kevin L. Hylton MS, Carol W. Shaw NP, Jamie L. Adams MD, Richard Barbano MD, Melanie K. Braun MD, Heidi B. Schwarz MD, B. Paige Lawrence PhD, Karl Kieburtz MD, MPH, Caroline M. Tanner MD, PhD, Briana R. de Miranda PhD, Samuel M. Goldman MD, MPH, International Parkinson's and Movement Disorder Society, https://movementdisorders.onlinelibrary.wiley.com/doi/full/10.1002/mds.29723 February 23, 2024,

[332] "Tetrachloroethylene (PERC), State of North Carolina, Department of Health and Human Services, https://epi.dph.ncdhhs.gov/oee/docs/perc_facts.pdf

[333] "EPA Sued Over Unregulated Water Pollution From Oil Refineries, Plastics Plants, Other Industries," Center for Biological Diversity, April 11, 2023, https://biologicaldiversity.org/w/news/press-releases/epa-sued-over-unregulated-water-pollution-from-oil-refineries-plastics-plants-other-industries-2023-04-11/

Pesticides

[334] "The Potential Endocrine Disruption of Pesticide Transformation Products (TPs): The Blind Spot of Pesticide Risk Assessment, Chenyang Ji, Qin Song, Yuanchen Chen, Zhiqiang Zhou, Peng Wang, Jing Liu, Zhe Sun, Meirong Zhao, Environment International, Volume 137, April 2020, https://www.sciencedirect.com/science/article/pii/S0160412019332647?via%3Dihub

[335] "IG Farben: A Lingering Relic of the Nazi Years," Edmund L. Andrews, New York Times, May 2, 1999, https://www.nytimes.com/1999/05/02/business/the-business-world-ig-farben-a-lingering-relic-of-the-nazi-years.html

[336] "Pesticide-Induced Diseases Database: Brain and Nervous System Disorders,"Beyond Pesticides, https://www.beyondpesticides.org/resources/pesticide-induced-diseases-database/brain-and-nervous-system-disorders

[337] "Genetically Engineered Crops, Glyphosate, and the Deterioration of Health in the United States of America," Nancy L Swanson, Andre Leu, Jon Abrahamson, Bradley Wallet, Journal of Organic Systems, 9 (2) 2014, https://www.organic-systems.org/journal/92/JOS_Volume-9_Number-2_Nov_2014-Swanson-et-al.pdf

[338] "Use of Genetically Modified Organism (GMO)-Containing Food Products in Children," Steven Abrams, Jaclyn Albin, Phillip Landrigan, Committee on Nutrition; Council on Environmental Health and Climate Change, Pediatrics, Dec 11, 2023, https://publications.aap.org/pediatrics/article/153/1/e2023064774/196193/Use-of-Genetically-Modified-Organism-GMO?autologincheck=redirected#

[339] "Pesticides and Childhood Cancer," SH Zahm, MH Ward, Environmental Health Perspectives, June 1998, https://www.ncbi.nlm.nih.gov/pmc/articles/PMC1533072/

[340] "Insecticide Fipronil and It's Tranformation Products in Human Blood and Urine: Assessment of Human Exposure in General Population of China," Lisha Shi, Yanjian Wan, Juan Liu, Zhenyu He, Shunqing Xu, Wei Xia, PMID: 33964773, DOI: 10.1016/j.scitotenv.2021.147342, National Library of Medicine, April 24, 2021, https://pubmed.ncbi.nlm.nih.gov/33964773/

[341] "Report: Pesticide Exposure Linked to Childhood Cancer and Lower IQ," Carina Storrs, CNN, September 14, 2015, https://www.cnn.com/2015/09/14/health/pesticide-exposure-childhood-cancer/index.html

[342] "2,4-D: The Most Dangerous Pesticide You've Never Heard Of," Danielle Sedbrook, NRDC, March 15, 2016, https://www.nrdc.org/stories/24-d-most-dangerous-pesticide-youve-never-heard

[343] Atrazine Continues to Contaminate Surface Water and Drinking Water in the United States, Mae Woo, Mayra Quirindongo, Jennifer Sass, Andrew Wetzler, April 2010, https://www.nrdc.org/sites/default/files/atrazine10.pdf

Lawsuit against the EPA

[344] US Court of Appeals, Petition for Review filed, Center for Biological Diversity and Waterkeepers Alliance and Other Groups v The EPA, April 11, 2023, https://biologicaldiversity.org/programs/environmental_health/pdfs/2023-04-11-Petition-for-Review-and-Cert-of-Service-FINAL.pdf

[345] "EPA Sued Over Unregulated Water Pollution From Oil Refineries, Plastics Plants, Other Industries," Tom Pelton, Center for Biological Diversity, April 11, 2023, https://biologicaldiversity.org/w/news/press-releases/epa-sued-over-unregulated-water-pollution-from-oil-refineries-plastics-plants-other-industries-2023-04-11/

PFAS

[346] "The Teflon Toxin,"Dupont and the Chemistry of Deception, Sharon Lerner, The Intercept, August 11, 2015, https://theintercept.com/2015/08/11/dupont-chemistry-deception/

[347] Pediatric Cancer Is On The Rise, With Some Types Becoming More Common," Northwell Health, December 26, 2023, https://www.northwell.edu/news/the-latest/pediatric-cancer-is-on-the-rise-with-some-types-becoming-more-common#:~:text=Northwell%20Health%20collaborated%20with%20Stacker,in%20how%20cancer%20is%20reported

[348] "Per- and polyfluoroalkyl substances (PFAS) exposure and thyroid cancer risk," van Gerwen, Maaike et al., eBioMedicine, Volume 97, 104831, https://www.thelancet.com/journals/ebiom/article/PIIS2352-3964(23)00397-3/fulltext

[349] EPA, Our Current Understanding of the Human Health and Environmental Risks of PFAS, https://www.epa.gov/pfas/our-current-understanding-human-health-and-environmental-risks-pfas

Pharmaceuticals

[350] "Pharmaceuticals in Water," Water Science School, USGS, June 6, 2018, https://www.usgs.gov/special-topics/water-science-school/science/pharmaceuticals-water

[351] "Diabetes Drug Makes Male Minnows More Female," Brian Bienkowski, Environmental Health News, Scientific American, April 28, 2015, https://www.scientificamerican.com/article/diabetes-drug-makes-male-minnows-more-female/

Phosphate Fertilizer

[352] "Battle over Phosphate Mining Roils Small Florida Town," Alan Toth, Laura Newberry, PBS News Hour, Oct. 31, 2018, https://www.pbs.org/newshour/show/battle-over-phosphate-mining-roils-small-fla-town

Plastic

[353] Microplastics Found Embedded in Tissues of Whales and Dolphins, Duke University, August 10, 2023, "https://www.sciencedaily.com/releases/2023/08/230810180115.htm
[354] https://www.rmit.edu.au/news/all-news/2016/august/microbeads-contaminate-fish-toxic-chemicals
[355] "Covid-19 Face Masks: A Potential Source of Microplastic Fibers in the Environment,"Oluniyi O. Fadare, Elvis D. Okoffo, Sci Total Environ. 2020 Oct 1; 737: 140279, https://www.ncbi.nlm.nih.gov/pmc/articles/PMC7297173/
[356] "Pandemic Face Masks Could Harm Wildlife for Years to Come,"James Ashworth, Science News, August 4, 2022, Natural History Museum, https://www.nhm.ac.uk/discover/news/2022/august/pandemic-face-masks-could-harm-wildlife-for-years-to-come.html
[357] http://www.abc.net.au/news/2017-05-21/scientists-warn-of-growing-cost-of-inaction-on-microfibres/8540606

Plastic Pellets
[358] The spread of plastics and oil in Sri Lanka from the wreck of M/V *X-Press Pearl*, *Woods Hole Oceanographic Institute, June 14, 2021*, https://www.whoi.edu/news-insights/content/sri-lanka-faq/
[359] "Nurdles: the Worst Toxic Waste You've Probably Never Heard Of," Karen McVeigh, The Guardian, November 29, 2021, https://www.theguardian.com/environment/2021/nov/29/nurdles-plastic-pellets-environmental-ocean-spills-toxic-waste-not-classified-hazardous

POPs

[361] http://www.epa.gov/international-cooperation/persistent-organic-pollutants-global-issue-global-response

PPCPs

[362] "Treatment Trends and Combined Methods in Removing Pharmaceuticals and Personal Care Products from Wastewater-A Review," Loganathan P, Vigneswaran S, Kandasamy J, Cuprys AK, Maletskyi Z, Ratnaweera H, Membranes (Basel). 2023 Jan 27;13(2):158. doi: 10.3390/membranes13020158. PMID: 36837661; PMCID: PMC9960457, https://www.ncbi.nlm.nih.gov/pmc/articles/PMC9960457/

Power Plants

[363] "Forest Biomass is a False Energy Solution," https://www.biologicaldiversity.org/campaigns/debunking_the_biomass_myth/pdfs/Forest-Bioenergy-Briefing-Book-March-2021.pdfCenter for Biological Diversity,
[364] https://www.riverkeeper.org/campaigns/stop-polluters/indian-point/radioactive-waste/
[365] https://projects.bettergov.org/power-struggle/

Radiation
[366] "Japan to Release Fukishima Water into the Ocean, "https://www.reuters.com/world/asia-pacific/japan-release-fukushima-water-into-ocean-starting-aug-24-2023-08-22/
[367] https://www.japantimes.co.jp/news/2017/07/14/national/science-health/tepco-says-decision-already-made-release-radioactive-low-toxic-tritium-sea-fishermen-irate/#.Wg9U5hNSx3k
[368] https://www.nrc.gov/docs/ML1703/ML17030A025.pdf
[369] https://projects.bettergov.org/power-struggle/leaks.html
[370] "Nuclear Plant Spills Radiation into Lake Michigan," John Upton, Grist Magazine, May 8, 2013, http://grist.org/climate-energy/nuclear-plant-spills-radiation-into-lake-michigan/
[371] https://www.nrc.gov/reading-rm/doc-collections/fact-sheets/3mile-isle.html
[372] Naturally Radionuclides in Public Drinking Water, https://www.epa.gov/radtown/natural-radionuclides-public-drinking-

water#:~:text=Many%20of%20the%20contaminants%20found,and%20can%20dissolve%20in%20water.

Road Salt
[373] "Go Easy on the Salt,"NRDC, Feb 11, 2016, https://www.nrdc.org/stories/go-easy-salt
[374] "Report: Indiana Has the Most Polluted Rivers, Streams of Any State, Rebecca Thiele, PBS WFYI Indianapolis, March 17, 2022, https://www.wfyi.org/news/articles/report-indiana-has-the-most-polluted-rivers-streams-of-any-state#:~:text=deemed%20%22impaired.%22-,Indiana%20has%20the%20most%20miles%20of%20rivers%20and%20streams%20deemed,coli%20and%20toxic%20algae.

Sewage
[375] NPDES CAFO Permitting Status Report: National Summary, Endyear 2013, May 14, 2024, https://www.epa.gov/system/files/documents/2024-06/cafo-status-report-2023.pdf
[376] "The Dangers of Sewage in Drinking Water," Spring Well Water Filtration, 800-589-5592, July 20,2022, https://www.springwellwater.com/sewage-in-drinking-water/
[377] "Bioswales," MMSD, Milwaukee Metropolitan Sewerage District, https://www.mmsd.com/what-we-do/green-infrastructure/bioswales

Styrofoam
[378] "Discovery and quantification of plastic particle pollution in human blood," Heather A. Leslie, Martin J.M. van Velzen, Sicco H. Brandsma, A.Dick Vethaak, Juan J. Garcia-Vallejo, Marja H. Lamoree, Environment International, Volume 163, May 2022, 107199.
https://www.sciencedirect.com/science/article/pii/S0160412022001258/

Sunscreen
[379] "Beware of Benzene: Shining a Light on Sunscreen Spray Contamination, EWG's Guide to Sunscreens, https://www.ewg.org/sunscreen/report/beware-of-benzene-shining-a-light-on-sunscreen-spray-contamination/?gclid=EAIaIQobChMIlf-H5pmQ_QIVgt7ICh3dHAhzEAAYASAAEgIGW_D_BwE
[380] "Reef Friendly Sunscreens," Surfrider Organization, https://www.surfrider.org/news/your-guide-to-reef-friendly-sunscreens-0,
[381] 7 of the Best Reef Safe Sunscreens, Rachel Schultz, May 23, 2024, National Geographic, https://www.nationalgeographic.com/lifestyle/article/best-reef-safe-sunscreen#:~:text=SurfDurt%20is%20made%20with%20non,water%2Dresistant%20for%2080%20minutes

Surfactants
[382] Fact Sheet: Nonylophenols and Nonylphenol Ethoxylates, EPA, Assessing and Managing Chemicals under TSCA, https://www.epa.gov/assessing-and-managing-chemicals-under-tsca/fact-sheet-nonylphenols-and-nonylphenol-ethoxylates
[383] http://www.panna.org/blog/dows-cancer-causing-garbage-chemical-drinking-water

TCP
[384] https://www.epa.gov/sites/production/files/2014-03/documents/ffrrofactsheet_contaminant_tcp_january2014_final.pdf
[385] "Groundwater Fact Sheet 123 -Trichloropropane,"California Water Boards, October, 2017, https://www.waterboards.ca.gov/gama/docs/coc_tcp123.pdf

Teflon
[386] https://www.democracynow.org/2018/1/23/dupont_vs_the_world_chemical_giant

Textiles
"Toxic Threads," Green Peace, Nov 20, 2012,
https://www.greenpeace.org/international/publication/6889/toxic-threads-the-big-fashion-stitch-up/

Train Derailments
[387] "The Dangers of Vinyl Chloride, Phosgene, and Dioxins," Jessie Paluch, Tru Law, June18, 2024, https://trulaw.com/the-dangers-of-vinyl-chloride-phosgene-and-dioxins/#:~:text=When%20vinyl%20chloride%20burns%2C%20it,weapon%20in%20World%20War%20I.

Vinyl Chloride
[388] "Vinyl Chloride," National Cancer Institute, https://www.cancer.gov/about-cancer/causes-prevention/risk/substances/vinyl-chloride#:~:text=Vinyl%20chloride%20is%20used%20primarily%20to%20make%20polyvinyl%20chloride%20(PVC,combustion%20product%20in%20tobacco%20smoke

Waste
[389] "Addressing the Plastic Crisis, why Vinyl Has to Go," Bill Walsh, Healthy Buildings Network, October 2021, https://healthybuilding.net/blog/586-addressing-the-plastics-crisis-why-vinyl-has-to-go#:~:text=Like%20most%20plastics%2C%20PVC%20is,chlorine%2C%20upwards%20of%2040%25.

[390] The Issue with Tissue, NRDC Natural Resources Defense Council, Feb 2019, https://www.nrdc.org/sites/default/files/issue-tissue-how-americans-are-flushing-forests-down-toilet-report.pdf

Window Cleaner
[391] http://nj.gov/health/eoh/rtkweb/documents/fs/0275.pdf

Xenobiotics
[392] https://www.merriam-webster.com/dictionary/xenobiotic

[393] "Xenobiotics: Chemical Transformation of Xenobiotics by the Human Gut Microbiota," Nitzan Koppel, Vayu Maini Rekdal, Emily P. Balskus, American Associaton for the Advancement of Science, June 23, 2017, sciencemag.orghttp://science.sciencemag.org/content/356/6344/eaag2770

[394] "Toxic Peripheral Neuropathies: Agents and Mechanisms, William M Valentine, Toxicology Pathology, January, 2020, https://www.ncbi.nlm.nih.gov/pmc/articles/PMC6901819/

TSCA
[395] "A Primer on the New Toxic Substances Control Act (TSCA) and What Led To It," Richard A. Denison, Environmental Defense Fund, https://www.edf.org/sites/default/files/denison-primer-on-lautenberg-act.pdf

[396] "Environmental Determinants of Chronic Disease and Medical Approaches: Recognition, Avoidance, Supportive Therapy, and Detoxification,"Margaret E. Sears, Stephen J Genuis, Journal of Environment Public Health, Jan 19, 2012, https://pmc.ncbi.nlm.nih.gov/articles/PMC3270432/

[397] http://www.nmfs.noaa.gov/pr/laws/mmpa/

[398] "Saving the Nation's Wetlands," Andrew James, Natural Resources Conservation Service, June 25, 2015, https://www.usda.gov/media/blog/2015/06/25/saving-nations-wetlands

Groundwater in Danger
[399] The Water Cycle, "The Cycling of Water," https://illinois.pbslearningmedia.org/resource/buac20-68-sci-ess-cyclingofwater/the-cycling-of-water/

[400] USGS, Groundwater Contaminants, https://water.usgs.gov/edu/groundwater-contaminants.html

[401] "Impacts of Pharmaceutical Effluents on Aquatic Ecosystems," Shola Kayode-Afolayan, Eze Ahuekwe, Obinna Nwinyi, Hydro Research Volume 5, 2022, Scientific African, September 2022, https://www.sciencedirect.com/science/article/pii/S2468227622001958

Lakes in Danger
[402] "Milwaukee Sewage Tunnel Overtaxed," Water World, June 21, 2004, https://www.waterworld.com/drinking-water-treatment/infrastructure-funding/article/16224679/milwaukee-sewage-tunnel-overtaxed

[403] Great Lakes Water Levels, Georgian Bay Association, http://www.georgianbayassociation.ca/water-levels/

[404] "Stopping Line 5: What's Going on Now, and What Happens Next?" Sierra Club, Wisconsin, April 14, 2024, https://www.sierraclub.org/wisconsin/blog/2024/04/stopping-line-5-what-s-going-now-and-what-happens-next

Animals in Danger
[405] "Nonpoint Source: Agriculture," EPA, https://www.epa.gov/nps/nonpoint-source-agriculture
Saving Whales
[406] "Ropeless Fishing Gear," Center for Biological Diversity,
https://www.biologicaldiversity.org/campaigns/ropeless-fishing-gear/index.html
[407] 'Scientists and Advocates Zero In On What Is Really Killing Whales," Dawn Kane, Grid Philly, October 2, 2023, https://gridphilly.com/blog-home/2023/10/02/scientists-and-advocates-zero-in-on-what-is-really-killing-whales/
[408] 'Scientists and Advocates Zero In On What Is Really Killing Whales," Dawn Kane, Grid Philly, October 2, 2023, https://gridphilly.com/blog-home/2023/10/02/scientists-and-advocates-zero-in-on-what-is-really-killing-whales/
[409] http://www.noaa.gov/media-release/gulf-of-mexico-dead-zone-is-largest-ever-measured

Oceans in Danger
[410] "Microplastics Deposited on the Seafloor Triple in 20 Years," Environmental Science and Technology, Universitat Autonoma de Barcelona, December 22, 2022, https://www.sciencedaily.com/releases/2022/12/221222101005.htm
[411] Resolution Adopted by the United Nations Environmnet Programme, March 2022, https://wedocs.unep.org/xmlui/bitstream/handle/20.500.11822/39764/END%20PLASTIC%20POLLUTION%20-%20TOWARDS%20AN%20INTERNATIONAL%20LEGALLY%20BINDING%20INSTRUMENT%20-%20English.pdf?sequence=1&isAllowed=y
[412] "Breaking the Plastic Wave: Top Findings For Reducing Plastic Pollution, Simon Reddy and Winnie Lau, Pew Trusts, July 23, 2020, https://www.pewtrusts.org/en/research-and-analysis/articles/2020/07/23/breaking-the-plastic-wave-top-findings
[413] "Plastics, EDCs, & Health, Jodi Flaws, Pauliina Damdimopoulou, Heather Patisaul, Andrea Gore, Lori Raetzman, Laura Vandenberg, Endocrine Society, https://www.endocrine.org/-/media/endocrine/files/topics/edc_guide_2020_v1_6chqennew-version.pdf

Red Tides
[414] Red tides on the Rise Worldwide, Laurie Ann Peach, Christian Science Monitor, July 21, 1992, https://www.csmonitor.com/1992/0721/21121.html
[415] Potential Disaster at Huge St. James Waste Pile Has Crews Racing to Prevent Massive Wall Collapse, David J. Mitchell, The Advocate, Jan 30, 2019, https://www.theadvocate.com/baton_rouge/news/article_3cf05134-233a-11e9-aa0f-17aeb020318d.html
[416] The Clock is Ticking on Florida's Mountains of Hazardous Phosphate Waste, Craig Pittman, Sarasota Magazine, April 26, 2017, https://www.sarasotamagazine.com/articles/2017/4/26/florida-phosphate
[417] About Radioactive Material from Fertilizer Production, EPA, https://www.epa.gov/radtown/radioactive-material-fertilizer-production
[418] What Does Big Sugar Have to Do With Florida's Red Tide, Biana Graulau, WTSP News, Sept 6, 2018, https://www.wtsp.com/article/news/local/what-does-big-sugar-have-to-do-with-floridas-red-tide/67-587820301
EPA Takes Over Mississippi Phosphates' Huge Mounds of Acidic Byproduct, Karen Nelson, Sun Herald, March 7, 2017, https://www.sunherald.com/news/local/counties/jackson-county/article137021948.html
[419] Mosaic Plant Sinkhole Dumpa 215 Million Gallons of Reprocessed Water into Floridan Aquifer, Christopher O'Donnell, Tampa Bay Times, Sept 17, 2016, https://www.tampabay.com/news/environment/water/mosaic-plant-sinkhole-dumps-215-million-gallons-of-reprocessed-water-into/2293845
[420] State Can Dump Water in Gulf, Dale White, Herald Tribune, April 4, 2003, https://www.heraldtribune.com/article/LK/20030404/News/605247753/SH/
[421] Red Tide is Devastating Florida's Sea Life, Are Humans to Blame? Maya Wei-Haas, National Geographic, Aug 8, 2018, What's more, recent exceptional red tide years seem to follow massive storms,

[422] Florida Red Tide FAQs, Mote Marine Laboratory and Aquarium, https://mote.org/news/florida-red-tide
Toxic Algae
[423] "Glyphosate Sprayed On GMO Crops Linked to Lake Erie's Toxic Algae Bloom," EcoWatch, July 5, 2016, https://www.ecowatch.com/glyphosate-sprayed-on-gmo-crops-linked-to-lake-eries-toxic-algae-bloom-1906543478.html

Wetlands

[424] "Protecting New York's Freshwater Wetlands is Now More Important Than Ever," Drew Gamils, Riverkeeper, https://www.riverkeeper.org/blogs/ecology/protecting-new-yorks-freshwater-wetlands/
[425] The Convention on Wetlands, www.Ramsar.org
[426] Small Wetlands, Big Benefit: How to Harness nature to Filter Agriculture Runoff," Nature Conservancy, April 15, 2024, https://www.nature.org/en-us/about-us/where-we-work/united-states/illinois/stories-in-illinois/constructed-wetlands-reduce-agricultural-runoff-study/
[427] "Urban Wetlands, Prized Land not Wasteland," Ramsar.org, https://www.ramsar.org/sites/default/files/documents/library/wwd18_handouts_eng.pdf
[428] "2024—First Year the US Expects More than 2M New Cases of Cancer," Sonya Collins, American Cancer Society, Jan 17, 2024, https://www.cancer.org/research/acs-research-news/facts-and-figures-2024.html

People in Danger

[429] President's Cancer Panel Report, page viii, Executive Summary, https://deainfo.nci.nih.gov/advisory/pcp/annualReports/pcp08-09rpt/PCP_Report_08-09_508.pdf
[430] "The Field Report: The Clean Water Act Has Failed to Curb Ag Pollution," Lisa Held, Civil Eats, March 22, 2022, www.civileats.com/2022/03/22/field-report-clean-water-act-regulations-curb-pollution-farms-cafos-runoff/
[431] See 277
[432] "Oil Refineries Release Lots of Water Pollution near Communities of Color, Data Show," Rebecca Hersher, NPR, January 26, 2023, https://www.npr.org/2023/01/26/1151464514/oil-refineries-release-lots-of-water-pollution-near-communities-of-color-data-show
[433] "'Disturbing': Weedkiller ingredient Tied to Cancer Found in 80% of US Urine Samples," Carey Gillam, The Guardian, July 9, 2022, , https://www.theguardian.com/us-news/2022/jul/09/weedkiller-glyphosate-cdc-study-urine-samples
[434] "Sources and Solutions: Agriculture," https://www.epa.gov/nutrientpollution/sources-and-solutions-agriculture
[435] "In Minnesota, Families Blame Farm Nutrient Contamination For Heavy Cancer Toll," Keith Schneider, October 3, 2023, Investigate Midwest, https://investigatemidwest.org/2023/10/03/in-minnesota-families-blame-farm-nutrient-contamination-for-heavy-cancer-toll/
[436] NPDES CAFO Permitting Status Report: National Summary, Endyear 2013, May 14, 2024, https://www.epa.gov/system/files/documents/2024-06/cafo-status-report-2023.pdf
[437] "DNR: Ethanol Plant Pollution Likely Harmed Public Health For Years Near Shell Rock," Jared Strong, Iowa Capital Dispatch, July 25, 2024, https://iowacapitaldispatch.com/2024/07/25/dnr-ethanol-plant-pollution-likely-harmed-public-health-for-years-near-shell-rock/#:~:text=An%20ethanol%2Dproducing%20facility%20in,Iowa%20Department%20of%20Natural%20Resources.
[438] "Quantifiable urine glyphosate levels detected in 99% of the French population, with higher values in men, in younger people, and in farmers. ," Grau D, Grau N, Gascuel Q, Paroissin C, Stratonovitch C, Lairon D, Devault DA, Di Cristofaro J. Environ Sci Pollut Res Int. 2022 May;29(22):32882-32893. doi: 10.1007/s11356-021-18110-0. Epub 2022 Jan 12. PMID: 35018595; PMCID: PMC9072501, https://pubmed.ncbi.nlm.nih.gov/35018595/#:~:text=Glyphosate%20was%20quantified%20by%20a,body%20mass%20index%20(BMI).
[439] "Explosion of Disease in America's Cancer Capital Could Have Same Root Cause As State's Economic Boom, Maiya Focht, Daily Mail, August 17, 2024, https://www.dailymail.co.uk/health/article-13663295/disease-america-cancer-capital-cause-state-economic-boom.html

[440] "Corn: Fall 2021," Iowa Ag News – Chemical Use, United States Department of Agriculture (USDA), National Agricultural Statistics Service, May 13, 2022, https://www.nass.usda.gov/Statistics_by_State/Iowa/Publications/Other_Surveys/2022/IA-Ag-Chem-Corn-2022.pdf

[441] "EPA Revisits Atrazine," Britt E. Erickson, March 1, 2010, Volumer 88, Number 9, Chemical and Engineering News, https://pubsapp.acs.org/cen/environment/88/8809gov1.html

[442] "Dead Zone," National Geographic, https://education.nationalgeographic.org/resource/dead-zone/#

[443] "Impacts of Environmental Pollution on Brain Tumorigenesis," Pagano C, Navarra G, Coppola L, Savarese B, Avilia G, Giarra S, Pagano G, Marano A, Trifuoggi M, Bifulco M, Laezza C, Int J Mol Sci. 2023 Mar 6;24(5):5045. doi: 10.3390/ijms24055045. PMID: 36902485; PMCID: PMC10002587, https://www.ncbi.nlm.nih.gov/pmc/articles/PMC10002587/

[444] "Agricultural exposures to carbamate herbicides and fungicides and central nervous system tumour incidence in the cohort AGRICAN," Clement Piel and Camille Pouchieu and Team, Environment International, September 2019

[445] "Fungicides Commonly Found on Citrus Linked to Breast Cancer Risk," Alexis Temkin, Environmental Working Group, May 10, 2021, https://www.ewg.org/news-insights/news/2021/05/fungicides-commonly-found-citrus-linked-breast-cancer-risk

[446] 446

[447] Pesticides and Herbicides, Breast Cancer Prevention Partners, https://www.bcpp.org/resource/pesticides-other/

[448] Deadly Pesticide Poses an Increased Risk of Hormone-Associated Reproductive Cancers in Women, Beyond Pesticides, July 13, 2023, Dichlorobenzene, https://beyondpesticides.org/dailynewsblog/2023/07/deadly-pesticide-poses-an-increased-risk-of-hormone-associated-reproductive-cancers-in-women/#:~:text=(Beyond%20Pesticides%2C%20July%2013%2C,of%20common%20endocrine%20(hormone)%2D

[449] "Ag Runoff Into Tap Water Linked to 12,000 Cancer Cases A Year", Julie St. Louis, Courthouse News Service, June 10, 2019, https://www.courthousenews.com/ag-runoff-into-tap-water-linked-to-12000-cancer-cases-a-year/

[450] "Association Between Pesticide Exposure and Colorectal Cancer Risk and Incidence: A ystemic Review, Eryn K Matich, Jonathan A. Laryea, Kathryn A Seely, Shelbie Stahr, L. Joseph Su, Pink-Ching Hsu, Ecotoxicol Environ Saf, Aug 2021, https://www.ncbi.nlm.nih.gov/entrez/eutils/elink.fcgi?dbfrom=pubmed&retmode=ref&cmd=prlinks&id=34029839

[451] "Nitrate," Cancer Trends Progress Report, National Cancer Institute, https://progressreport.cancer.gov/prevention/chemical_exposures/nitrate#:~:text=Studies%20have%20shown%20increased%20risks,results%20in%20increased%20NOC%20formation.

[452] "High Prevalence of Pentatrichomonas hominas infection in gastrointestinal cancer patients," Zhang N, Zhang H, Yu Y, Gong P, Li J, Li Z, Li T, Cong Z, Tian C, Liu X, Yu X, Zhang X,. Parasit Vectors. 2019 Aug 28;12(1):423. doi: 10.1186/s13071-019-3684-4. PMID: 31462294; PMCID: PMC6714378, https://www.ncbi.nlm.nih.gov/pmc/articles/PMC6714378/

[453] 453

[454] "Nitrate," Cancer Trends Progress Report, National Cancer Institute, https://progressreport.cancer.gov/prevention/chemical_exposures/nitrate#:~:text=Studies%20have%20shown%20increased%20risks,results%20in%20increased%20NOC%20formation.

[455] 1,4-Dichlorobenzene, 15th Report on Carcinogens, National Toxicology Program. 15th Report on Carcinogens [Internet]. Research Triangle Park (NC): National Toxicology Program; 2021 Dec 21. 1,4-Dichlorobenzene: CAS No. 106-46-7, https://www.ncbi.nlm.nih.gov/books/NBK590902/

[456] "Can Weed Killers Containing Glyphosate Cause Cancer,"Beth Sissons, Medical News Today, September 20, 2021, https://www.medicalnewstoday.com/articles/does-roundup-cause-cancer

[457] "Health Effects of Neonicotinoids on an Agricultural Community, Jocelyn Rodriguez-Paar, University of Nebraska Medical Center, December, 2022, https://digitalcommons.unmc.edu/cgi/viewcontent.cgi?article=1229&context=coph_slce#:~:text=Some%20neonicotinoids%20have%20been%20shown,and%20thiamethoxam%20causing%20liver%20cancer.

[458] (449)

[459] "Woman's Grapefruit-Size 'Liver Cancer' Tumor Was Actually A Parasite," A. Pawlowski, Today Show, Feb 13, 2020, https://www.today.com/health/woman-s-grapefruit-size-liver-cancer-tumor-was-actually-giant-t173901
[460] Pesticide Exposure and Lung Cancer Risk, Teera Kangkhetkron, Chudchawal Juntarawijit, F1000 Research, Jan 4, 2024, https://www.ncbi.nlm.nih.gov/pmc/articles/PMC10904940/#:~:text=Some%20studies%20also%20linked%20individual,associated%20with%20lung%20cancer%2014%20.
[461] "Pesticide Use and Cutaneous Melanoma in Pesticide Applicators in the Agricultural Health Study," Leslie K. Dennis, Charles Lynch, Dale Sandler, Michael Alavanja, Environmental Health Perspectives, June, 2010, https://www.ncbi.nlm.nih.gov/pmc/articles/PMC2898858/
[462] "Can Weed Killers Containing Glyphosate Cause Cancer,"Beth Sissons, Medical News Today, September 20, 2021, https://www.medicalnewstoday.com/articles/does-roundup-cause-cancer
[463] NHL, "The association between non-Hodgkin lymphoma and organophosphate pesticides exposure: A meta-analysis," Liqin Hu, Dan Luo, Tingting Zhou, Yun Tao, Jingwen Feng, Surong Mei, Environmental Pollution, Vol 231 Part 1, December, 2017, https://www.sciencedirect.com/science/article/abs/pii/S0269749117307170
[464] "Certain Pesticides Linked with Pancreatic Cancer," Medscape, Aug 3, 2024, https://www.medscape.com/viewarticle/certain-pesticides-linked-risk-pancreatic-cancer-2024a100069f?form=fpf
[465] Arsenic: The Cancer-Causing Element That's All Around Us, Columbia University Medical Center, May 8, 2024, https://www.columbiadoctors.org/news/arsenic-cancer-causing-element-thats-all-around-us
[466] "Long-Term Exposure to Nitrate in Drinking Water May Lead to Higher Risk for Prostate Cancer, Hannah Clarke, Urology Times, March 9, 2023, https://www.urologytimes.com/view/long-term-exposure-to-nitrate-in-drinking-water-may-lead-to-higher-risk-for-prostate-cancer#
[467] "Nitrate," Cancer Trends Progress Report, National Cancer Institute, https://progressreport.cancer.gov/prevention/chemical_exposures/nitrate#:~:text=Studies%20have%20shown%20increased%20risks,results%20in%20increased%20NOC%20formation.
[468] "Cancer Health Effects of Pesticides, Systematic Review," Bassil KL, Vakil C, Sanborn M, Cole DC, Kaur JS, Kerr KJ,. Can Fam Physician. 2007 Oct;53(10):1704-11. PMID: 17934034; PMCID: PMC2231435, https://www.ncbi.nlm.nih.gov/pmc/articles/PMC2231435/
[469] "Domestic Use of Pesticides During Early Periods of Development and Risk of Testicular Germ Cell Tumors in Adulthood: A French Nationwide Case-Control Study," Aurélie M. N. Danjou,[1] Olivia Pérol,[2,3] Astrid Coste,[2,3] Elodie Faure,[2,4] Rémi Béranger,[5] Helen Boyle,[6]Elodie Belladame,[2] Lény Grassot,[2] Matthieu Dubuis,[2] Johan Spinosi,[7] Liacine Bouaoun,[1] Aude Fléchon,[2] Louis Bujan,[8,9]Véronique Drouineaud,[9,10] Florence Eustache,[9,11] Isabelle Berthaut,[9,11,12] Jeanne Perrin,[9,13,14] Florence Brugnon,[9,15,16]Barbara Charbotel,[2,17] Joachim Schüz,[1] Béatrice Fervers,[2,3] and For the TESTIS study group, Environmental Health, Oct 28, 2021, https://www.ncbi.nlm.nih.gov/pmc/articles/PMC8554827/
[470] "Water, Health, and Environmental Justice in California: Geospatial Analysis of Nitrate Contamination and Thyroid Cancer," Adrianna Q Tariqi, Colleen Naughton, Environmental Engineering Science, May, 2021, https://www.ncbi.nlm.nih.gov/pmc/articles/PMC8165459/
[471] "Researchers Examine Link Between Pesticides and Thyroid Cancer Risk in Central California Area, Avital Harari, MD, UCLA Health, Aug 18, 2022, https://www.uclahealth.org/news/release/researchers-examine-link-between-pesticides-and-thyroid
[472] "Parasites that can Lead to Cancer," American Cancer Society, https://www.cancer.org/cancer/risk-prevention/infections/infections-that-can-lead-to-cancer/parasites.html
[473] http://www.nejm.org/doi/full/10.1056/NEJM200007133430201#t=article
[474]Epigenetic diet: impact on the epigenome and cancer, Tabitha M. Hardy and Trygve O. Tollefsbol, Department of Biology University of Alabama
https://www.ncbi.nlm.nih.gov/pmc/articles/PMC3197720/
[475] "How Nanoparticles May Drive the Spread of Cancer," Anna Sandoiu, Medical News Today, Feb 4, 2019, https://www.medicalnewstoday.com/articles/324352

Carcinogens

[476] "President's Panel: 'Eat Organic, Ward Off Cancer," Marion Nestle, The Atlantic, May 12, 2010, https://www.theatlantic.com/health/archive/2010/05/presidents-panel-eat-organic-ward-off-cancer/56552/
[477] http://www.toxipedia.org/display/toxipedia/Cholinesterase+Inhibitor
[478] https://www.prwatch.org/news/2017/07/13269/poison-papers-expose-collusion-industry-regulators-hazardous-pesticides-chemicals
Endocrine Disruptors
[479] Endocrine Disruptors, National Institute of Environmental Health Sciences, https://www.niehs.nih.gov/health/topics/agents/endocrine
[480] Hormonal System, Health Direct Australia, https://www.healthdirect.gov.au/hormonal-system-endocrine

Neurotoxins

[481] "Air Pollution Linked to Dementia Cases," National Institutes of Health, September 5, 2023, https://www.nih.gov/news-events/nih-research-matters/air-pollution-linked-dementia-cases
[482] "Common Herbicide Exposure Linked to Worse Brain Function in Adolescents," Lily Ramsey LLM reviewed, News Medical Life Sciences, Oct 12, 2023, https://www.news-medical.net/news/20231012/Common-herbicide-exposure-linked-to-worse-brain-function-in-adolescents.aspx
[483] "The Association Between Pesticide Exposure and the Development of fronto-Temporal Dementia-Cum-Dissociative Disorders: A Review, Carlos Alfonso Flores-Gutierrez, Erandis Dheni Torres-Sanchez, Emmanuel Reyes-Uribe, Juan Heriberto Torres-Jasso, Mireya Oila Reyna-Villela, Daniel Rojas-Bravo, Joel Salazar-Flores, Brain Science, August, 2023, https://www.ncbi.nlm.nih.gov/pmc/articles/PMC10452640/#:~:text=Pesticides%20such%20as%20dieldrin%2C%20rotenone,or%20Alzheimer's%20disease%20%5B21%5D
[484] "Fungal Infection in the Brain Produces Changes Like Those Seen in Alzheimer's Disease," Science Daily, Baylor College of Medicine, Oct 16, 2023, https://www.sciencedaily.com/releases/2023/10/231016163107.htm
[485] "Nitrosative Stress Molecules in Multiple Sclerosis, A Meta-Analysis," Moritz Forseter, Chritopher Nelke, Saskia Rauber, Hans Lassmann, Tobias Ruck, Maria Pia Sormani, Alessio Signori, Hans-Peter Hartung, Patrick Kury, Sven G. Meuth, David Kremer, Biomedicines, Dec, 2021, https://www.ncbi.nlm.nih.gov/pmc/articles/PMC8698769/
[486] "*Clostridium perfringens* associated with dairy farm systems show diverse genotypes," Rui Andre Nunes Dos Santos [a], Jiryes Abdel-Nour [b], Cathy McAuley [b], Sean C. Moore [c], Narelle Fegan [c], Edward M. Fox, May 16, International Journal of Food Microbiology, 2022, https://www.sciencedirect.com/science/article/pii/S0168160522004056
[487] "The Association Between Pesticide Exposure and the Development of fronto-Temporal Dementia-Cum-Dissociative Disorders: A Review, Carlos Alfonso Flores-Gutierrez, Erandis Dheni Torres-Sanchez, Emmanuel Reyes-Uribe, Juan Heriberto Torres-Jasso, Mireya Oila Reyna-Villela, Daniel Rojas-Bravo, Joel Salazar-Flores, Brain Science, August, 2023, https://www.ncbi.nlm.nih.gov/pmc/articles/PMC10452640/#:~:text=Pesticides%20such%20as%20dieldrin%2C%20rotenone,or%20Alzheimer's%20disease%20%5B21%5D
[488] "Clarification of the molecular mechanisms underlying glyphosate-induced major depressive disorder: a network toxicology approach," Li, J., Bi, H.. *Ann Gen Psychiatry* **23**, 8 (2024). https://doi.org/10.1186/s12991-024-00491-4, https://annals-general-psychiatry.biomedcentral.com/articles/10.1186/s12991-024-00491-4#citeas
[489] "What You Need to Know About Chlorypyrifos, Earth Justice, April 9, 2024, https://earthjustice.org/feature/chlorpyrifos-what-you-need-to-know
[490] "Pesticide Exposure at Work Linked to Risk of Heart Disease, Stroke," American Heart Association News, Sept 25, 2019, https://www.news-medical.net/news/20231012/Common-herbicide-exposure-linked-to-worse-brain-function-in-adolescents.aspx
[491] "Potential health Effects of Pesticides," Penn State Extension, June 30, 2022, https://extension.psu.edu/potential-health-effects-of-pesticides#:~:text=Signs%20and%20symptoms%20of%20acute%20exposure%20for%20several%20herbicide%20active%20ingredients.&text=Irritating%20to%20skin%2C%20mucous%20membranes,Bizarre%20or%20aggressive%20behavior.
[492] "Neuropsychiatric Disorders in Farmers Associated with Organophosphorus Pesticide Exposure in a Rural Village of Northwest México," Serrano-Medina A, Ugalde-Lizárraga A, Bojorquez-

Cuevas MS, Garnica-Ruiz J, González-Corral MA, García-Ledezma A, Pineda-García G, Cornejo-Bravo JM.. Int J Environ Res Public Health. 2019 Feb 26;16(5):689. doi: 10.3390/ijerph16050689. PMID: 30813607; PMCID: PMC6427808, https://www.ncbi.nlm.nih.gov/pmc/articles/PMC6427808/

[493] "Early exposure to agricultural pesticides and the occurrence of autism spectrum disorder: a systematic review," Bertoletti ACC, Peres KK, Faccioli LS, Vacci MC, Mata IRD, Kuyven CJ, Bosco SMD.. Rev Paul Pediatr. 2022 Sep 9;41:e2021360. doi: 10.1590/1984-0462/2023/41/2021360. PMID: 36102405; PMCID: PMC9462403, https://www.ncbi.nlm.nih.gov/pmc/articles/PMC9462403/

[494] "Autism-like Behaviors in Male Juvenile Offspring after Maternal Glyphosate Exposure," Yaoyu Pu, Li Ma, Jialjing Shan, Xiayun Wan, Bruce D. Hammock, Kenji Hashimoto, Clinical Psychopharmcology Neuroscience, Aug 31, 2021, https://www.ncbi.nlm.nih.gov/pmc/articles/PMC8316667/

[495] "The Plastic Brain: Neurotoxicity of Micro- and Nanoplastics,"Minne Prust, Jonelle Meijer, Remco H.S. Westerink, Part Fibre Toxicol, June 8, 2020, https://www.ncbi.nlm.nih.gov/pmc/articles/PMC7282048/

[496] "Toxic Neuropathy," The Foundation for Peripheral Neuropathy, https://www.foundationforpn.org/causes/toxic-neuropathy/

Reproductive Toxins
The Endocrine Disruption Exchange, TEDX, https://endocrinedisruption.org/about-tedx/theo-colborn-ph.d.-president/

Proposition 65
[497] American Cancer Society, Propostion 65, https://www.cancer.org/healthy/cancer-causes/general-info/cancer-warning-labels-based-on-californias-proposition-65.html

Respiratory & Digestive Toxins

[498] ToxFAQs for Glyphosate, Toxic Substances Portal, ATSDR Agency for Toxic Substances and Disease Registry, https://wwwn.cdc.gov/TSP/ToxFAQs/ToxFAQsDetails.aspx?faqid=1489&toxid=293#:~:text=Glyphosate%20has%20been%20associated%20with,likely%20to%20develop%20respiratory%20effects.

[499] "Adverse health effects of emerging contaminants on inflammatory bowel disease," Chen X, Wang S, Mao X, Xiang X, Ye S, Chen J, Zhu A, Meng Y, Yang X, Peng S, Deng M, Wang X.. Front Public Health. 2023 Feb 24;11:1140786. doi: 10.3389/fpubh.2023.1140786. PMID: 36908414; PMCID: PMC9999012, https://www.ncbi.nlm.nih.gov/pmc/articles/PMC9999012/

[500] "Genetically Engineered Crops, Glyphosate and the Deterioration of Health in the United States,"Nancy L. Swanson, Andre Leu, Jon Abrahamson, Bradley Wallet, Journal of Organic Systems, Volume 9 No.2 2014, https://www.organic-systems.org/journal/92/abstracts/Swanson-et-al.html

Toxic Substances
[501] https://deainfo.nci.nih.gov/Advisory/pcp/annualReports/pcp08-09rpt/PCP_Report_08-09_508.pdf

[502] "Neurotoxicity of Pesticides," Richardson JR, Fitsanakis V, Westerink RHS, Kanthasamy AG, Acta Neuropathol. 2019 Sep;138(3):343-362. doi: 10.1007/s00401-019-02033-9. Epub 2019 Jun 13. PMID: 31197504; PMCID: PMC6826260, https://www.ncbi.nlm.nih.gov/pmc/articles/PMC6826260/

[503] "Major pesticides are more toxic to human cells than their declared active principles." Mesnage R, Defarge N, Spiroux de Vendômois J, Séralini GE, Biomed Res Int. 2014;2014:179691. doi: 10.1155/2014/179691. Epub 2014 Feb 26. PMID: 24719846; PMCID: PMC3955666, https://www.ncbi.nlm.nih.gov/pmc/articles/PMC3955666/

[504] Sierra Club, Wisconsin Chapter, https://www.sierraclub.org/wisconsin/line-5

SOLUTIONS

[505] "Stormwater 101," Wisconsin Stormwater Week, https://www.wistormwater.com/stormwater-week-topics/stormwater101

[506] "Plants That Clean Water," Kellogg Garden Products, https://kellogggarden.com/blog/gardening/plants-that-clean-water/

[507] https://www.rodalesorganiclife.com/home/diy-insect-spray-covers-most-pests

[508] Dr. Samuel Epstein, Politics of Cancer, www.preventcancer.com/losing/acs/wealthiest_links.htm

[509] "Regenerative Agriculture: The Key to Solving the Climate Crisis," Hunter Lovins, Climate and Capital, Feb 15, 2023, https://www.climateandcapitalmedia.com/regenerative-agriculture-the-business-that-could-offset-all-human-emissions/

[510] "Alkaline Water: Miracle or Marketing?", Arthritis Foundation, Linda Rath, April 25, 2023, https://www.arthritis.org/health-wellness/healthy-living/nutrition/alkaline-water-benefits

[511] "Hydrogen-rich Water As A Modulator of Gut Microbiota?" Sergej M. Ostojic, Journal of Functional Foods, Vol 78, March, 2021, https://www.sciencedirect.com/science/article/pii/S1756464621000098#:~:text=HRW%20may%20induce%20protection%20of,%2C%20weight%2C%20and%20fluid%20loss.
[512] "Reducing Environmental Cancer Risk," What We Can Do Now,US Dept of Health and Human Services, National Institutes of Health, National Cancer Institute,President's Cancer Panel, April 2010, https://deainfo.nci.nih.gov/advisory/pcp/annualreports/pcp08-09rpt/pcp_report_08-09_508.pdf
[513] "NASA Research Illuminates Medical Uses of Light," NASA Spinoff, May 19, 2022, https://spinoff.nasa.gov/NASA-Research-Illuminates-Medical-Uses-of-Light
[514] "Red Light Therapy: Benefits, Side Effects and Uses, Kimberly Dawn Neumann, Forbes Health, Jan 12, 2024, https://www.forbes.com/health/wellness/red-light-therapy/
[515] "Undercover Video Shows Shocking Animal Cruelty at Eggland's Best Supplier,"Michael Addady, June 22, 2016, Fortune, https://fortune.com/2016/06/22/animal-cruelty-video/
[516] The Hateful Eight: Enemy Fats That Destroy Your Health, Dr. Cate, https://drcate.com/the-hateful-eight-enemy-fats-that-destroy-your-health/
[517] "Hormones in Dairy Foods and Their Impact on Public Health—A Narrative Review Article," Hassan Malekinejad, Aysa Rezabakhsh, Iranian Journal of Public Health, June 2015, https://www.ncbi.nlm.nih.gov/pmc/articles/PMC4524299/
[518] "Opposition to the Use of Hormone Growth Promoters in Beef and Dairy Cattle Production," American Public Health Association, Nov 10, 2009, https://www.apha.org/policies-and-advocacy/public-health-policy-statements/policy-database/2014/07/09/13/42/opposition-to-the-use-of-hormone-growth-promoters-in-beef-and-dairy-cattle-production
[519] "Recombinant Bovine Growth Hormone (rBGH)," American Cancer Society, https://www.cancer.org/cancer/risk-prevention/chemicals/recombinant-bovine-growth-hormone.html
[520] "Organic Consumers Association Takes Legal Action Against Eggland's Best Eggs," Jackie Mitchell, Quality Assurance and Food Safety Magazine, March 21, 2024, https://www.qualityassurancemag.com/news/organic-consumers-association-takes-legal-action-against-egglands-best-eggs/
[521] http://www.historycommons.org/entity.jsp?entity=michele_merkel, https://www.cbsnews.com/news/dissent-at-the-epa/
[522] "America's Children and the Environemnt, Environment and Contaminants, Drinking Water Contaminants, https://www.epa.gov/americaschildrenenvironment/environments-and-contaminants-drinking-water-contaminants
[523] EPA, Office of Water, https://www.epa.gov/aboutepa/about-office-water
[524] http://www.epa.gov/laws-regulations/basics-regulatory-process
[525] http://www.epa.gov/laws-regulations/summary-clean-air-act
[526] http://www.nmfs.noaa.gov/pr/laws/mmpa/
[527] http://www.epa.gov/laws-regulations/summary-national-environmental-policy-act
[528] https://www.nps.gov/history/local-law/anti1906.htm
[529] http://npic.orst.edu/reg/laws.html
[530] http://www.nrdc.org/food/files/safety-loophole-for-chemicals-in-food-report.pdf
[531] https://www.edf.org/health/policy/chemicals-policy-reform
[532] http://www.epa.gov/laws-regulations/summary-comprehensive-environmental-response-compensation-and-liability-act
[533] http://www.epa.gov/laws-regulations/summary-resource-conservation-and-recovery-act
[534] http://www.epa.gov/laws-regulations/history-clean-water-act
[535] http://www.epa.gov/laws-regulations/summary-safe-drinking-water-act
[536] https://www.epa.gov/hydraulicfracturing
[537] https://www.usbr.gov/history/borhist.html
[538] [538] http://ozone.unep.org/pdfs/Montreal-Protocol2000.pdf
[539] https://www.state.gov/e/oes/eqt/chemicalpollution/83009.htm
[540] http://chm.pops.int/TheConvention/Overview/tabid/3351/
[541] Kyoto: http://unfccc.int/kyoto_protocol/items/2830.php
[542] https://ec.europa.eu/clima/policies/international/negotiations/paris_en
[543] "Kunming-Montreal Global Biodiversity Framework Explained," World Wildlife Fund, www.wwf.panda.org

INDEX

ADHD 74
ALS 37,
AMR 37, 38,103
Antimicrobial resistance
Abdominal fat 44
Activated Carbon 6,7,78,174,250
Adrienne Anderson 53
Agricultural Runoff i, 2, 34, 35, 36,39, 81,85, 126, 152, 194 199,200,206,207,211,212,215, 224,226,228,235
Allergies 19,57, 65, 69, 71, 78, 103, 171, 273, 288
Aluminum 22, 37, 69, 104, 119, 120, 170, 233, 289,
Alzheimer's 19, 37, 74,114, 119, 234, 235,
Ammonia 14,39, 56, 58,65, 77, 83,87,90,95,112,117,127,128, 163,237,245,269
Ammunition 2,40,108
Anemia 23, 25, 30,50,57,63, 65,69,78,286,287,291,293,
Animal Health 51, 86, 124,141,189,190
Antibiotic Resistance 37, 42, 73,85, 103,
Antimicrobial Resistance 37
Apoptosis 100
Arsenic 7,10,22,40,52,69, 94, 98, 104, 107,198,223, 228.233,287
Arthritis 93,94,
Asthma 63, 115,
Atherosclerosis 56-57, 75
Atrazine 51
Autism 19, 104, 115, 233-235
Atrazine 36, 41, 80, 81, 100, 102, 145, 146, 151, 213, 217, 223, 225, 228,285,291
BDA 2, 56,78,
BPA, BADGE, BPS 5, 44-47, 110, 119, 156, 160, 244, 245, 255
BTEX 50
Bacteria and Pathogens 4,35, 37,38,42,43, 56,77, 83,85,87, 128,130,134,197,202,
BADGE 44, 46, 47,110,156,255
Behavioral changes 50, 69, 100, 104,107,111,113,120,149,161, 170,171, 233, 234, 237, 238
Benzene 50,55, 65,74,95,
97, 98,103,110,119,141, 147, 155, 156, 161, 169, 170, 171,176,178,180, 228, 291, 292,293, 294,295,297
Berkey Filter 7,94,250, 251,301
Big Ag 2, 21,85,143, 224,
Bile duct cancer 42, 57
Biodiversity iv,18,21,86,90, 124,127,192,238187-217,
Biosolids 2, 21, 37, 38, 51-53, 150, 154, 167,168,194, 213,298
Biotech 2, 85,86, 120,140, 142,198,
Birth Defects 41,44, 51, 54, 69, 73,75, 78,79, 97,104, 115,140,149,156,175,223,236, 238,241,281
Bladder damage 57, 78,99,140,
bladder, bile duct cancer 42, 57, 228
Blindness 39,42,173
Blood Brain Barrier -BBB 37, 82,121,146,170, 239
Blood Vessels 57, 65,78
Blue baby syndrome 27, 28, 126- 127
Boil Water 4
Bone damage, cancer 93
Bone disease 37,
Bottled Water 3-6, 17, 64, 93, 99,107-109,110, 114, 166,212,244,250,263, 268,301
Brain Cancer 59, 140, 179
Brain damage 29, 104 115,
Brain function 40
Brain infections 42,
Breast Cancer 51, 53-54, 151,
Bromine 54, 78
Building supplies 55
CAFOs 2, 34, 3538, 73, 83, 166, 217, 285
Cadmium 2, 23, 69, 98, 104, 233, 288
Camp Lejeune 2, 137
Cancer i, 6, 19-21, 30, 31, 35, 39, 41, 42, 44, 45, 50, 51, 56-57, 58,59, 63-65, 69, 70-76, 77, 78, 80, 81, 83-84, 88, 92, 93, 97-99, 100- 104, 111, 112, 119, 120-121, 125, 126, 127, 139, 142-144, 155, 166, 169, 170, 171, 175- 177, 193, 217, 222, 223, 224,

352

225, 228-229, 231, 236, 238, 244, 268, 286-293
Cancer Accelerant 74,
Cancer Alley 112
Cancer Clusters 139, 177
Carbon Block Filter 4, 6, 7, 8, 54, 110, 250, 301,
Carcinogens 13,
Carcinogenic 59, 82, 84,
Cardiovascular damage 41, 44, 74, 237, 291
Chagas disease 42
Chemical castration 41, 150,
Chemical Contaminants 16
Child development 44,
Childhood Cancer 19, 84,143, 144, 149
Chloramines 65, 86
Chlorine 4, 14, 39, 42, 54, 56-58, 65, 66, 69,76-79, 116, 143, 144, 154,171,178,179,181, 246
Chloroform 2, 56, 65,72, 77-79
Chlorpyrifos 59-62, 144, 145, 228
Cholesterol, increase 22, 51, 148, 287
Cholinesterase inhibitors 62, 230
Chromium 6: 2, 63,64, 176, 217
Chronic Fatigue Syndrome 115
Clean Water Act 10, 13, 23, 62
Clean Water and Health 9,
Cleaning Products 74
Climate Change 11, 21, 86, 90, 112,126, 127, 128,148, 195,202,210, 260,318
Climate Crisis i, 36, 136,
Coal 2, 23, 26-28, 53,67-69, 94,113, 115, 213, 217, 244, 260
Coal Ash 67-69
Cognitive problems 69, 113,
Colon Cancer 19, 57, 73, 101,102
Colorectal 57
Concentration difficulty 107, 234
Conserving Water 5, 18,
Coral Reef, *harm to* 120, 170-172, 188, 205
Cosmetics 48, 70-72, 282
Cyanobacteria 2, 85, 87
DBPs 2, 15, 58, 59, 77-79
Damage DNA 67, 78, 120, 156, 171, 287,
Dead Zones 126, 151, 192, 206, 207, 216, 217, 226
Dementia, memory effects 19, 37, 59, 120, 234, 235,
Dental fluorosis 93
Depression 100, 113, 194, 235,
Dermatitis 24, 69, 288
Developmental Delays 53, 69, 78, 117, 187
Diabetes 19, 46, 74, 150, 273
Dichlorobenzene (p-DCB)74, 228
Digestive disorders 52,
Dioxin 2, 31, 52, 75-76, 85, 181, 205, 212-213, 217, 230, 231, 294,
DNA Damage 156, 287,
E. Coli 42,
EPA 88, 90, 93, 95-97, 102, 107, 109, 110, 112, 113- 117, 122, 124, 128, 137, 139, 140, 144, 146-147, 148, 149, 152, 164, 167, 173, 174, 175, 182, 184, 188,198, 200, 203, 207, 211, 220, 221, 230, 241, 242, 243, 247, 250, 259, 279, 284- 298
EPA lawsuit 146-147
Early Puberty 74
Earth. 53,54,55, 59,67, 68, 72
Emerging Contaminants 70, 80,161, 173, 281,285
Endangered Species 101,123-124
Endangered Species Act 191, 283, 308
Endocrine Disruptors (EDCs) 2, 5, 41, 44, 65, 71, 80, 88, 100, 103, 105, 119,144, 145, 148,155, 169, 171, 176, 194, 200, 213, 227, 231-232, 245, 249, 269
Endometriosis 75, 231
Epilepsy 37, 76, 111, 139, 141, 143, 156, 234,235, 239
Epoxy 46, 110, 179
Esophagael cancer 58, 125, 228
Ethanol 2 81, 222,224, 225, 260,
Ethylene Glycol 71, 82, 95, 97, 156, 178, 182
Exxon Valdez Oil Spill 132-134,
FDA 35, 45-49, 54, 70, 72, 73, 82, 102,103, 114, 115, 119, 121, 171, 184, 267, 279, 281, 282, 309, 310
Factory Farms 14, 34-38, 83-84,

85, 189, 211, 221, 222,224, 282, 298
Federal Water Pollution Control Act Amendments 11,12, 311
Feminization 41, 150
Fertility 41, 44, 150
Fertilizer Industry Unregulated Pollution 157-158
Fertilizer runoff 35, 85-87, 128, 192, 198, 213, 214
Fertilizer, synthetic 2, 21, 36, 39, 85, 86, 90, 105, 124, 125, 126, 127, 128, 139, 152, 198, 207, 211, 217, 223, 228, 259
Filter Your Water Chart 22
Firefighters 89
Fireworks 22, 104
Flame Retardants 14, 88, 89, 91, 160, 176, 200, 213, 231,234, 255, 298
Fluoride 92-94, 104, 160, 228, 233, 249, 250, 289, 298, 316
Food Packaging 2, 44, 47, 48, 82, 133, 134, 148, 149, 175, 180, 184, 208, 254, 259, 274, 282
Food Quality Protection Act 60, 307, 308
Fossil Fuels 2, 21, 104, 198
Fracking 2, 50, 67, 68, 87, 95-97, 112, 129, 132, 198, 200, 212, 213, 217, 235, 298, 312
Furans 76, 160
GRAS 2, 49, 80, 101, 256, 309, 310
Gallbladder 237
Gastrointestinal problems 23, 25, 30, 35, 63, 69, 104, 115, 183, 237, 288, 289, 294,
GEN X. 13, 99, 148, 149, 175, 213
GMOs 2, 34, 85, 86, 87, 140, 183, 272, 274, 317, 282,
Glyphosate 36, 80, 81, 90, 100-102, 142, 198, 221, 222, 223, 228, 235, 237, 239, 246, 285, 295, 317
Greenhouse Gas 81, 87, 125, 127
Groundwater 6, 7, 22-31, 41, 63, 68, 95-97, 124, 128, 129, 134, 136, 164, 166, 167, 185, 196-198, 216
Groundwater Contaminants 22-31
Gut microbiome 100, 234, 237
Halocetic Acids 77, 78
Hand Sanitizers 44, 44-46, 65, 74, 103, 144, 173, 254
Hazardous Waste 2, 15, 40, 51 53, 66, 68, 94, 95, 96, 98, 124, 134, 152, 153, 174, 213, 311
Headaches 30, 50, 100, 107, 110, 182
Heart Attack 56, 57, 78
Heart damage 41, 56, 57, 69
Heart Disease 75
Heavy Metals 2, 7, 10, 51-53, 58, 67, 70, 71, 72, 80, 83, 95, 97, 104, 107, 110, 119, 120, 134, 162, 166, 170, 177, 198, 200, 205, 213, 215, 220, 227, 233, 235, 237, 238, 248, 249, 252, 268, 316, 318
Herbicides 2, 20, 30, 40, 80, 85, 86, 100, 102, 105, 135, 138, 139-141, 183, 185, 197, 213, 223, 234, 237, 239, 244, 252
High blood pressure 23,51,56, 107, 289
High cholesterol 22, 51, 56-57, 148, 287
Honeybee Colony Collapse 122
Hormonal Changes 74, 100, 104, 142, 169, 176, 210, 232, 233
Hormone Disruptor 136, 254
Hydrogen 1, 3, 57, 66, 83, 87, 116, 237, 251, 266
Hyperactivity 44, 74, 234
Hypothyroidism 136
Immune system problems 44, 47, 65, 74, 75, 103, 104, 148, 171, 231, 233, 238, 272, 296, 297,
Immunological disorders 50
Increase speed of cancer 120
Indiana water quality 166
Infertility 41, 42 74, 75, 148, 171, 210, 223, 231, 238
Insecticides 2, 20, 30, 59, 123, 124, 140-145, 197-198, 217, 223, 230, 235, 237,
Intestinal cancer 139
Iodine, suppresses absorption of 109, 150
Iodoacids 86
Ion Exchange 6,7, 8, 110
Iowa Cancer 35, 84, 166, 222, 224-225
Joint pain 102, 117
Keystone Pipelne 134
Kidney damage 22, 23, 24, 25,

27, 29, 31,41, 42, 63, 65, 69,
73, 74, 78, 79, 82, 93, 94, 99,
104, 107, 115, 137, 139, 156,
175, 176, 182, 228, 233, 286-
297
Kidney disease 37, 69, 94, 104,
   156, 233
Kidney cancer 51, 60, 151, 236
Lakes 3, 17, 60, 76, 83, 84, 116,
   126, 129, 157, 163, 165, 166,
   181,188,192, 193, 196, 199-
   202,210, 213, 215-217, 249
Landfills 2, 24,25,53, 67, 97,
   115, 118, 136, 159,169, 290,
   291, 296
Landscaping 114
Laws 301-314
Lead 2, 22, 26, 47,52, 57, 69, 72,
   94,95, 98, 106-111,112, 233,235
Lead pipes 106-111
Learning disabilities 113, 117, 150,
   160-161
Lethargy 113
Leukemia 50, 74,97,144, 179, 228
Liver cancer 57, 175, 179
Liver damage 22-25, 27, 29, 30, 31,
   41, 44, 51,57, 65, 69, 73, 79, 82, 88,
   93, 99, 114, 118, 135, 137, 176
Liver disease 42, 104,233
liver enzyme 51
Liver enzyme changes 60,
Liver failure 63
Liver health effects 87, 97
Low birth weight 72,
Lower IQ 40, 59, 69, 75, 92, 94, 104,
   223
Lung cancer 19, 69, 73,101, 102,
   119, 126, 137, 140, 179
Lung Disease 69,
Lung problems 78,
Lymph disease 42,
Lymphoma 74, 138,144,145,228
MS 135, 137, 235,
MX 2, 56, 77, 78
Malaria 42
Manganese 2, 5, 26, 69, 80, 95, 104,
   113,114,197,198, 223,233,235
Manganism 113
Memory 54, 59, 107, 122,141,
   233, 234, 235
Memory loss 234, 235
Mental health affects 113, 114,
141, 238,
Mercury 77, 79, 80, 94, 98, 104,
   115-117, 162, 199,213, 217, 223,
   233, 290
Metabolic Dysfunction 82
Methemoglobinemia 28, 125
Microbeads 70, 72, 154-156, 161,
   194, 200, 205, 209, 217, 244
Microplastics 51, 117, 154, 156,
   157, 208,
Miscarriages 44, 57, 78
Mitochondrial dysfunction 100,
   235, 239
Monocropping 34, 85, 86, 194
Nanoparticles 2, 21,46,49, 80, 112,
   119-122, 142, 157, 161, 170, 171,
   205, 229, 233,237, 238, 282, 300,
   302
Nasal problems 63
Natural Gas Facilities, Fracking 59
Nausea 233
Neonicotinoids 26,101, 122,123,
   141, 142, 239,
Neuropathy 183, 234 235
Newborn death 51
Nerve disorders 54, 107
Nervous System Damage,
   Disorders 87, 102, 117, 125,
   155, 176, 179, 182, 223, 230, 233,
   234, 235, 237, 238, 239
Neurological Disorders 59, 102,
Neuromotor changes 123
Neurotoxins 13, 50, 59, 68, 72, 75,
   79, 80, 88,100, 104, 105,106, 113,
   114, 115,119, 137, 143-145, 169, 177,
   183, 213, 223, 227, 233,234-235, 238,
   269
Nitrate 18, 67, 90, 137
Nitrosamines 70
Nitrification 77
Nitrous Oxide 87, 124, 125, 127
NOAA 204
Non-Hodgkins Lymphoma 82
Nuclear Waste 14
Nurdles
Nutrient pollution 140
Nutritional deficiencies 52
Obesity 53, 60, 112, 160-161
OCD behavior 123
Oceans 14, 70, 117, 133, 155, 156,
   157, 158, 166, 180, 181, 192, 193,
   200, 205-210, 215, 245, 248, 285,

Oil Refineries 50, 146, 147, 233
Oil Spills 14, 68, 131-133, 134, 194, 205, 206, 212, 213, 217, 249,
Organic Fertilizer 86, 87,
Organophosphates 59, 141, 142, 228, 230, 235, 239
Ott, Dr. Rikki 133
Ovarian Cancer 41, 71, 74, 228, 236
Ovarian Toxin 82
Oxygen 1, 3, 7, 28, 57, 121, 126, 151, 170, 180, 187, 188, 204, 206, 207, 226,
Ozone Disinfection 26
Ozone Layer 21, 56, 72, 117, 169, 171, 176, 260, 317
PFAS 13, 14, 51-53, 71, 80, 99, 148-149, 159, 166, 175, 176, 177, 181, 198, 213, 223, 228, 245, 255, 260, 269, 275, 302,
Packaging Waste 135-136
Paper Ind 75- 76,181, 213, 217,
Paper Mills 2, 75- 76
Paraquat 102, 137 144, 145, 228, 235,
Parasites 4, 35, 42, 43, 51, 52, 83, 199, 202, 228, 237,
Parasitic infection 42, 167,
Parkinson's Disease 37, 74, 102, 112,135, 137, 142, 234, 235, 239,
 Parkinson's- like- 123
Pathogens in water 52,
PERC, Perchloroethylene 13,137, 151, 235,
Perchlorate 136, 178, 213, 228, 235,
Periodic Table 299
Personal Care Products 121, 131, 149, 155,161, 173, 184, 200, 202, 213, 216, 234, 249, 256, 300,
Pesticide unregulated 157-158
Pesticides 13, 152-259
Petrochemicals 2,112, 134, 157
Petroleum 50, 23,68,98, 133, 134, 139, 154, 155,179, 288, 291, 296, 297, 298, 312
Pharmaceuticals 2, 20, 30, 50, 51, 53, 54, 59, 78, 79, 80, 114, 115, 147, 150, 161, 183, 184, 200, 202, 213, 229, 231, 282,
Pharmaceutical Pollution 13, 89
Phosphorous 151
Phosphate fertilizer 65, 94, 151-152, 211, 212, 213,

Phosphate Mining 87, 151-152, 197, 207,
Phosphates 151, 161, 268 316
Phthalates 2, 13, 45, 154, 155, 176, 244, 318,
Pipelines 14 Spills- 2, 68, 97, 132-133, 195, 198, 200, 205, 217, 245, 255
Pitcher Filters 7, 8, 243, 249
Plastic 2, 5, 17, 24, 25, 30, 31, 45, 46, 47, 48, 50, 51, 70, 72, 75, 79, 110, 117-118, 133, 143, 154-159, 221, 223, 231, 244, 245, 254,259,268, 289, 296, 297, 316
Plastic Pellets 147, 155, 156,158, 194, 202, 208, 210,
Plastic Pollution 117, 157, 204, 206, 210, 245
Plasticizer 31, 44, 155, 231
Pool Owners 57
Power Plants 2,14, 37, 41, 67, 68, 75, 114-115, 134, 162, 163, 164,
Precautionary Principle 121, 158, 280, 300
Pregnancy complications 107, 236, 57
Premature death 114
President Kennedy ii-v, 12, 302
Presidents Cancer Panel Report 6, 20, 83, 229, 238, 244, 268,
Propylene Glycol 80
Prostate Cancer 51, 53, 82
Protozoa 2, 4, 42, 228, 237
Quats, Quaternary 71,144, 200
Rachel Carson ii, 12,
Radiation 87, 163, 164, 207, 228,
Radon 87, 152, 164, 225, 228
Raw Sewage 166-167,199, 202, 223
Red Tides 96
Refineries 108, 114, 143, 145, 146, 221, 223, 233, 287, 288, 290, 295,
Reproductive Problems 54, 59, 72, 78, 108
Reproductive Toxins 24, 30, 59, 63, 65, 69,73, 75, 82, 93, 104, 120, 146, 170, 179, 182, 233, 237, 238, 268, 281, 84, 91, 113, 117
Respiratory Distress 69
Respiratory Paralysis 59
Reverse Osmosis 4, 6-8, 18, 54, 58,

78, 94, 110, 136, 243,249, 250, 262,
Rivers 12, 21 60, 68, 76, 83, 84, 128, 138, 144,147, 150, 157, 165, 166, 181,185, 192, 196, 212-213, 216-217, 248, 313
Roundup 73, 194, 214, 221, 224, 225, 236, 239, 317,
Safe Drinking Water 31,
Schaeffer, Eric 220,
Scleroderma 138
Seizures 42, 93
Sewage Sludge 36, 51-53, 149, 254
Skeletal fluorosis 93
Skin cancer 57
Smog 81, 112, 116, 171
Stomach cancer 25, 31, 35, 40, 43, 57, 58, 63, 69, 81, 92, 111, 118, 124, 126, 223, 228, 237, 266, 271, 283, 287, 294, 295,
Stroke 56- 57, 78, 235
Styrofoam 88, 118, 119, 135, 136, 154, 155, 169, 178, 180,181, 183202, 209, 210, 217
Surfactants 14, 101,130, 142, 151, 173, 239,
Synthetic Fertilizer 2, 21, 36, 39,85,86, 90,125,126, 127,128, 141, 198, 211, 216,221,223,228,260
2,4-D 102, 137, 144, 145, 235, 237, 292
2-Butoxyethanol 65, 182
Teflon 2, 51, 99, 148-149, 175, 255
Testicular Cancer 23, 51, 74, 175, 228, 236
TCE 151
Thyroid Toxin 54, 88, 93, 100, 138, 144, 175, 176

Thyroid Cancer 74, 144, 148,
Toxic Algae 81, 85-87, 90, 105, 126, 151,152, 192, 199, 200, 215, 216, 217, 275
Toxic Substance Control Act 121, 173, 182, 184, 313, 314,
Trichloromethane 79
Trihalomethane 77-79, 286
Ulcers 69, 175
Union of Concerned Scientists 112
USDA 84, 91, 194, 195, 225, 241, 242,248, 279, 282, 298
United Nations 19, 21, 76, 210,
Untreated Animal Waste 35,36, 38
Untreated Sewage. 60, 166
Uterine Cancer 74, 223, 228, 236
Vertigo 63
Warming Temperatures 21, 35, 83, 86, 108, 125, 126, 128,148, 156, 204, 217,
Waste Water Treatment 2, 28, 150, 214,
Water contaminant 13, 14
Water Filters 1, 6,7,8, 110, 250, 301
Water Health 3, 13, 55, 135
Water Shortage 5, 16-18, 21
Water Softener 4, 7, 10
Well Water 6, 7, 10, 105, 139, 166, 167, 197, 221, 244, 268,
Weight gain 51, 88, 148, 273,
Wildlife Services 194, 282
Window Cleaner 65, 66, 80, 182, 252, 300,
World Health Organization 92,113
Xenobiotics 183
Yeast infection 42

America the Beautiful

O beautiful for spacious skies, For amber waves of grain,
For purple mountain majesties above the fruited plain!
America! America!
God shed His grace on thee,
And crown thy good with brotherhood from sea to shining sea!
O beautiful for pilgrim feet Whose stern impassioned stress, A
thoroughfare for freedom beat across the wilderness!
America! America!
God mend thine every flaw,
Confirm thy soul in self-control, Thy liberty in law!
O beautiful for heroes proved in liberating strife,
Who more than self their country love, and mercy more than life!
America! America!
May God thy gold refine
Till all success be nobleness, and every gain divine!
O beautiful for patriot dream that sees beyond the years,
Thine alabaster cities gleam undimmed by human tears!
America! America!
God shed His grace on thee,
And crown thy good with brotherhood from sea to shining sea!
Oh beautiful for halcyon skies for amber waves of grain
For purple mountain majesties above the enameled plain!
America! America!
God shed His grace on thee,
Till souls wax fair as earth and air and music-hearted sea!
America! America!
God shed His grace on thee,
Till paths be wrought through wilds of thought
by pilgrims foot and knee!
Oh beautiful for glory-tale
Of liberating strife, when once and twice
for man's avail Men lavished precious life!
America! America!
God shed His grace on thee,
Till selfish gain no longer strain The banner of the free!
America! America!
God shed His grace on thee,

Written by Katherine Lee Bates; (1859-1929),
(*www.purpleheart.org*)

Prepare to Rise Presents,
The Book that'll Save Your Life!

FILTER YOUR Water Now!

Human Health is affected by contaminants in Water. Discover what to do to protect your family and heal from disease-- & save the planet in the process!

A must read book!

www.ingramcontent.com/pod-product-compliance
Lightning Source LLC
Chambersburg PA
CBHW051524020426
42333CB00016B/1763